your HEART

TREAT IT LIKE YOU LOVE IT

YOUR RESOURCE BOOK for a HEALTHY HEART

GERRY MADDOUX, M.D.

Medical Illustrations / Yvonne Wylie Walston, CMI
Cover Illustration / Jeanne M. Hendrickson

Cover and text design by Jeanne M. Hendrickson

Cover photo by iStockPhoto

Sea Script Company
Seattle, Washington

ISBN: 0-9785436-4-5
Library of Congress Control Number: 2006940541

First Printing February 2007

All ideas, thoughts, and treatments on conditions, devices, and medications in this book are those of the author based on his experience and opinions. No treatments, devices, medications or recommendations are to be used by the reader except as prescribed by or with the consent of the reader's personal medical professional.

Printed in Hong Kong

Sea Script
SEA SCRIPT COMPANY
www.seascriptcompany.com
info@seascriptcompany.com
206.748.0345

CONTENTS

INTRODUCTION

1 of every 2 men and 1 of every 2.4 women in America die of crdiovascular disease!

Cardiovascular disease is the leading cause of death in the U.S. after age 25. Diseases of the heart and blood vessels constitute, by far, the largest percentage of health care problems in the civilized world today.

***Your Heart, Treat It Like You Love It* is written for you.**
You have an opportunity to change your destiny!

When we purchase a new automobile or stereo system, we receive a detailed instruction manual pointing out the item's features, its safe handling methods and maintenance, and how to get help should something go wrong. But unlike a car or stereo system, we're set on earth without an operator's manual!

Your Heart, Treat It Like You Love It is a resource book that covers almost every conceivable cardiovascular problem currently known. With this book, you have the chance to be proactive in your health care and to work *with* your doctor in determining the best treatment for you.

The Dos and Don'ts of Your Heart

This is not a "scare book" and it's not a lecture either. This is a "why, how to, and why not" book. It's an honest effort to give the average person with little or no medical education, a primer on *preventive maintenance* of the heart and blood vessel systems. If and when a disease of the heart and blood vessels strikes you or someone you love, you will have a resource book to use as an adjunct to whatever your doctor tells you or tells the person you care about. This book offers you helpful hints about your health, what to watch out for, and how to gently demand strict standards of care from your health care professionals.

Your Proactive Role in Partnership with Your Physician

It's not surprising that this elaborate and complex heart and blood vessel system of ours is particularly susceptible to breakdowns that alter or stop operation, especially in our current stress-filled world. And unlike any other organ in the body, if the heart has a problem, it needs to mend on the run. If and when a breakdown of the heart happens to you or someone you love, there is reason for great hope due to our current medical tools. You and your loved ones don't need to die before your time.

We have experienced huge developments in cardiac treatment. When they do have cardiac problems, the aging poulation and the oncoming baby boomers will increasingly carry medical devices or drugs around in their bodies. Some may have defibrillators, vena cava filters, or transplanted hearts; others may be on elegant new medications to control blood pressure, congestive heart failure, or hyperlipidemia.

This incredible surge in medical understanding about how to repair the heart and blood vessels and improve the quality and length of life comes at a time when there are fewer doctors per capita. We're simply becoming an older population. The greatest percentage of people who develop congestive heart failure do so as a simple process of aging. The heart just gets "stiffer" with age and this leads to congestive heart failure. With this demographic shift comes a greater need for doctors specializing in the heart and blood vessels and a greater need for you to take a proactive approach to your health care and treatment.

The physician population has not kept up with the graying of America. During the next few years when more than 75 million baby boomers turn 60, the system is going to be stretched beyond capacity. There will not be enough cardiologists in the world to discuss with each patient all of the nuances of his or her specific disease, how to treat it, procedures and potential risks, and medications and potential interactions. We are no longer in a medical world where the doctor sits in a chair across the desk from you and explains everything in great detail. There are more details to explain about each problem—to more people who have that problem—than at any time in history. And, unfortunately, there aren't enough hours in the day for physicians to have enough one-on-one time with each patient.

We have often received excellent and skilled care in the hospital or doctor's office only to exit that unique environment with no clue about what to watch out for after leaving and when to call for help. If we are to exert any control over our medical health, we have to become educated about our situations and enter into a partnership with the medical profession.

The Need for This Book

I recently traveled with a college education tour in Italy. There were several elderly people with coronary disease due to cholesterol plaques within arteries, atrial fibrillation, congestive heart failure, previous stents to prop open arteries, or coronary bypass. These are common problems in the above-60 crowd. I'm always amazed by how little many of these people know about their problems! These are the same people who can give you a very detailed account of their businesses or their investment portfolios.

On that trip to Italy, word got around that I was a cardiologist. After dinner the first night in Assisi, an elderly gentleman hobbled across the lobby of the hotel carrying two glasses of red wine, clearly headed in my direction. He sat down heavily. One glass was for me. I soon learned that it was what the old country doctors use to call "payment in kind." This nice gentleman proceeded to tell me about his pacemaker, his congestive heart failure, and his coronary and renal stents. He knew almost nothing about his condition and treatment and certainly nothing about the six or so drugs he was taking. He was frightened. The 16 hours of travel the day before had not been kind to him and he had new symptoms. His primary question was how to adjust his medication to take care of these new symptoms.

In further conversation, I learned that he was the same guy who had started three well-known companies and built them from the ground up. I asked him how it came to be that he knew so little about his health care. (I knew for a fact there were excellent cardiologists where he lived.) He threw up his hands in frustration and said, "My doctor never has time. It's not his fault. There are just too many of us to deal with." He's right. During the course of that trip, two other elderly people, both as successful in their worlds as the first gentleman, sought me out. Both were scared, each with his or her individual problem that had become worse several thousand miles from home.

Near the end of the trip, they approached me as a group, a little cadre of the walking wounded. The first man spoke up. He told me I had a knack for putting their problems in perspective so they could understand them. (Keep in mind that I had nothing but time during that trip; I could take all the time I wanted with them.) They suggested I write a book outlining care and treatment of various common heart and blood vessel problems so that folks could read it at their leisure and learn more about their conditions. They were especially interested in a book that would direct them on how they could adjust their medications or modify their diets and activities when they got into trouble. I admired what a brave bunch this group was, carrying over a half dozen prescribed medications and continuing their lives and their fun in spite of the constant looming threat of disaster. They urged me to write the book as a "traveler's medical manual" for the heart. When I began writing this book, however, it dawned on me that you don't have to travel from your own house to feel overwhelmed by the medical system or to become frightened about your problem. Meeting these folks and an awareness of the need for information on care of the heart and blood vessels led to this book.

Your Heart, Treat It Like You Love It is the culmination of over 30 years in the trenches as a cardiologist discussing problems with patients and what it means to them as they go about their lives. **Because I'm not your physician, it's important for you to go over any recommendations I make in this book with your doctor.** He or she will welcome any tool that helps you better understand the treatment they're providing.

Most of us like something we can refer to over and over again as the need arises. This heart resource book has been written to empower you, the owner of an elaborate heart and blood vessel system, to enter into partnership with the health care community. Use it in good health!

—Gerry Maddoux, M.D.

FOREWORD

Your Heart, Treat It Like You Love It is primarily written to help you understand your heart and blood vessel health and to help you to be proactive in preventing disorders of your heart and blood vessels. Secondarily, it is written to help you become an active partner with your health care professionals in understanding and treating your existing heart and blood vessel disorders.

I am not your doctor. **No suggestion or recommendation in this book should be taken without the consent of your personal physician.** This book is to provide you the information you need to discuss your concerns with your doctor.

The opinions expressed in this book are my own. Speak to your physician regarding your specific problem and your unique needs and care. If his or her opinion doesn't agree with an opinion expressed in this book, take your doctor's advice. If you are still concerned, seek a second opinion from a professional in the field. Ask the questions, expect to be answered.

I included a chapter on how to quickly evaluate and implement emergency measures if you are with someone when they collapse. **Speak with your health care professional or take emergency medical courses offered within your community before the need arises.**

Medicine is dynamic, ever evolving, and what I say today may change tomorrow. This is true of the treatments—drugs, tests, procedures, surgeries, and devices—as well as the ongoing research. Do not use them or have them done without the authorization of your doctor.

The information in this book will not diagnose or treat your problem (only your doctor can do that) but is intended to help you understand your problem or prevent you from having a problem.

ACKNOWLEDGEMENTS

A special thank you to my professor of cardiology, Dr. S. Gilbert Blount, Jr. Dr. Blount not only taught us all the principals of recognizing and treating diseases of the heart and blood vessels, but also showed us a compassionate way of interacting with the patient as a person.

I owe much to my wife, Mia. Her love and encouragement drove me forward when I faltered.

This book would not be a reality without the professional assistance of my editors, Pamela Brink and Cliff Carle, who offered wonderful insight; the beautiful illustrations by Yvonne Walston, a medical illustrator par excellence; and the cover design and illustration by Jeanne Henrickson, who nicely interpreted my vision of a heart held dear. Last, but not least, I owe tremendous gratitude to my publisher, Beth Farrell. She believed in the importance of my message and stuck with me along the way to make the book the best that it can be.

This book is dedicated to the many patients I have treated over the past 30 years and to people everywhere who want to participate in their own health care with understanding and confidence. It is also dedicated to those doctors whose primary focus is providing us with the best care available.

We will all be patients at one time or other and we do our best only when we understand what we have to deal with.

Your Heart, Treat It Like You Love It

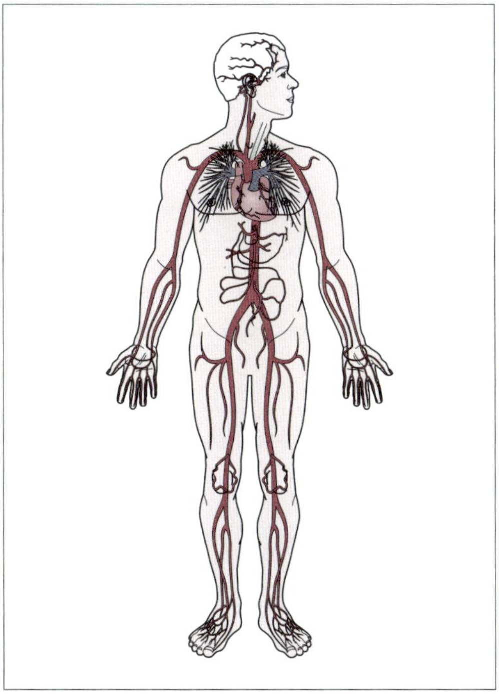

PREVENTIVE MAINTENANCE

Preventing Problems with the Heart and Blood Vessels

I THINK THAT, DEEP DOWN, all of us harbor concerns that we're going to have something go wrong with our heart or blood vessels. However, there are so many conflicting ideas out there from one time to another that it is easy to just throw up our hands and live the way we've always lived. The American novelist, John Dos Passos, wrote, "Apathy is one of the characteristic responses of any living organism when it is subjected to stimuli too intense or too complicated to cope with." It turns out that there actually are some great formats available for study so that we can live a heart-healthy life and feel better at the same time. The following is the skeletal backbone of such a format.

Food and Drink

Probably the best way to stay heart-healthy is to lean down and stay lean. How do you do that? By eating the right foods and the right number of calories coupled with a moderate amount of exercise. This sounds like everything else you've heard for the last dozen years; however, I'm going to walk you through this so you can learn it, refer back to it, and stick with it.

That said, there are certain people who will continue to battle to keep weight off. This is not a case of just eating right and exercising consistently because a lot of what we are has to do with the bacterial microflora culture in our gut. The other variable is determined by our genetic composition: energy efficient, holding onto every single calorie ingested, or poorly fuel efficient, requiring vast amounts of food just to hold our weight steady. Your unique population of bacteria probably has a lot to do with how much of your food is absorbed and converted to energy stores, some in the form of fat, and possibly which diseases you are prone to develop as well. We are all bacteria-free in the womb. We take on our first bacteria as we slide out to face the new world. From then on, we are partially captive to whichever bacteria set up housekeeping in our gut. If we receive a barrage of antibiotics early in life, we will have a certain population preponderance; if we receive few, it will be different. We also influence the bacterial population within our gastrointestinal tract with a variety of medications, increasing in number as we age. There may be, as some have suggested, a fat gene. This is speculative. We know, however, that there are fat-causing microbes that reside within some people's gastrointestinal tract.

On balance, your tendency to gain weight or not is determined mainly by four major factors:

1. Genetic composition regarding fuel economy.
2. Kinetic energy expended.
3. Total caloric intake.
4. Microflora in the gut, influencing efficiency of absorption of food as caloric contribution.

We can't fashion our genetic code. We can alter the amount of kinetic energy expended with our level of exercise, and we can modulate our caloric intake. As time goes on, I think we will be able to fine-tune the microflora population in the gut—optimizing the good guys, eliminating the bad—so that we can enjoy both our food and good health.

The Atkins Diet people did a terrific job of pointing out that if you limited carbohydrates, you could lose weight and keep it off. The dilemma is which carbs are good, which are bad, and what to eat to maintain a balanced diet and also to lose weight. I admired Dr. Atkins. I took exception with one aspect of his diet. He suggested that you could eat about as much fat as you wanted, as long as it was paired with an equivalent amount of protein. In my experience, you can't eat unlimited amounts of fat. Furthermore, there are some good fats and some very bad ones. Saturated fat is bad for you and it is never going to be good for you no matter how much protein you pair with it.

It has been well documented that fish, particularly salmon, are an excellent source of protein and also contain large quantities of omega fatty acids, which help protect against developing fatty plaque, the cholesterol deposit within coronary and other arterial vessels. Salmon is rich in fat, but it is good fat. In fact, it is great fat, as it will raise your HDL-cholesterol, the good fraction. There are some caveats, especially these days. Be sure your fish are caught in the wild and are not farm-grown, as the latter can possess large amounts of toxins. The fish farm industry is not well regulated. An occasional farm-grown fish won't hurt you. Just don't have a steady diet of them. Every place that serves only farm-grown salmon will reassure you that the government carefully regulates the amount of mercury and other toxins that can be found in them. The problem is we don't really know what "safe" levels are in these foods. We've never really been in this spot before—with increasing amounts of several toxins within foods—and no one really knows what long-term exposure will do to you, as there is a lot of individual variation in terms of sensitivity. In summary, unless one is a strict vegetarian, fish should be a main staple for protein; however, farm-grown fish should be kept to a minimum.

This concept fits in well with the so-called Mediterranean diet. This is the diet primarily consumed by those living in proximity to the Mediterranean Sea and is rich in olives and olive oil, fish, grains, fresh vegetables, and copious amounts of fruits. One caveat is in order. Olive oil is a great source of good fat, one that will raise the good cholesterol fraction. However, when you use it for frying at high temperatures, it changes its composition and turns into a very bad fat. One should choose an alternative oil for frying, such as canola or avocado oil. The Mediterranean diet is, for the most part, a very heart-healthy diet.

At the other end of the spectrum, the worst food one can eat is not butter, as you might suspect, but one that is rich in partially hydrogenated vegetable oil. This has been routinely found in chips and crackers, as well as a variety of other foods. These are the infamous *trans-fats* (trans fatty acids) that are so ubiquitous in the Western diet. There is simply no metabolic pathway that allows the human body to process and eliminate these terrible trans-fats—and they very aggressively cause plaque formation (arteriosclerosis or hardening of the arteries).

Back when we were in one of the major food fads—low-fat or non-fat—the food production industry quickly learned that they could easily produce "non-fat" foods and slap it on the label even as foods rich in trans-fats flew under the radar screen of the FDA. In other words, trans-fats didn't count as fat grams and the product didn't have to be labeled as containing them. Consequently, I have had many patients who thought they were doing exactly the right thing, but had a terrible progression of their arteriosclerotic problem because they were consuming a lot of trans-fat-rich food. These foods, the "non-fat" ones, were also frequently high in sugars. These were really great products if one wanted to become overweight and arteriosclerotic at the same time!

Thankfully, since January 2006, food distributors are required by law to label the amount of trans-fats that are contained within a particular food. However, fast food places do not have to. It seems incredible to me that, in this age of heightened awareness of obesity in children and young adults, with its attendant complication of diabetes and arteriosclerosis down the road, these places are not regulated with regard to disclosure of trans-fats. The biggest concentration of trans-fats in the world is found in none other than the infamous (and the very famous) french fry! One should avoid this tasty morsel like the Black Plague! It turns out that the longer the frying oil is used, the higher the quantity of trans-fats in the fries. They taste great; they just aren't great for you. They will not only make you fat, they will eventually make you sick, as the trans fatty acids are incorporated into the phospholipid membrane of cells. They accelerate the development of atherosclerotic disease and increase the incidence of sudden cardiac death.

How do you protect yourself? Look at each potential purchase and if it lists "partially hydrogenated vegetable oil" as an ingredient, don't buy it. Soon you will learn which foods contain this and will steer around them.

If you want a safe cracker, Edward & Sons Brown Rice Snaps are safe and they taste great. You can buy them in most health food stores and in many grocery stores. They come in many flavors; Tamari Sesame is my favorite. These are made from tamari (soybeans, water, and a little salt), sesame seeds, and brown rice. They are wheat-free, low in sugars, fat-free, all natural, and great to use with soy cheese, hummus, or other foods for a good snack.

Nuts constitute another great source of protein that happens to also be an effective hunger-killer. They are all loaded with fats, but again, these are the good fats—largely omega-3 fatty acids. I happen to think that the much-ignored walnut is the best, simply because it also seems to have intrinsic anti-arrhythmic properties. In other words, while we all have extra beats coming from our hearts and these become more frequent with age, walnuts seem to decrease that frequency. Additionally, they are a great source of fiber and promptly kill that wolf-like hunger that makes us gorge.

Walnuts, almonds, pecans, and pistachios, as well as their poor cousin, the much-maligned peanut, are all great sources of protein and are full of good fats. One can't make a meal of them as they are loaded with calories. Still, it's much better to grab a half-handful of nuts a few times a day rather than a high carbohydrate food. Make sure to avoid eating a large amount of salted nuts, since that will cause you to hold onto water and can raise your blood pressure. In certain circumstances, especially in the aged, they can precipitate congestive heart failure.

Some nut processing plants add some "bad" oils as taste enhancers. These are cottonseed oil or peanut oil. I have always been leery of peanut oil. People say it's good for you. However, when I was doing research on coronary artery disease many years ago, the quickest way we could induce high-grade coronary artery disease in pigs was to feed them peanut oil. I haven't forgotten that. I recommend you stay away from it.

Speaking of taste enhancers, this seems a good time to introduce *monosodium glutamate* (MSG), another well-known additive used to add flavor. Obviously, the good chefs don't need to use this. The poorer the chef or the lower the quality of food, the more apt one will find MSG in it. It is not particularly good for anyone. There are certain people for whom it is sheer poison causing palpitations, a racing or irregularity of the heartbeat, and other adverse symptoms. There have actually been documented cases of death when MSG was used in large amounts in food ingested by individuals who had a fair amount of alcohol to drink, the so-called "Chinese Restaurant Syndrome." If you sense that you might be sensitive to MSG, ask your server to check. Even if they are offended, you're paying the bill and deserve to know that there is nothing in the food that might make you ill. Again, it makes no sense to me that restaurants are not required by law to tell you, the consumer, if they use this poison in their food preparation. So far, they are not.

Another great source of protein is soy cheese. I'm not against dairy cheese in small quantities. However, it is full of saturated fat, and I still think it's not healthy. My good friend, Dr. Robert Vogel, has shown a marked increase in forearm arterial resistance following high-saturated fat intake, a strong suggestion that this diet adversely affects the health and function of the artery. If you want to have a nibble of a good dairy cheese occasionally, be aware that you are ingesting your limit of saturated fats right there! As a dairy cheese, the very best is low-fat cottage cheese (1–2%). It is a great snack, especially mixed with low-carb yogurt, nuts and blueberries, raspberries, or strawberries.

Soy products are made from soybeans and are very high in good protein. However, the down side is that they possess a material for which many people do not have a good enzyme system; therefore, some have to curtail the amount they eat in order to prevent gastrointestinal distress, such as bloating and stomach ache. This is variable and each person will have to carefully add soy milk, cheese, or other products containing soy until their specific tolerance is reached.

There are many great products out there made with soy. One of my personal favorites is the soy sausage. They are great with Egg Beaters and in omelets and are not particularly made to taste like meat. Soy is a particularly good protein and seems to have a large number of health benefits. The trick is being able to tolerate them.

Egg Beaters is an absolutely great invention. It offers a large amount of protein without risk of salmonella and is free of most, if not all, of the pesky saturated fats and cholesterol that come with regular eggs. The downside is that it contains xanthan and guar gum material that cause constipation. Again, you have to find an individual tolerance. Egg whites don't have this substance in them and this is a better-tolerated food for me. I believe that the yolk of the egg is actually important as a dietary substance. I eat about a half-dozen regular eggs a week. Our brain and nervous system are comprised more of fat than anything else, and the yolk contains good brain food. I don't want to live to be a hundred but have a shell of a brain, so I try to mix regular eggs with Egg Beaters or egg-whites in a recipe that is tasteful to me, gives me a lot of protein in the morning when I am just getting revved-up, yet spares me a huge cholesterol load.

No one can live just on the foods I've mentioned, and shouldn't. I'm not trying to limit your diet; I'm trying to point out what is healthy, what is not, and let you pick and choose. I want to reemphasize that the Mediterranean diet is hard to beat and as those of you who have visited one of the Mediterranean countries can attest, these people don't suffer when it comes to good food!

Unless you make your own bread, you're going to have a tough time finding the right bread. A great bread that won't add to your waistline is the so-called "Bible Bread." It goes by the name Ezekiel 4:9 and takes its name from the scripture: "Take also unto thee wheat, and barley, and beans, and lentils, and millet, and spelt, and put them in one vessel, and make bread of it." It so happens that when one actually does that, a complete protein is created that very closely simulates that found in milk and eggs. It contains all of the essential amino acids, is free of flour and oil, and has a great taste. This is literally "bread protein!"

Many of you will have noticed by now that I've left out meat. I'm not opposed to meat; it's a great way to get protein into your diet. You need to limit the amount you eat because it's generally full of harmful fats. Buy very lean cuts of meat and eat it only in moderation. I'm quite sure that quantity is the strongest determinant in our obesity epidemic. A good rule of thumb for a normal-sized person is to portion your protein to the size of a deck of cards.

Chicken and turkey are usually low in fat. I have been concerned about some of the additives that poultry producers use; however, it's better regulated than it was. When "organic" is on the label, they are a good source of protein.

Man does not live by protein alone. We also need some carbohydrate. This has become the dirtiest word in America and for all the wrong reasons. Processed carbohydrate, such as simple sugar, is terrible for us in significant amounts. It goes right to the blood stream where it produces a big sugar rush. There is absolutely nowhere for it to go but toward the manufacture of fat tissue unless a person is exercising vigorously and it is burned on the spot. If you are hiking the Grand Canyon, it's fine to eat simple sugar. Simple sugar causes the outpouring of insulin in order to handle the sugar load. A big sugar hit will be met with an equally large insulin surge. Then, as the glucose level in the blood stream falls, you're very hungry again and, in many cases, shaky from low blood sugar. You grab some more high-sugar foods and the cycle repeats. This is the surest way to obesity and diabetes.

Complex carbohydrates are another matter. These require some enzymatic processing by the body and it takes a while before glucose hits the blood stream. Not only that, it doesn't enter the blood stream as a big jolt, but enters over a period of time. You have to be careful with even these types of carbs, however. Basically, you should get these carbs from foods that offer trade-off benefits. These are either vegetables or fruits that offer strong antioxidant benefits.

Vegetables, such as broccoli, Brussels sprouts, asparagus, spinach, green beans, and to a lesser extent (because of higher carbohydrate loads) corn and carrots represent good complex carbohydrates. All of these vegetables have one thing in common: They are high in antioxidants. We all hear this term and know that it is supposed to be "good for you." What is this exactly? There is no easy answer. First, let me define what the "bad things" are that we are going after with antioxidants. Oxidation is a necessary part of metabolic pathways, the way you process your food and generate energy. However, inappropriate oxidation is harmful. For example, the process that makes butter rancid is oxidation. Free radicals are compounds that occur as a result of oxidation within all cells. These free radicals cause injury to cells, leading to aging and disease. They also damage blood vessels and participate in the process leading to arteriosclerosis. As an aside, they may also play a big role in degenerative diseases, such as Alzheimer's and dementia, as well as cancer. They are bad actors! Each of us has an individual genetically determined rate of production of free radicals as we go about our everyday life. For reasons that we do not totally understand, the concentration of free radicals within a cell increases with age and they probably are, indeed, a large part of the aging process. Large amounts of free radicals are dangerous and deleterious to our health.

Now that we've defined what we're going after, we can define antioxidants. Simply put, antioxidants are chemical substances that give an electron to a free radical, converting it to a harmless molecule. The more free radicals we can convert to harmless molecules, the better off we are, as the less damage we have incurred within our cells and vital organs. We need heaps of antioxidants, more as we get older because we produce more free radicals with age.

Now I have to introduce something that I know will be met with boos and, after you taste it, disdain if not disgust. This is wheat grass juice. One ounce contains as much good stuff as two and a half pounds of vegetables. I like vegetables; however, knowing that we produce more free radicals as we age—requiring more vegetables to neutralize them—one of the ways I get enough antioxidant power is by drinking a couple of ounces of wheat grass juice two or three times a week. You can get it at many smoothie and juice counters these days. One that is growing like wildfire is Keva Juice, which began in New Mexico. You'll be able to get wheat grass juice in any city very soon if Keva Juice keeps growing. Wheat grass juice doesn't taste great. I use a mango juice "chaser" and it does just that—it chases away the grass taste and you have your fix for the day. You can also make your own wheat grass juice at home.

Other sources of good carbohydrates are dark fruits. They are also rich in antioxidants. A good rule of thumb for both vegetables and fruits: the darker they are, the stronger the antioxidant power. Therefore, the best are blueberries and blackberries, closely followed by strawberries and raspberries. It has been shown that daily consumption of blueberries is the only thing that can clearly slow down the deterioration of motor function (the performance portion of our nervous system) with advancing age. I figure if they are that fabulous for the nervous system, they must be good for the heart as well. And that has turned out to be exactly the case. The reason is at least partially due to the fact that they possess a family of polyphenols that chemists call condensed tannins, also found in cranberry, elderberry, and pomegranates. Actually, grape nectar has the highest concentration of these condensed tannins, a fact discovered by the French and one that may partially explain the "French Paradox." This is the relatively low incidence of coronary artery disease in the French even though their diet is rich in fats and more of them smoke than Americans. Along that line, condensed tannins found in grapes have even been found to be effective in preventing some of the free-radical damage induced by tobacco usage. Since the French have, in the past, consumed more wine than Americans, this may be the explanation. For those of you who are non-drinkers, there is a great grape seed extract that is even richer in these antioxidants than red wine. It can be found in any good health food store. It is known as resveratrol.

I know that a lot of you like cereal for breakfast. Many are loaded with sugar and have very little nutritive value. A great one is Kashi Heart-to-Heart. It is made up of oats, a good source of fiber that can drop your cholesterol; it is low in sugar and salt; and it contains several natural antioxidants, including some that we've just talked about. One of them even contains blueberries, the miracle fruit.

I could go on and on about the power of antioxidants. It is impossible to overemphasize the importance of these foods. It is basically the only way I know to combat the age-dependent accumulation of disease-causing free radicals within our cells.

While also a great source of fiber and potassium, bananas and apples are much less rich in antioxidants and produce a greater suger load. Again, as with everything, it is better to eat these fruits several times a day in very small portions, rather than a big bowl at one time.

The reason for this multiple small portion schedule is the so-called glycemic index, which has been calculated for every food. It is, simply put, the level of blood sugar–production tendency for that particular food. Therefore, if one has strawberries mixed with low-carb yogurt, cottage cheese, and walnuts, it will possess a lower glycemic index than if the fruit were ingested alone. Keep this in mind when preparing your snack.

You also have to pay great attention to what you drink. Sodas are simply sugar with a particular taste modifier and water added. They are the worst of the "butt and belly foods." Non-caloric sodas obviously do not possess this tendency, but I'm still wary of drinking much of them due to artificial sweeteners. I don't have any good data. I'm just concerned about using something that is man-made to sweeten my drink. I'm also down on high fructose corn syrup, as it really will lay on the pounds. It's everywhere! Just trying to go down the isle of your grocery store, buying nothing that contains it, will take some time.

The best source of fluid is good, pure water. Obviously, there is a great concern about our daily water source and generally for good reason! Ground water has become grossly contaminated by factory effluent and farm fertilizers in many parts of the country, and I think most people are getting pretty leery of city water. Otherwise, bottled water would not be such a huge market. When you travel, it seems that every single person is toting a bottle of water. I'm one of them! I'm sure that at least some of that water actually does come from some pristine mountain spring somewhere. I also suspect that much of it doesn't. I first thought this when my 17-year-old daughter laughingly noted that Evian is "naïve" spelled backwards! I'm sure this is merely a coincidence; I'm fond of Evian water.

A great source of water that you know is good for you is one that is readily accessible in great quantities at a low price. This can be achieved by using a device called Waterwise, which processes your regular tap water. It removes everything harmful from it, and you have a pure source of water without lugging bottles of water home from the grocery store at great expense. You can store several gallons in containers for emergency use as well.

Unfortunately, I'm not particularly fond of water. I do, however, like green and black tea, but fairly weak. This gives me extra water throughout the day. It has been shown that green tea, in particular, will help curb your longing for food, especially carbs. The rule of thumb is to drink roughly eight glasses of water a day. This is quite a bit of water. However, our cells possess very high water content. When they become dehydrated, they don't work well. If you want to try an experiment, take a word contest when you have had only coffee and a couple of glasses of water all day long, then maybe an alcoholic drink, which completes the task of true dehydration. Do it again when you have had eight glasses of water during the day. The brain cells, like all cells, work better when they are happily hydrated. Nonetheless, eight glasses is a lot and very arbitrary. It boils down to this: You need more water when you eat protein or when you exercise. The end product of protein metabolism is blood urea nitrogen (BUN). It makes urine yellow. The goal is to keep your urine near colorless, regardless of how much protein you eat. This is the only way to be sure that you are properly hydrated. This may mean that some days you drink 6 glasses of water, others 10 or even 12.

Coffee is a strong antioxidant. Additionally, tea, especially green tea, contains phenolic compounds that are strong antioxidants (more of the condensed tannin class). Just make sure you also drink enough pure water that is free of harmful elements.

Now we come to a crucial item: dessert. It just so happens that the "food of angels" (better known as chocolate), if in concentration greater than 70%, is a very acceptable dessert. It is a strong antioxidant, as it also contains those great phenolic compounds. In this concentration, chocolate possesses very little simple sugar. It particularly has a good glycemic index, if taken in conjunction with almonds and walnuts. In addition to tasting great, the unsaturated fat in walnuts, almonds and dark chocolate will actually raise your HDL-cholesterol, which is the good stuff (the higher, the better).

I have seen patient after patient on a very low-fat diet demonstrate an extremely low HDL, only to increase it substantially by simply adding in nuts and dark chocolate along with olive oil and salmon, in moderation. Don't forget the "moderation" part, as these are calorie-rich foods. I personally raised my HDL from 26 to 49 with just this change. For years, I ran five miles a day and kept this same paltry HDL. If I ran ten miles a day, I lost weight, but would only raise my HDL to 27 or 28. Since people with such low HDL-cholesterol levels are much more likely to develop coronary artery disease (have heart attacks) and possibly even die suddenly, I was not very happy with my seemingly unfixable situation. If one finds a fix, and it has the added benefit of actually tasting good, it is cause for major celebration.

For those unfortunate people who cannot eat chocolate for dessert, raspberries and blueberries mixed with low-carb yogurt and low-fat cottage cheese is a good alternative. And, of course, we all must simply give in occasionally and have the dessert of our choice. Better yet, share one with a friend.

Now, a final word about food and drink. By the time we reach 50, many of us have a roll around the middle though this is not inevitable. If you look inside the abdomen, the stomach in a moderately obese person is about twice the normal size compared to lean people. Additionally, the little muscular and fibrous tissue sphincter that keeps the stomach inside the abdomen becomes stretched. This produces the typical esophageal hiatus hernia that is the cause of so much misery. Loss of the gastroesophageal sphincter allows part of the stomach to protrude into the chest. The typical person simply eats too much at one time! Over the years, if this over-eating persists as a habit, the stomach stretches. The gastroesophageal sphincter gets larger and less competent, and gastric acid refluxes into the lower esophagus. The esophagus hates acid, preferring an alkaline pH. This acid literally burns the inside of the esophagus and the result is truly miserable. The pain from this so frequently mimics the chest pain of heart attack that it drives people crazy, as many folks have both reflux and heart disease.

Chronic reflux, in addition to the discomfort and the confusion introduced as to whether that discomfort is due to reflux or to heart pain, is harmful to you. It is one of the main contributors to developing a Barrett's esophagus, a pre-malignant process in the esophagus. I am no gastroenterologist; however, the main treatment for this is prescribing a proton pump-inhibitor. These are okay if taken now and then. However, they work by preventing the production of stomach acid. We know that you actually need stomach acid for break-down of food and, additionally, it reduces your chances of carrying the bacteria that cause ulcers. Obviously using one of these pills all the time is not the answer for millions of people. They work; they reduce stomach acid and, as such, can relieve your symptoms of heartburn within minutes. However, unless we just want to add another expensive pill to our cabinet (already full by age 60) many of us need to search for an alternative method of preventing reflux, such as changing how we eat and drink.

If you gauge the amount of food you eat at one time, don't ever gorge, drink a lot of good water, avoid carbonated beverages, and let your stomach shrink down to the size that it was intended to be, you'll be amazed at the result. These tenets—along with abstinence from food or drink for a couple of hours before retiring to bed—will fix about 75% of reflux. And in the process, they will save you a heap of money that you would ordinarily spend on pills. I personally know a couple of gastroenterologists who treat their own heartburn in just this way, taking a proton pump-inhibitor only rarely. Despite all best efforts, there is going to be a group of you out there who simply have to take one of these pills (such as the "purple pill" that receives so much advertising attention) every single day to prevent harmful reflux. The reason for changing how we eat and drink is not to get everyone off anti-reflux medications, especially those who might go on to develop esophageal cancer if allowed to continue to reflux constantly. However, I don't think we want every single adult over age 40 on a daily pill to prevent reflux! Using the above information, a great percentage can prevent significant day-to-day reflux the natural way. If you do your best and you still have reflux, you need a medication for it.

The feeling of fullness (satiety) is a result of at least two interrelated mechanisms. There is a satiety center in the brain that reacts very slowly to food intake. The stretch of the stomach sends signals to the brain that one is "full." If you eat quickly, by the time you receive the "full-up" signal by either mechanism, you are way past your needed intake. The take-home message is to eat slowly, eat an amount that looks like enough, and don't go back for more. Then allow your reflex center time to react to what you have done. Talk to someone during dinner and take your time. Eat like the Europeans. Also, if you drink a fair amount of water throughout the day and have a salad first and wait a while before the main course, you will not be so hungry and will not wolf down so much food.

I mentioned in the Introduction that this was not going to be a diet book. It isn't. I just didn't see how I could provide you with a book directed toward heart and blood vessel disease without saying something about food and drink that is good for you and, alternatively, food that is bad for you. This list is not complete. It's merely a primer. For more details, please go to what I believe is the best diet book for good cardiovascular health in the world, *The South Beach Diet Book*. It's written by a cardiologist. I've never met him but consider the book an excellent resource and recommend it to my patients. There is enough flexibility within the diet to allow you to still enjoy your food.

I'm often told, "But doctor, eating is a large part of my social life" or more recently, "But you can't take the spirit of community out of eating." I don't mean to do this.

However, I remember Johnny Carson's comment after he had peripheral vascular surgery for a blocked artery in his leg. He said something like, "Some people live to eat. Others eat to live. I have, by necessity, just joined the latter group." I have not attempted to dictate to you what you should eat. I have merely attempted to tell you what is good for you and what is bad. It's your decision.

Have you ever known a cowboy? They're usually great people, very laconic; don't like vegetables but love horses, dogs, children, and pickup trucks, just like the song says. They eat steak. And, of course, they like potatoes. I was raised on a ranch so I've known a lot of cowboys. They have strong ideas about everything including what they want for supper. My dad was sort of a cowboy. I was once asked to come up with a "heart-friendly cowboy diet." I knew roughly what that meant. It meant that these guys weren't going to be eating much salmon, for one thing. This was a request by a large rancher, a patient of mine who had suffered a heart attack. He hired a vast number of cowboys and wanted to provide them with good nutritious food. I went over the list I just gave you. He wanted a meal-by-meal account. This was difficult, as I do not eat meat. I grew up on a ranch but I just don't like meat and never have. Nonetheless, I wrote out a menu for breakfast incorporating real eggs mixed with egg whites. Believe it or not, I got quite a few of them hooked on soy sausages though quite a few continued to eat bacon or meat sausage. They all got hooked on Pom juice (made from pomegranates), which possesses very strong antioxidants; and they already liked coffee, also high in antioxidants. They didn't go for green tea! I guess there is a limit, after all. The cook made sure they had access to nuts, carrots and celery, and fruit throughout the day; and they all started drinking much more water. In the evening, they all ate lean beef, which they had in abundance, but some substituted green vegetables for potatoes. They decreased their bread intake by half. They took to the chocolates pretty well, too. After listening to my spiel, almost 50% stopped using tobacco in any form. Is this group of cowboys going to live longer? I don't know for sure, but I strongly suspect that they will live better—with fewer heart attacks and fewer early retirements because of bypass surgery or blocked leg arteries. I was told that all of them still think they have a pretty good diet and enjoy it just as much as before. One of them, in a strong Texas drawl, asked me if he would live longer if he followed these rough guidelines. My reply (attempting to match his drawl) was, "Well, Red, I'm not sure you're going to live longer, but it's certainly going to seem longer."

I haven't been called on to write a plan for truckers, another group with a notoriously high incidence of arteriosclerosis. I want them, and all of you, to educate yourselves about food and drink that is good for you. Then you can blend it into your personal preferences. I know very well that you can't take a bunch of cowboys and feed them tofu. You probably can't get them to drink wheat grass juice either. The gradual incorporation of at least some of these concepts into your own diet will allow you to enjoy better health of the heart and blood vessels.

Now for some sobering comments to the over-60 crowd. We're all told, "We are what we eat." We aren't. We are what we *absorb*. A disturbing bit of information is that many of us don't absorb break-down products of food across the gastrointestinal tract very well after a certain age, and this is as variable as how quickly our hair turns gray. You may remember that I made some early comments about the gastrointestinal microflora, the bacterial population in the gut. Well, we tend to change the preponderant components of our microflora as we get older. Part of this has to do with all the medications we take. The usual American over age 65 takes an average of six prescription medications, one of which is usually a proton pump-inhibitor that I mentioned earlier for treatment of heartburn. If you take this on a regular basis, it changes your gut microflora population. Stomach acid is important; when you prevent it from being formed, the population of bacteria changes. Many other medications, including the ubiquitous non-steroidal anti-inflammatory drugs, do the same thing.

The key word for those of us who are over age 60 becomes *bioavailability*, which translates into the efficiency of the gut in transporting essential fatty acids and amino acids across its barrier and into the bloodstream. It turns out that many great foods, such as proteins and good fats, have a low index of bioavailability when you change as you have after five decades of hard living. I have absolutely no doubt that a great number of the degenerative processes that we face in our last couple of decades have a lot to do with this altered bioavailability of essential amino acids and fatty acids at just the time when we need them the most for preservation of cellular integrity. In some of us, the incorporation of antioxidants is equally impaired at precisely the time when oxidative stress (the injury inflicted by increased levels of free radicals) is at its highest. These two things—cellular integrity and antioxidation of free radicals—if properly implemented, should prevent many of the degenerative processes we face as we age. We'll never achieve this without, in some cases, obtaining bioavailable compounds to fill this nutritional gap. In my view, a future of good health means not filling a prescription for treatment of a degenerative disease, but filling a prescription for the nutritional deficiencies that led to this problem. In one instance, this may mean a balanced amino acid complex. In another, it may mean an intensely concentrated antioxidant capsule. I pray that a large portion of our health care dollar that is now going to buy all of these prescription drugs goes instead toward determining what your unique metabolic needs are so that you can maintain optimal cellular integrity and antioxidation.

REMINDERS

1. Restrict carbohydrates, especially simple sugars. Pay attention to the glycemic index.
2. Small amounts of high protein food (such as nuts) taken a few times a day, will help suppress the appetite. So will green tea.
3. Watch your intake of high-fat foods and be sure to avoid trans-fats.
4. Drink a lot of good, pure water.
5. Save your carbohydrate load for those foods that offer you a trade-off antioxidant effect.
6. My mom's dictum from many years ago still holds: "Eat breakfast like a king, lunch like a prince, and dinner like a pauper."
7. We are what we absorb. The bacterial components of the gastrointestinal tract change with time and overuse of prescription medicines. This means that bioavailability of amino acids and fatty acids is frequently altered by age 60.
8. The usual correct protein load is the size of a deck of cards.

Teeth Care and Heart Disease

We all know that every tooth is precious; however, our teeth may be even more precious than the average person would suspect. Through a number of studies, it's been established that the incidence and amount of *arterial* plaque (cholesterol deposits in arteries) in patients with coronary artery disease (so-called hardening of the arteries) is directly related to the number and health of their teeth. In other words, you are more apt to develop coronary artery disease if you have gum disease than if not.

The degree of arteriosclerosis gets worse as you lose teeth. The person with no remaining natural teeth routinely has more advanced coronary disease than the person with a number of remaining teeth. This problem with gum disease seems to be related to promoting a constant inflammatory state within the body. Since arteriosclerosis is first an inflammatory disease, a harmful cycle is readily produced by gingivitis, gum disease, and subsequent loss of teeth. Therefore, it is especially important that you brush often and floss!

Making dietary changes away from simple sugars and more toward protein will go a long way in reducing the ideal environment for bacterial growth between the teeth. Bacteria love sugar, just as we do. The less sugar we ingest, the lower the population of bacteria in the gums and between the teeth.

However, a high-protein diet comes with its own price by creating a different set of hygienic social consequences. A very high-protein diet frequently causes ketosis in the blood stream due to the breakdown of all that protein. This is noticeable on the breath and doesn't smell good. So—brush, floss, and use mouth wash. Above all, drink large amounts of water if you follow an especially high-protein diet.

REMINDERS

1. **The more teeth you keep, the less risk of coronary heart disease.**
2. **Arteriosclerosis starts as an inflammatory process. Try to prevent gingivitis.**
3. **If you are a high-protein fanatic, be prepared. You may have bad breath!**

Exercise

It is especially important that we exercise all of our muscle groups daily. You don't have to stay on the bike for an hour. It is more important to get some aerobic exercise, during which you raise your heart rate and oxygen consumption substantially, mixed in with some strengthening exercises. Why? It gives you cardiopulmonary conditioning but also raises the catabolic rate (the rate at which you burn calories during a routine day). It's best to do this in the morning so that your catabolic rate is increased throughout the day. If you exercise too close to your bedtime, it's easy to retire with a high endorphin level. Sleep comes poorly in that state. The endorphins are a group of hormones secreted during intense exercise. They stimulate one's senses, and the circulating blood stream level takes a while to revert back to normal.

Walking is a terrific exercise and will drop most people's blood pressure several points, if done on a regular basis. So is swimming. If you want to perform all of your exercises inside, a Bowflex machine and a stationary bike are really all you need for a complete gym, and they'll fit into a very small space. Drink plenty of good water before, during, and after exercise. Exercise every day unless you are ill.

Today, many people are practicing yoga and Pilates. As the population ages, we're going to look for gentler, more sophisticated ways to work the body and incorporate this into the discipline of the way we think. I suspect we'll see more and more people turn to some sort of "spiritual" exercise rather than the repetitive exercises that can injure already well-used joints. There's a place for both.

Performed on a regular basis, exercise will cause an increase in the population of mitochondria within your muscle cells. These are the cellular machinery packets that produce energy. The more of these you have, the better off you are, for they allow you to be a more efficient "machine." Additionally, your heart rate will come down as will as your blood pressure. Your endorphin level increases and with that, your mood is elevated. Your HDL cholesterol may increase, which is a good thing. More importantly, you will be able to gain—and maintain—control of your weight.

REMINDERS

1. **Make exercise a daily event.**
2. **Don't try to perform just one form of exercise. Exercise all your muscle groups.**
3. **Mix aerobic and anaerobic exercise with meditative exercise, such as yoga.**

Meditation and Sleep

It's very important, especially in these stressful times, to set aside quiet time every day. The more I travel and study the history of a particular region, the more I think that every period in history has contained a fair amount of stress. A quiet, peaceful, simple, and non-threatening time of yesteryear is mostly a splinter of our memory and was, at best, brief or imagined. We will not get back to that time, even if we sell everything, give up our day jobs, and move to the country.

In lieu of this imagined peaceful world, we have to cultivate a sense of inner peace. This is peace within our soul. Everyone does this differently. I rise early, read the *Daily Word*, think about peaceful things such as my garden, try to find something of beauty to watch or listen to, and read the teachings of the Dalai Lama. The book *Live in a Better Way* is my favorite. It has a great chapter on controlling anger, which is a problem with a lot of people, especially men. These simple words fit in with any religion and should not offend anyone. In fact, I once considered writing a book titled *Buddhism for Baptists* and then thought better of it.

If you're religious—most of us are in one form or another—reading scripture from the Bible, Koran, Torah, or the teachings of the prophets of your particular religion may give you inner peace. It takes a surprisingly short amount of time to get a daily fix of tranquility and it does a world of good. It's also a good time to take stock of what you're doing with your life and to commit to a positive fulfilling attitude.

I so often see such huge displays of anger (thankfully, not all of which is directed at me) that I wonder if those people know the concept of karma. *Our life follows our thoughts!* It's that simple. If we think good, positive thoughts about our life, our actions, and the needs of others, our life will be positive. Conversely, if we have negative thoughts, negativity will prevail and we'll be more likely to have a serious illness.

Depression is a debilitating condition. I am increasingly convinced that depression is a coronary risk factor and a potent one at that. If you cannot fix depression by reading, exercising, and positive influences, you need chemical help until other treatments can be studied and incorporated. If the depression turns out to be due to an irreversible chemical problem—such as a low serotonin level, a necessary neurotransmitter—you should have continued professional help coupled with a drug to raise your serotonin to a favorable level.

Sleep is as important as meditation and exercise. The ancients thought that each hour of sleep before midnight was worth at least two after midnight. It seems to be true. Most adults need eight hours of sleep a night. Knowing that Einstein and other great thinkers may have subsisted on only four or so hours of sleep per night has done the rest of us a disservice. The theory that to be bright and competitive, we must get by on caffeine and little sleep seems to be the dictum for the day. Trust me, it's counterproductive. The person who is well rested is much less likely to make mistakes and is more apt to be friendly, charismatic, and productive than the sleep-deprived one. From a purely cardiac standpoint, you're in a bad spot if you're under constant stress, pouring out huge quantities of harmful stress hormones all of the time. These markedly accelerate the formation of plaque within arteries.

Learning how to work hard, play hard, get plenty of rest, control your anger, meditate, and relax can literally save your life. If you must take something as a sleep aid, melatonin (a strong antioxidant) is about the only truly safe one. It is especially good to use for jet lag.

REMINDERS

1. Get plenty of sleep. Adults need eight hours per night.

2. Meditation is essential. Try to relax and calm the mind several times throughout the day.

Vitamins and Additives

I think a daily vitamin is very helpful. I previously commented on the harmful effects of oxidative stress and free radicals. We produce more free radicals as we age over 50, and we produce even more when we exercise. The Cooper Clinic in Dallas has formulated a number of supplements, each formatted for your age and level of activity. These are reliable and are also inexpensive. Fat-soluble vitamins can be harmful but only if taken in large quantities. Most water-soluble vitamins will just give you expensive urine if your body doesn't need them. Excess vitamin B6, a water-soluble vitamin, can cause neuropathy and nerve damage. A good daily vitamin such as CentrumSilver is not harmful and will take care of many of the deficits that you may have created by a certain dietary indiscretion.

If you're taking a statin (a common drug that reduces cholesterol) then you should also take CoEnzyme Q10, as the blood level of Q10 is depleted by statin drugs.

If you're a vegetarian, it's important to take some form of calcium. The same is true for B12, which comes only from meat, eggs, and dairy products.

There is currently no clear-cut unequivocal evidence that taking zinc, selenium, or vitamin C prevents heart disease. There are, however, certain individuals who possess high levels of homocysteine, an amino acid shown to be an accelerant of arteriosclerosis. This can be treated with folic acid but only when taken in combination with B6 and B12.

I think that a well-balanced diet is the best strategy. Don't jump on the fad-diet bandwagons. You need some good fat, such as that found in fish, eggs, olive oil, and nuts. I'm very concerned that ultra-low-fat diets may eventually cause nerve damage and even brain damage. For more on this, there's a helpful book by Dr. David Perlmutter titled, *The Better Brain Book*. He has some excellent comments on vitamins, mainly from the standpoint of good brain function as we age. Obviously, the worst thing we could do would be to protect our heart but destroy our brain.

REMINDERS

1. Anyone on a statin drug should also take CoEnzyme Q10.

2. B vitamins are excellent as supplements, especially as we age.

3. *The Better Brain Book* by Dr. David Perlmutter is a great resource for information on vitamins and supplements for good brain function.

> **4.** You can get many of the vitamins you need by drinking an ounce or two of wheat grass juice each day.
>
> **5.** The older we are and the more exercise we perform at this older age, the more free radicals we produce. I recommend combating the process with a proper supplement.

Fish Oil

I receive a huge number of questions about fish oil. People are concerned about the mercury levels in fish, and they should be, for such levels are increasing all over the world. Most people just don't like the taste or smell of fish.

I think the jury is in on the fish-based omega-3 polyunsaturated fatty acids. These are primarily EPA (eicosapentaenoic acid) and DHA (docosahexaenoic acid). These fish-based compounds significantly reduce cardiovascular deaths. They do this by reducing the degree of inflammation within the linings of the blood vessels (the endothelium), preventing clotting and other adverse conditions. If plaque rupture and vessel clotting do occur, they also seem to reduce sudden death by an electrical process.

If you decide to take EPA and DHA concentrated capsules, be sure that they are free of heavy metals, dioxin, and PCBs, all of which are found in increasing levels in fatty fish. If you decide to obtain your omega-3 fatty acids from ingestion of fatty fish, make sure you don't routinely eat farmed fish, as the industry is not very well supervised and the levels of these neurotoxins are higher than I personally would like to ingest on a regular basis.

> ### REMINDERS
>
> **1.** EPA and DHA are polyunsaturated fatty acids that had been shown to reduce cardiovascular mortality.
>
> **2.** It's good to supplement once or twice a week fatty fish consumption with a fish oil capsule on non-fish days.
>
> **3.** Keep fatty fish contaminants to a minimum. They are neurotoxic.

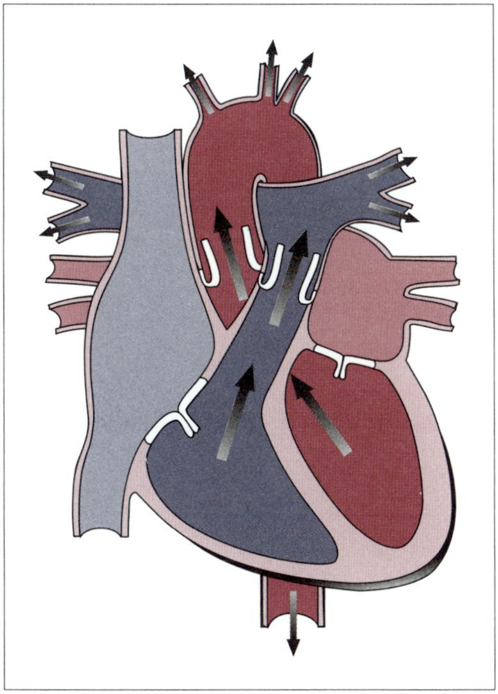

STRUTURE AND FUNCTION OF THE HEART AND BLOOD VESSELS

How It's All Put Together

THE HUMAN HEART IS BASICALLY a four-chambered, muscular structure containing four valves. Just like a house, the heart possesses its own unique electrical and plumbing systems. The primary function of the heart is to serve as a pumping station to provide the body with blood. The business of the heart and blood vessels can be summed up in one very important four letter word: flow. All of this—the marvelously complex heart, the endless miles of arteries and veins, the interspersed capillaries—have but one purpose: to provide adequate blood flow to each and every one of the billions of cells of the body, no matter what the conditions, no matter what the demands, no matter what the age. We'll explore the make-up of this incredible system, without which there would be no life, no brain or meaning in life, and no soul.

An Overview

The upper chambers of the heart are thin-walled, sparsely muscled receiving chambers (reservoirs). They are separated from the lower more muscular chambers, the ventricles, by valves. The left ventricle is the main pump, thickly muscular, while the right ventricle pumps against a much lower pressure and is thinner walled. Blood flows within an endless loop. Oxygen-rich red blood is pumped by the left ventricle through arteries to all parts of the body. Oxygen is given off by the hemoglobin molecule to the cells via a maze of capillaries, tiny spidery vessels between the smallest artery and the smallest venule. When oxygen is given off, it is swapped for carbon dioxide, the end product of cellular metabolism and energy expenditure. This "blue blood" is taken back to the right atrium via the veins. Blue blood, kept separate from the red, moves through the heart and is pumped to the lungs through the pulmonary artery. It is called an artery, even though it carries blue blood, because it comes off a pump—the right ventricle—and carries blood to a structure, in this case, the lungs. This blue blood reaches the lungs via smaller and smaller arteries until we once again get to tiny blood vessels. These vessels offer carbon dioxide from the hemoglobin molecule to the alveolus (the tiny air pocket in the lung) in exchange for oxygen. This red blood returns to the left atrium into the left ventricle and the cycle continues. (Figure 1)

Such a trip recurs between 60 and 150 times a minute depending on your level of activity. It is all made possible by the electrical stimulation of the heart, opening a couple of valves here, then there, an incredible choreography of motion in response to soundless electrical signals. We take it all for granted, but the heart "listens" to each of our emotions and actions, speeding up as needed, slowing when possible, ushering us through the complexities, heartbreaks, joys, and explosions of life with seldom a whimper. But this system, like any complex system, does and will break down, especially if we treat it badly.

The Electrical System of the Heart

There is a population of extremely well-specialized cells located in the upper portion of the right atrium. This is the chamber that receives blue blood (spent blood with oxygen removed) from all parts of the body. This specialized "node" of cells, called the sinus node, is responsible for initiating the electrical "spark" that subsequently spreads throughout the heart and causes the muscle to contract, pumping blood to all parts of the body. This occurs through a spontaneous intentional leak of ions across the

Figure 1 Main Arteries of the Body

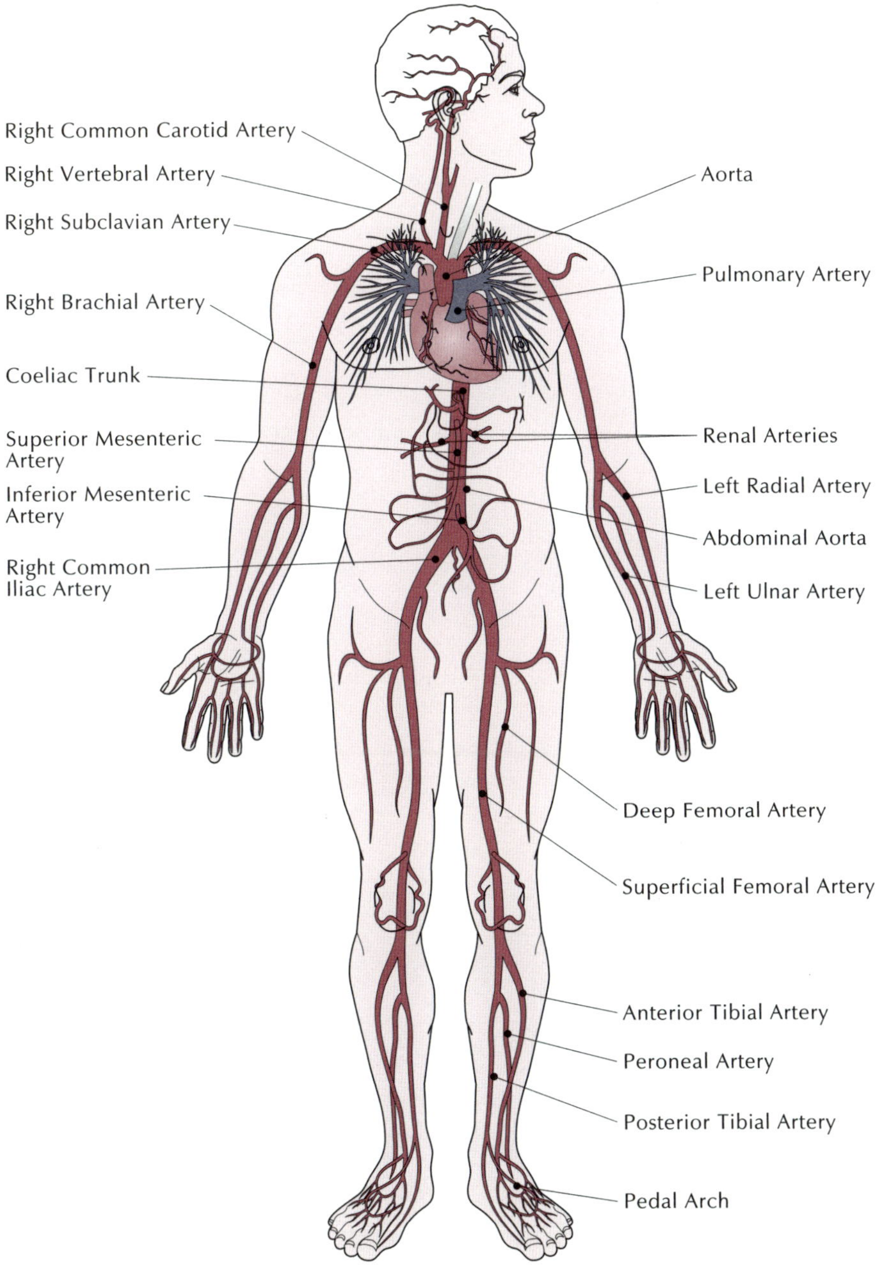

cell membrane. This spark of electrical current spreads synchronously throughout both upper chambers of the heart (the atria) so that they contract together. They pump blood into the main pumps of the heart, the lower chambers (the ventricles). The right ventricle pumps blue blood to the lungs where it will pick up oxygen. The left ventricle pumps red oxygenated blood out the giant blood tube, the aorta, to all parts of the body.

It may surprise you to learn that there are actually *three* intrinsic "pacemakers" within the heart. (Figure 2) In addition to the kingpin pacemaker mentioned above (the sinus node), there is the junctional pacemaker just below the level of the tricuspid and mitral valves (the valves that separate the upper and lower heart chambers) in the middle of the heart. A third pacemaker resides within the ventricular muscle.

The latter two are subservient. The junctional pacemaker and the ventricular pacemaker willingly follow the electrical cadence set by the sinus node. It is only when the sinus node fails that the junctional pacemaker assumes a lead role. Likewise, it is only when both the sinus node and junctional pacemakers have failed that a ventricular focus becomes the electrical captain of the heart.

Figure 2 Electrical System

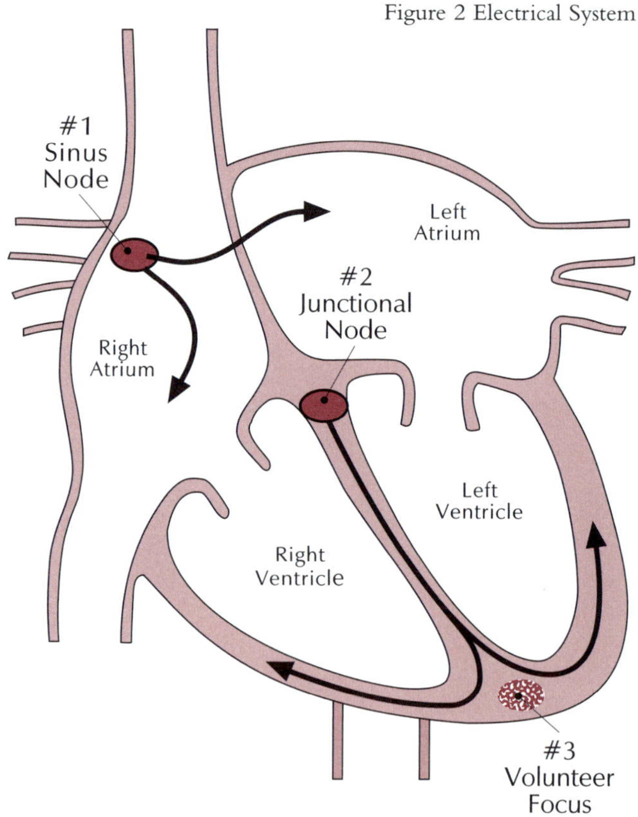

The sinus node is subject to the influences of various extrinsic signals. This area is literally and figuratively bombarded by signals, arriving in the form of nerve fibers that transmit what the rest of the body is experiencing. These influences come predominantly from the structure that possesses the notion it is in charge, namely, the brain. For example, if an individual is frightened, "fight or flight" hormones are released and the heart rate speeds up dramatically. If, on the other hand, the individual is in deep slumber, the heart rate will fall, as those hormone concentrations have decreased in the blood stream and there are frequently no disturbing signals from the body. When you have a nightmare, however, the heart rate increases more and more the closer you get to falling off the boulder and into the deep canyon. With excercise, the heart rate also rises. With lethargy or simple inactivity, it falls. The heart rate is much lower in a well-conditioned athlete since the mitochondria population (the energy-producing packets within all cells) in the muscles everywhere is so well-developed and the heart is so much more effective.

If one ingests a product that has a stimulative effect, such as caffeine or alcohol, the heart rate will increase. The heart rate rises mainly in response to these "fight or flight" influences, whether secondary to exercise, fear, or anger. The heart rate falls mainly in response to signals transmitted via the vagus nerve, the modulating nerve sending rate-lowering messages to the heart. This vagal system is activated by straining down, such as by inflating a balloon, by lifting, or by initiating a bowel movement. Some vagal tone is always present.

The sinus node is the most responsive to its owner's thoughts and actions, speeding or slowing to fit the need. On the other hand, the second tier "pacemaker," the junctional pacemaker, works at a fixed rate of about 40. There is little we can do to speed the junctional pacemaker when it assumes electrical control over the heart. At the sinus node level, the influence exerted by the vagus nerve is frequently overcome by excitatory stimuli of one sort or another. Not so with the junctional region. Here we are more apt to see just slowing influences.

In other words, the sinus node, subject to all sorts of messages—sometimes occurring all at once—runs the heart rate. This rate may vary from 60 to 160 beats per minute. If the sinus node fails, the junctional node, a collection of electrical cells with some semblance of automaticity, will emerge reluctantly as the pacemaker of the heart. It will pace the heart at a rate of about 40 beats per minute with very little rate variation. If it too fails, the ventricular pacemaker (the lowest spontaneous pacemaker) will maintain life with its intrinsic rate of about 25 to 35 beats per minute. This is a built-in survival mechanism, an electrical cascade of responsibility that allows for survival of the individual even though the dominant and even the intermediate pacemakers in the heart have failed.

As it makes its way throughout the heart, this electrical activity inscribes the unique pattern that we see on an electrocardiogram. Many electrical abnormalities can be detected merely by close scrutiny of this recording. Obviously, with an electrical system this intricate, coupled with all of the things that we humans do to rev it up or tone it down, there is going to be an occasional malfunction. This malfunction, as it happens, becomes more likely as we make our passage through life.

The Valve System of the Heart

There are four valves within the heart. These are the structures that compartmentalize the blood, holding it securely within a particular chamber. We will take this in stepwise fashion, following blood through the heart. Keep in mind, however, that the upper chambers pump in synchrony, and then the lower chambers pump in synchrony.

Blue blood, from which oxygen has been removed at the tissue level, returns to the right upper chamber, the right atrium. (Figure 3) It enters from vessels draining the head and upper extremities via the *superior* vena cava. Blood arrives from vessels draining everything below the heart via the *inferior* vena cava. The right atrium is a holding chamber, acting largely as a reservoir. When the electrical activity activates the atria, they pump together, the right atrium pumping blue blood into the major pump of the right heart, the right ventricle. When this is accomplished, the tricuspid valve, the first valve the blood encounters in its trip through the heart, closes. When the right ventricle pumps blood toward the lungs, this valve prevents escape of blood back into the atrium. The valve at the other end of this forward passage, the pulmonic valve, then opens and allows for the bulk of this blood that has entered the right ventricle to now be pumped into the pulmonary arteries, the giant arteries carrying blood to the lungs. When the right ventricle relaxes, the pulmonic valve closes, acting as a check valve to prevent blood that has been handled from escaping back into its pump.

Figure 3 Cut-away of Heart and Vessels

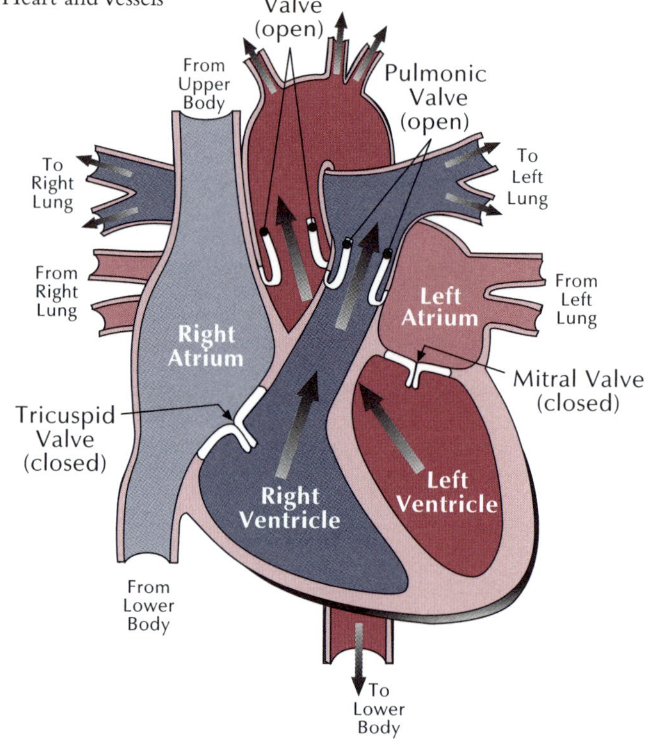

Red blood, which has taken up oxygen from the lungs, enters the left atrium when it is relaxed. As the atrium pumps, blood is pushed across the wide-open mitral valve into the major pumping station of the left heart, the left ventricle. When the left ventricle contracts, the mitral valve closes, preventing leakage of blood back into the left heart reservoir (the atrium). As the left ventricle contracts, blood opens the aortic valve, pumping red blood into the giant blood conduit (the aorta) which in turn carries it to every organ in the body.

As you can tell, each valve needs to be performing its task efficiently for this synchronized choreography to work. Grasp the concept that the electrical system activates the heart muscle and the muscular pump moves the blood forward. The upper chambers contract together and the lower chambers contract together. The valves prevent back-flow of blood that has been handled, always ensuring the forward passage of blood, with minimal leakage across the valves.

The tricuspid and the mitral valves, sometimes called the *atrioventricular valves* because they are situated between the atria and the ventricles, are somewhat similar in anatomic features. The mitral is much more intricate and made up of valve tissue attached to a ring (annulus) within the opening. This mitral valve tissue is quite extensive. If we excise the mitral valve and smooth it out on a bench, the area of the tissue is about three times that of the mitral valve ring. It is supported by roughly 32 delicate strings—fine, slender threads of connective tissue extending from the valve tissue to protrusions of the ventricular muscle—called papillary muscles. This mitral valve is exceptionally complex, and not only does the amount of valve tissue need to be just right but the support strings (the chordae tendinae) need to be just the correct length for this valve to work efficiently. As the left ventricle contracts, the papillary muscle contracts along with it. This tenses the chordae, holding the mitral valve in place with the leaflet tissue snugging one section against another in a process called coaptation. Closed in this fashion, the valve tissue is similar to an accordion.

The aortic valve and the pulmonic valve are similar to each other in structure. They are much less intricate than the atrioventricular valves and are made up of three leaflets. These leaflets open, then close, with this encounter of tissue forming a juncture called a commissure.

The Heart Muscle

The heart muscle is unique. The atria, while containing muscle that is capable of contracting, are only endowed with a scant amount of muscle compared to the ventricles. This is because the atria only have to pump blood into the ventricles at very low pressure under normal conditions. The ventricles are the main pumping chambers and therefore possess predominantly muscle cells which are arranged in a unique fashion. These muscle fibers lay neatly one beside the other so that they form an organized unit of labor. This composition of fibers, taken together as they spiral around the heart, is called a syncytium. Because the right ventricle pumps against a peak pressure of only about 15–25 mmHg (millimeters of mercury, a form of blood pressure measurement, just like that measured with a blood pressure cuff), it is relatively thin-walled as compared to the greater work horse, the left ventricle. The left ventricle must pump against the blood pressure we measure within the arm with a cuff, ideally about 120/80 mmHg.

Muscle fibers contract in response to a stimulus, such as electricity, by fiber shortening. Remember the twitch of the frog leg in biology class when it was shocked by a spark of electric current? The same applies to the heart muscle cells. Only they do it all together, thousands and thousands of them spiraling about the lower chambers, involving both the right and the left ventricles. When the fibers shorten, the cavities encased within this muscle fiber network—the right and left ventricles—get smaller. When this happens, the blood has to go somewhere. It goes out the valves at the distal end of each ventricle—blue blood to the lungs, and red blood to the organs.

The left ventricle is the main pump of the heart, pumping oxygen-rich blood into the aorta with each beat. The geometric configuration of the ventricle is of paramount importance in this task. The left ventricle looks kind of like a football with one end cut off. When all of these spiraling muscle cells contract, the heart actually twists as it empties its contents, then untwists when it relaxes. This was first recorded by Leonardo da Vinci in the 16th century (along with everything else, it seems). This "wringing" geometric change is extremely important in the proper function of both ventricles, but especially so with the left.

Just like the skeletal muscle fibers in the legs or elsewhere, these heart muscle fibers always require a certain maintenance amount of blood to supply them with oxygen and nutrients. The harder they work, the faster they go, and the more aggressively they contract, the more oxygen and nutrients they require and the more the blood source has to increase to satisfy them. The result of all of that work is lactic acid, carbon dioxide, and other end products of metabolism.

As an aside, it is obvious why one frequently has so much pain when a heart attack occurs. Blood flow to a portion of the heart muscle ceases due to an obstruction, but the muscle keeps on valiantly trying to do its job, producing lactic acid as it does so. This build-up of lactic acid is similar to that which accumulates in the leg muscles when you climb stairs, and it burns in much the same way.

These muscle cells all contain mitochondria. These are the energy-generating packets within any cell. If the muscle cell is insulted, for example, by a virus or by inadequate blood flow, these mitochondria will start to falter. We have found by performing biopsies on skeletal muscle, that three months worth of repetitive work is necessary to develop the maximal population of mitochondria, while only three days of relative inactivity will allow that same population to start to wane. This hardly seems fair but it is reality.

The Plumbing System of the Heart

The plumbing of the heart consists of the arteries that carry red oxygenated blood to the hard-working heart muscle cells. This is a big task. These muscle cells can't simply stop and rest. They keep at it 24/7. In fact, if you are 50 years of age with a mean heart rate of 60 beats per minute, your heart muscle cells have each contracted 1,576,800,000 times! A lot of blood has been pumped. The pump is totally dependent upon its supply of blood directed to the muscle via the arterial conduits bringing constant supplies of oxygen and nutrients. It will not tolerate even a brief interruption of supply.

Remember that all arteries carrying blood to various organs originate from the aorta, the giant blood tube emerging from the heart. The very first arteries that come off the aorta do so just above the heart and carry blood to the heart muscle. They are called the coronary arteries and there are three: the left anterior descending that travels down the front of the heart, the circumflex that carries blood around to the back side of the heart, and the right coronary artery that supplies the bottom portion of the heart. (Figure 4)

Figure 4 Coronary Arteries

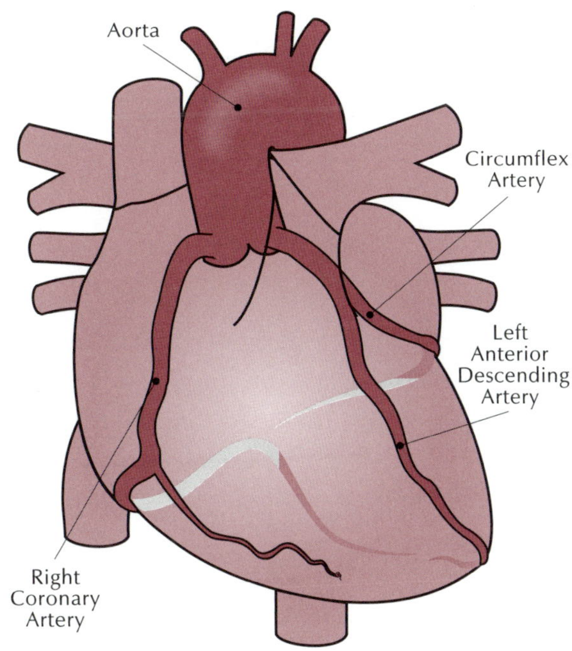

In most people, the left anterior descending coronary artery is by far the most important in that it supplies the most territory. It also supplies tremendously important structures, albeit for different reasons. It supplies the apex (tip) of the heart. Since the heart twists and shortens as it squeezes, the apex plays a vital role in this geometric form. If one loses the apex, the pumping action of the heart becomes markedly altered. The left anterior descending also supplies the septum, the partition that separates the lower chambers. Through this septum goes the electrical system connecting the upper chambers to the lower. One can readily see that if the left anterior descending artery is lost, not only is a lot of muscle in jeopardy but vital structures can be damaged, potentially resulting in electrical catastrophes.

The coronary arteries carry blood to the heart muscle primarily during the time when the heart muscle is relaxed, called diastole. During systole, when the muscle cells contract, coronary blood flow tapers off.

Structure and Function of Arteries

Figure 5 Cut-away of Artery

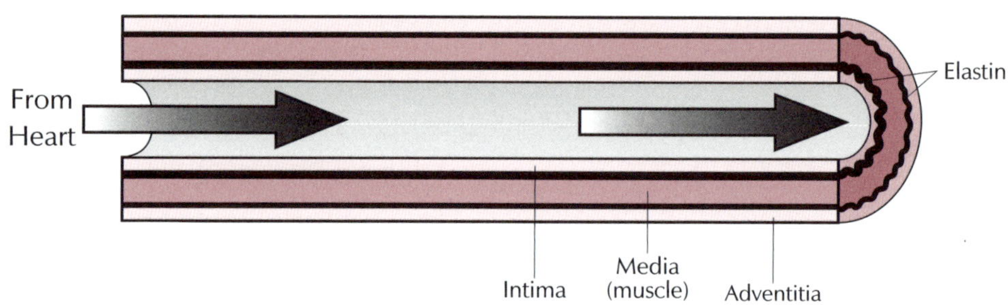

The structure of arteries is unique and is the same for all arteries of the body. (Figure 5) The thin, inside lining is called the *intima*. The middle portion, called the *media*, is comprised of smooth muscle and elastic fibers. These act to provide "tone" to the artery. Within the innermost lining of the arteries is the exceptionally important *endothelium*, the vast one-cell thick manufacturing system of nitric oxide that relaxes the walls of the artery, as well as millions of other production responsibilities, all of which influence the well-being of the artery and ultimately, its owner.

Each artery in the body is invested with a plethora of nerve fibers. These give instructions to the arterial wall as to whether more or less blood is needed to be carried through the arterial conduit. The elastic fiber in the media of the artery gives recoil to the artery when it has been distended. The muscle fibers can relax, enlarging the artery, or inversely, can contract, causing the artery to become smaller. The amount of blood that is carried down the lumen of the artery is dependent upon this mechanism.

The outer layer of any artery is comprised of connective tissue, a protective covering called the *adventitia*.

Structure and Function of Veins

Figure 6 Cut-away of Vein

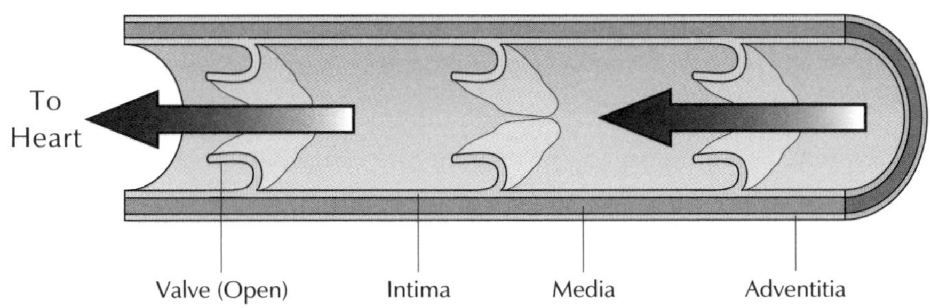

The veins are the structures that carry spent (oxygen-depleted) blood back to the heart from any organ in the body. They all converge upon the superior vena cava, carrying blue blood back to the heart from the head and arms, and the inferior vena cava, draining the lower extremities. Contrasted to arteries, the veins are thin-walled, flimsy-looking structures. (Figure 6) The larger ones possess valves, appearing as chevrons within the vein.

Blood is returned to the heart via the venous system primarily due to a milking action exerted by the surrounding muscles. For example, the longest venous structure in the body is that draining the legs. If you are immobile, such as on a long airplane trip, blood tends to pool in the leg veins, and it is not unusual to find that your legs have swollen during the journey. This is because pressure has built up at the lowest point, the feet and ankles, pushing water into the surrounding tissues.

When you get up and move about, the muscles in the legs contract, milking blood up toward the heart by literally squeezing the walls of the veins within this muscular compartment. When blood is pushed upward, the valves open. When a column of blood

Figure 7 Oxygen Exchange in Capillary

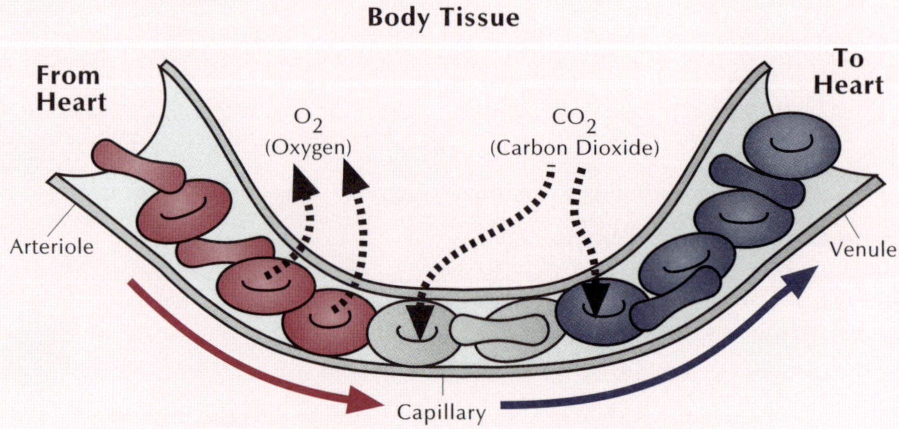

has made its way upward, the valve closes, holding that column in place until another column of blood comes along to push it higher yet. This awkward and unseemly mechanism gets the job done. However, it should come as no great surprise that after 50 or 60 years of performing this silent thankless task, some of these structures don't look so great and they don't work as well as they once did. For example, these valves may start to break down creating varicosities, better known as varicose veins.

Wear and tear is not usually the trouble, however. The real trouble frequently comes in the form of some sort of insult. This insult, usually a result of surgery, trauma, inactivity, or cancer, causes activation of the clotting mechanism throughout the body. This, in turn, causes clot to form inappropriately, frequently with serious consequences.

Capillaries

No discourse on the structure and function of the circulatory system would be complete without at least a nod to the little vessels that actually deliver the oxygen and nutrients to the tissues. These are the capillaries, often excluded in our rush to define the function of their larger parent vessels. They are the end result of the ever-diminishing size of vessels off the arterial side of things, as well as the smallest and earliest vessels on the venous side, carrying oxygen-depleted blood back to the heart. In 1619, Sir William Harvey described so many things correctly in his famous treatise, *De Motu Cordis.* Amongst them was his discovery of the existence of these tiny networks connecting the arteries to the veins, dropping off oxygen to the cells in the bargain. (Figure 7)

REMINDERS

1. The electrical system within the structure of the heart consists of three pacemaker systems stacked so that each lower pacemaker has a slower rate than the one above it. Both the junctional and ventricular pacemakers are subservient to the upper pacemaker, the sinus node.
2. This lead pacemaker, the sinus node, is subject to a multitude of stimuli which serve to speed the heart rate in response to the body's need or simply due to stimulants that we humans like to use. It is also subject to influences that would serve to slow the heart rate. The mid-heart pacemaker is usually more responsive to slowing influences, and the lower pacemaker is autonomous, running at a set, very slow, rate.
3. The valves within the heart are there to function with one purpose only: to prevent blood that has been pumped from one chamber to another from leaking back into the previous chamber.
4. The heart muscle is unique, spiraling around the heart. The twisting motion and configuration of the heart is intricately involved in the efficiency of the pumping chambers.
5. The plumbing system of the heart consists of three coronary arteries running on the surface of the heart, sending perforator vessels down into the muscle to provide oxygen and nutrients to the heart muscle. The heart muscle can't rest. Therefore, these arterial conduits need to constantly bring blood to the muscle.
6. All arteries within the body have the same composition and design. It is important for each artery to have a mechanism for getting smaller or larger—carrying less or more blood and oxygen correspondingly—to fit the metabolic needs of the structure it serves. This is done through an investment of nerves carrying messages regarding the level of need, and hormones in the blood stream, causing local changes in the caliber of the arteries.

7. The arteries throughout the body must work within a high-pressure environment. The same blood pressure measured with a cuff around the arm is transmitted throughout the arteries. This makes them uniquely susceptible to arteriosclerosis, a deposition of cholesterol within the wall of the artery, the nemesis of modern society.
8. Veins, on the other hand, carry blood within a very low-pressure environment. This rather sluggish flow makes the blood within them more likely to clot. This is the major form of trouble within the venous system.

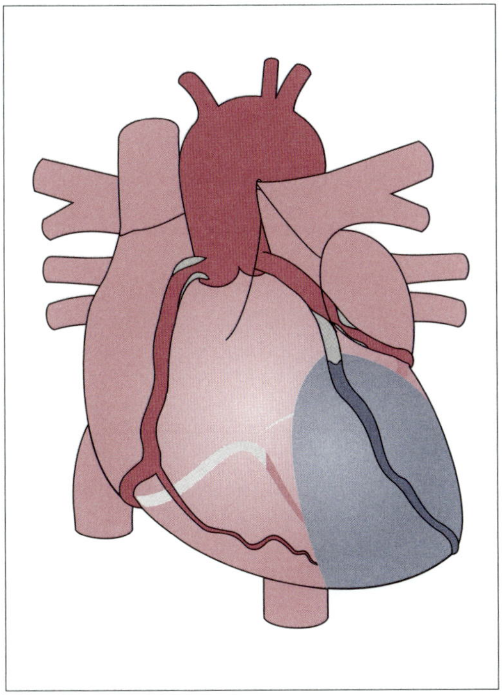

3 HEART ATTACK!

A Heart Artery Has Closed

CORONARY ARTERY DISEASE (CAD) IS THE number one killer in America. Almost half of adult men will die of cardiovascular disease. Of great surprise to many is that the fate of American women is not much different. In fact, while the death rate from cardiovascular disease has fallen slightly in men, it has risen in women. In polls, if women are asked from which disease they are most prone to die, they routinely answer, "breast cancer." Cardiovascular disease including stroke, heart attack, and congestive heart failure actually claims more women's lives in the U.S. than all forms of cancer put together! It's such a strong mortality influence that cardiovascular disease becomes the predominant mortality in women after age 25.

However, the diagnosis of CAD certainly does *not* imply a coronary death is in your future or that a *myocardial infarction* (MI or heart attack) will occur at some point. There is a huge amount of "silent" CAD out there. In fact, it is mostly silent. *The purpose of this book is to keep it silent and suppressed.* But when trouble strikes, and it inevitably will in some of us, the purpose of this book is to tell you how and when to get help.

CAD is the deposition of cholesterol beneath the inner-most lining (the *intima*) of the artery supplying the heart muscle. This is an insidious process that, depending on the incidence, severity, and multiplicity of known risk factors, may begin at an early age and may progress with absolutely no warning. Women are relatively protected by hormonal influences until menopause. Therefore, this is traditionally an earlier disease in men by 10 to 15 years. After this gender-induced moratorium, the women unfortunately catch up with the men at warp speed.

The well-built muscular man standing beside you at Home Depot or the pretty vivacious woman at Starbucks may well have CAD. As the saying goes, "Looks can be deceiving." Several years ago, my secretary was a muscular, fit young lady who was very calm and looked like the last person in the world who would be a candidate for a heart attack. I moved to a different city when she was about 35 years old. Some 15 years later, I was shocked to learn that while standing in the screening line at a large city airport, she suffered a cardiac arrest. As is common for women with CAD, she had experienced some mild discomfort in the epigastrium (the area just below the breast bone) but not in the chest, jaws, or arms. She thought little about it; it only seemed a nuisance. The discomfort recurred in the airport security line, but this time it was more severe. She then developed sweating and lightheadedness. She asked the security officer if they had an external defibillator because she thought she was having a heart attack and might be having a cardiac arrhythmia. She could feel her heart beating wildly inside her chest and was worried that she might black out.

Just after they laid her down on the floor, she lost consciousness, had a seizure, and was promptly defibrillated by the airport security personnel. She was immediately taken to a hospital where a cardiologist promptly diagnosed the problem as an acute occlusion of the left anterior descending coronary artery, and deployed a stent, reestablishing blood flow to the heart muscle downstream. They saved her life at the airport. The procedure performed by the cardiologist saved the bulk of her heart muscle supplied by that artery. Since this is usually the most important coronary of the three vessels supplying the heart muscle, and since large heart attacks in the distribution of this artery are so closely linked to life-ending or life-changing results, this story had a magnificent ending.

Most CAD is silent. There is no warning bell going off. In this young lady's case, there was a very strong family history of CAD and she had chronically elevated serum cholesterol, but it was being treated. She had never smoked and she religiously worked out every day. She had no symptoms that were typical of CAD. Her symptoms, as is the case with so many women, were atypical. We were taught in medical school that heart pain due to inadequate arterial blood supply (*angina*) would be crushing pain in the center of the chest radiating into the arm (left more than right) or jaws. All too frequently, this is simply not the case in women. They are more likely than men to have pain in the area just below the sternum and are more likely than men to have sweating and nausea as associated symptoms. Even men seldom fit the classic textbook caricature that we learned. This is truly a silent disease in most people until some stimulus causes it to explode onto the scene like an uninvited guest at a wedding!

In this story, my secretary's experience working in a cardiac office gave her a headstart so that she knew something was dreadfully wrong. The assessment of the situation she gave to the security staff may have saved precious minutes and even brain function.

It is important for you to become empowered with knowledge of cardiac and blood vessel disease not only because it is the number one killer in today's society, but because it is primarily up to you to detect it and take care of it. For example, even if this young lady had been seen by her doctor a week before this event, she may not have had the work-up necessary to preempt this emergency. In the city where I work, which is blessed by having good doctors, I can tell you that she likely would not have had her problem detected. However, if she had known that she had silent CAD, her cholesterol would have been addressed much more vigorously and, hopefully, she would have had a test to determine if she were a high-risk individual for a heart attack. I would like to reemphasize one important point: This prevalent disease develops over years, remaining silent in the great majority of people until a triggering event occurs. We will explore just what this trigger might be.

Lipid (fat) material can be deposited in the wall of any artery in the body. It is never deposited within the walls of veins, just arteries, as these are the high-pressure conduits in the body. The coronary arteries carrying red, oxygenated blood to the heart are by far the most vulnerable of any of the arteries in the body. When we speak of atheromatous material, plaque, or an arterial lesion, we are speaking of the same thing: this complex deposit of fat material and its conglomerate parts within the arterial wall.

Years ago, we thought this plaque material was inert and that the deposits occurred slowly until the vessel became completely clogged and a heart attack occurred due to the abrupt stoppage of blood delivery to the heart muscle. We now know that the cellular composition of the plaque, along with activity of the innermost cell layer within the artery, determines whether this process remains silent or becomes vicious and destructive. Here's how it happens:

Plaque Formation

The initiation of this plaque formation can be precipitated by one or several causes. First, the plaque almost always occurs in an area of the coronary circulation where turbulence is strongest, just like debris accumulating at the split of a raging mountain stream. We call this effect—the drag force acting on the inside of the blood vessel—the shear stress. We know that arteriosclerosis (the laying down of plaque) is most prominent in those areas where there is directional change in the pattern of flow. There is also frequently some degree of inflammation present at that site, but this may well be coupled with a high LDL-cholesterol ("bad" cholesterol), a low HDL-cholesterol ("good" cholesterol), high triglycerides (a blood stream fat generated from sugar), or a high homocysteine (a pesky, arterial-destructive amino acid) level. In fact, all of these may be present. Additionally, the individual may be diabetic or pre-diabetic and insulin-resistant. He or she may smoke and may have raging high blood pressure. We know that these factors all lead to the formation of arteriosclerosis, this slow plaque accumulation. However, to muddy the waters, sometimes none of these abnormalities or habits is obvious. Approached statistically, each of these risk factors produces an additional likelihood that such a plaque will develop within the arteries. Tobacco, *any* kind of tobacco usage, incites injury to the inside of the blood vessel. This focus of injury continues to accumulate plaque material long after the injurious cause has been removed. In other words, plaque begets plaque.

Figure 8 Coronary Artery with Partial Obstruction

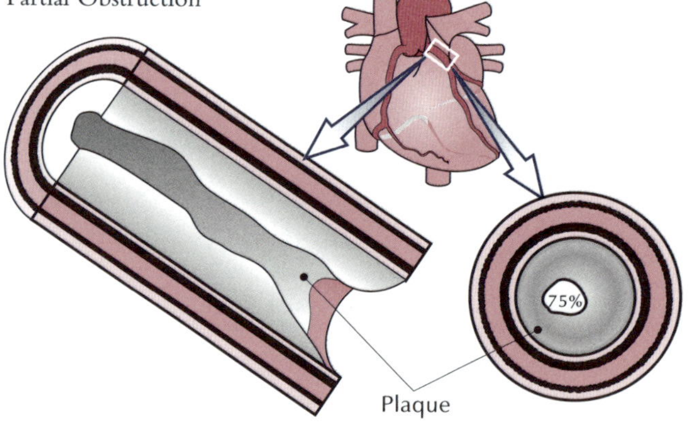

While this material may be distributed throughout the entire artery, and usually is, the major focus is frequently fairly discreet due to some early damage in one particular susceptible area of the artery. (Figure 8) If the plaque build-up continues until it poses a partial obstruction to blood flow, we refer to it as a *stenosis,* and with angiography (outlining the wall of the artery with contrast material that stands out on x-rays), we grade the severity by the apparent degree of blockage. When that stenosis becomes so severe that it restricts flow to the downstream heart muscle to the extent that it is not receiving sufficient nutrients and oxygen, we refer to this situation as *ischemia.*

We know that anything less than a 50% stenosis never causes ischemia, even under circumstances of exertion, accompanied as it is by increased oxygen demands by the heart. We also know that a 75% stenosis will likely cause ischemia only with exercise or stress. Since there is continuous adjustment of the tension within the wall of the coronary artery, as is true in all arteries of the body, there may well be considerable variation in the size of the lumen (the inside channel where blood travels) of the artery. This depends on environmental and emotional influences such as stress, activity, eating, or sleeping.

What are these coronary plaques made of? We said earlier that instead of being inert, they are dynamic structures made up of an array of changing elements. A plaque consists of a glob of lipid (fat material) within an environment that with time usually accumulates some degree of calcium. The older the plaque, the more likely it is to possess calcium and in progressively greater concentration. Calcium is usually a more predictable component in men than in women. However, it is the cellular composition that really makes the difference between a dormant and an aggressively changing plaque.

Each plaque possesses a unique number and predominance of these cellular elements. All of this—lipid core, cells, and usually, calcium—is contained by a thin connective tissue covering, the fibrous cap. This enclosing cap is made from collagen fibers similar to thin scar tissue. This very flimsy-looking fibrous cap is what keeps the plaque from splitting open and wreaking havoc. It is the only structure that stands between tranquility and disaster, and that is exactly why we treat it with so much respect.

There are basically two main cell types within this plaque material. The fibroblasts are thin flat cells that look like oat seeds. They migrate to the surface and produce materials to rebuild and reinforce the protective fibrous cap. These fibroblasts are the good guys. Therefore, we yearn for a strong predominant population of them. The macrophage is more of a scoundrel. These are large somewhat misshapen cells that produce enzymes such as metalloproteases that attack the composition of the fibrous cap. In significant numbers and accompanied by increased activity within the endothelium of the artery (the inside single-cell layer), they can become assertive enough to cause erosion or rupture of the fibrous cap. This sets the stage for a heart attack.

So far, three factors have been defined that set the stage for plaque rupture:

1. A lipid-laden core.
2. A thinned-out fibrous cap, usually with abundant macrophages right under the surface.
3. A preponderance of inflammatory cells.

Unfortunately, we have no way of clinically detecting this disturbing and sometimes rapidly evolving situation. This sequence leads to the formation of *vulnerable plaque*, so named because these have been identified as the plaque most likely to rupture. Pathologists noticed a population of these plaques in people who suffered a heart attack. Specifically, they observed that the culprit plaque that caused the heart attack was eroded and a clot had formed next to it. However, another phrase we like to use is "plaques travel in packs." Other members of the "pack" were of the above-described variety and also ready to pop. We currently have no good way to recognize the presence of these vulnerable plaques, but we're getting closer with the multi-slice CT angiogram and MRI angiography. The pathologists' discovery of vulnerable plaque is of great interest, as it is almost certainly the "pre–heart attack" plaque, the one that is ripe for erosion and rupture.

The spectrum of events leading up to a heart attack is made even more complex by influences upon the endothelium, the one-cell thick inside layer of the artery where so many messengers are assembled. These can dictate health or havoc within the artery.

Early Detection

Obviously, we would like to detect this process before a heart attack occurs. Early detection is always the best thing, no matter what we are dealing with. This is doubly true with a heart attack. When someone comes into the emergency room with a fatal heart attack, we frequently lament, "If only we had seen him yesterday!" Yesterday, his vulnerable plaque was ready to rupture but he was still asymptomatic. While it is true we cannot yet identify a vulnerable plaque, we can indirectly determine its presence. For example, there are many markers of inflammation that we can measure. The high-sensitivity *C-Reactive Protein* (hsCRP) along with traditional coronary risk factors constitute the best early detection signals available. Again, all of the known coronary risk factors—smoking, abnormal blood lipids, high blood pressure, family history of heart attack or stroke, diabetes, obesity, and sedentary lifestyle—are *additive*. The more you have, the more likely you are to have silent coronary artery disease. When we see evidence of inflammation tied to one or more or these conventional risk factors, we are very concerned that a vulnerable plaque—ready to rupture and cause a heart attack—may be potentially forming. When we see a high CRP but a normal lipid profile (not a common finding), we still treat it with a statin drug. We have only a couple of drugs that we feel have any influence over this inflammation. A statin drug (the same drug we use to treat elevated LDL-cholesterol) is considered the best, though an angiotensin-converting enzyme-inhibitor and platelet drugs are thought to exert positive influences as well. If we try to separate out those individuals who are at most risk of having a vulnerable plaque ready to morph into an ulcerated plaque as a precursor to a heart attack, they are the ones with either a very high LDL-cholesterol or a very low HDL-cholesterol (or both) coupled with high hsCRP levels. If this were reliably precise, we would have a great way of finding the "pre–heart attack" individuals. It is not precise, however, and there are many variations. This is where coronary screening of those with coronary risk factors—no matter what the combination—comes into play.

As a person's list of known atherosclerotic risk factors grows, so should the need to perform non-invasive tests to determine if the disease of arteriosclerosis has already planted its roots. If so, how deeply? These tests are discussed in detail in Chapter 10 on *Silent Coronary Artery Disease and Angina.*

Plaque Rupture, Coronary Occlusion, and Heart Attack

There are many factors that bring about rupture of a plaque within a coronary artery. We know now that as the fat material enters the wall of the artery, a protein called a cytokine is secreted. Cytokine causes two things to happen:

1. Misshapen cells called macrophages develop from a cell type within the bloodstream (monocytes) and become part of the plaque system.
2. The area of the artery involved becomes "sticky." The enzymes produced by these macrophages play a substantial role in determining what happens to the plaque.

If enough of these enzymes are produced, they may well cut through the fibrous cap, allowing for rupture of the plaque into the lumen of the blood vessel. In other words, the plaque cracks open. This plaque erosion or ulceration is the cause of almost all heart attacks.

We know that something dynamic sets this plaque up for rupture. The vulnerable plaque concept is extremely important. For example, it is not unusual to find an ulcerated *carotid* (the artery leading to the brain) plaque system in a patient with a ruptured coronary plaque and a recent heart attack. It seems, then, that the signal sent to activate a plaque in a coronary artery may not just be a "local" phenomenon, but may well be due to a more generalized signal. An even more likely explanation is that the body's chemistry has brought about this life-threatening change in the integrity of plaques within the arteries of the body, causing plaque rupture here and there.

Whatever the reason, we refer to the unstable and activated plaque within a coronary artery—leading to a threatened heart attack—as an *acute coronary syndrome.*

These lipid-laden plaques are important. While many plaque systems possess a great deal of calcium, some of these vulnerable plaque systems do not. This is especially true in women, who tend to calcify less and later than men. This is one of the reasons that when a woman complains of symptoms that might represent ischemia, a multi-slice CT angiogram is ordered straightaway. It will frequently detect these lipid-laden plaque

FFigure 9a Stable Plaque

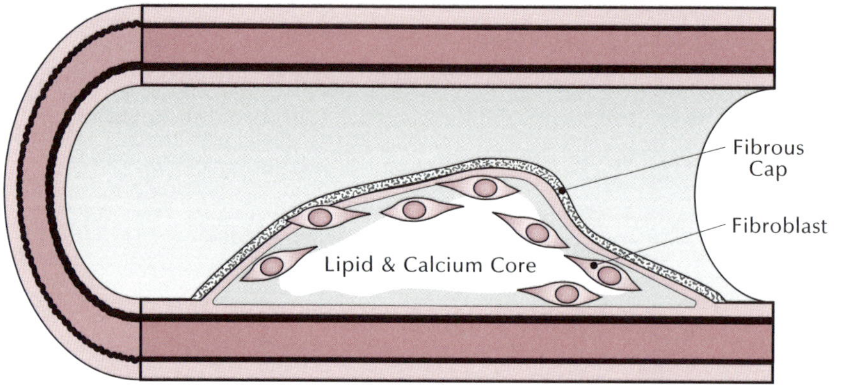

Figure 9b Vulnerable Plaque

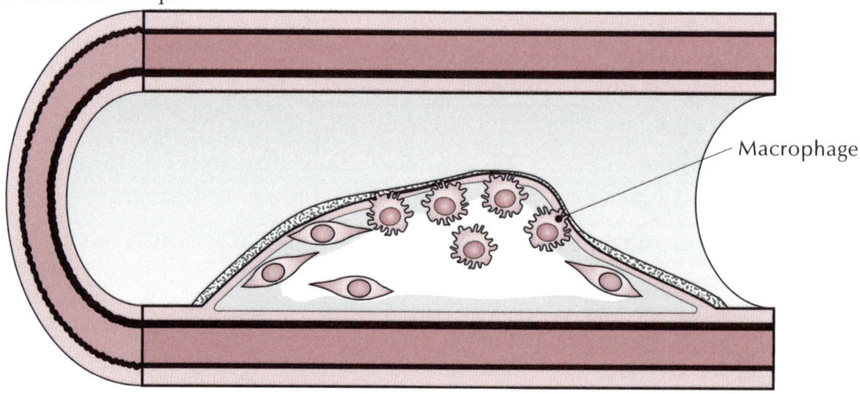

systems, while a test that merely measures calcium deposits within the coronary artery misses the situation completely. Nonetheless, it is not just these non-calcified plaques that rupture. Plenty of heart attacks occur due to plaque erosion of a heavily calcified plaque. Whether calcified or not, plaque erosion and rupture is the first in the sequence of events in the transition from a vulnerable plaque to a heart attack.

Figure 9c Ruptured Plaque

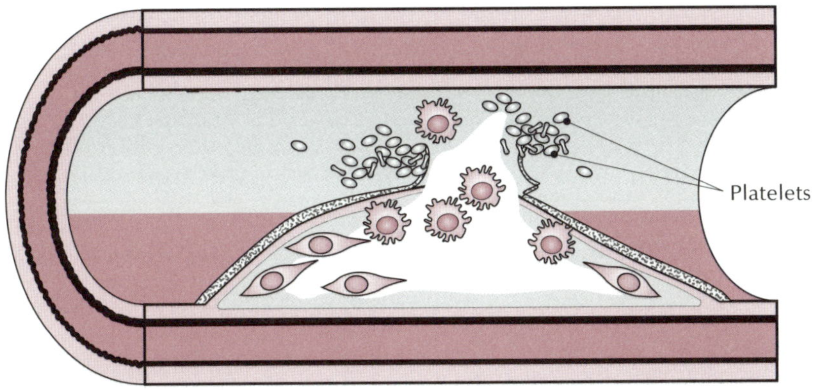

Platelets within the blood stream are the first line of defense in the event of any injury that might cause interruption of the integrity of a blood vessel. There are approximately 250,000 to 500,000 platelets per cc (about a million in a teaspoon of blood). In the event of an injury, such as a ruptured spleen in an automobile accident, they become activated and rush to the site of the injury. There they start to clump—like holding hands with each other—to initiate the clotting process. They are the first responders. Unfortunately, platelets cannot think and have no way of knowing whether their owner has been involved in an automobile accident or has merely ruptured a coronary plaque system. In the first process, they may save your life; in the second, they may help end it.

The collective platelets serve as a loosely organized system that is easy to disperse. However, as time goes on, other elements such as fibrin (the architectural framework of a clot) form within the platelet plug. With each passing minute, the clot becomes more

Figure 9d Clot Formation

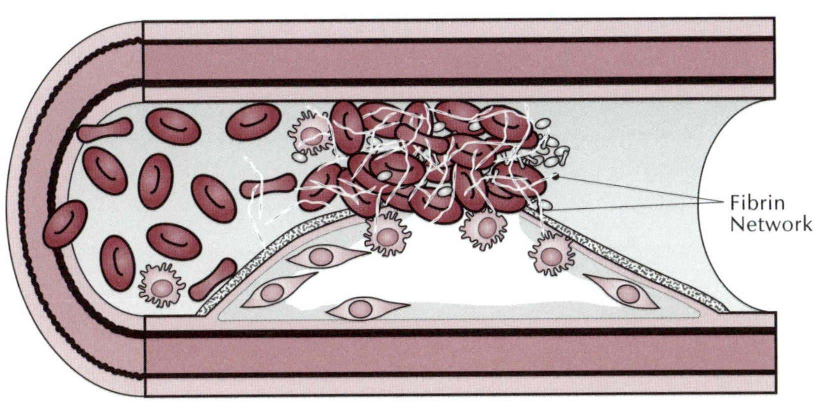

and more organized, denser and tougher, due to a reworked, more sophisticated fibrin network. The clot also becomes more and more difficult to dissolve. When the structure of the clot becomes tightly reinforced, flow down the coronary artery is completely obstructed, and the downstream heart muscle cells start to suffer because of lack of oxygen and nutrients. Lactic acid, the same stuff that makes your leg muscles burn when you climb stairs, begins to accumulate in the heart muscle tissue. This is because the contracting heart muscle cells continue to work as diligently as they can, pumping blood to all parts of the body. However, the waste products of energy production, lactic acid, cannot be washed away because in-coming blood flow to this afflicted segment of heart muscle has ceased. This is the beginning of a heart attack. (Figure 9a,b,c,d, pages 42–43)

Something dramatic triggers this cascade of events. All at once, a perfectly stable plaque began its silent course of destruction. We now believe that inflammatory cytokines are at least as important as the macrophage cell in this process. Cytokines act like hormones, signaling certain events. The cytokine messenger can help you if you have an infectious disease; it signals for help from all of the infection-fighting white cells in the body. In the wall of the coronary, within the complexities of the coronary plaque, lies the macrophage sending out erosive enzymes, constantly interacting with the signals sent by these inflammatory cytokines. Unfortunately, the cytokines signal that it is time to rev up and clot off this artery. This is only one example of a cellular mechanism inflicting damage on its owner due to a primitive reflex action.

Time is Muscle

Early identification and treatment is of utmost importance in dealing with a heart attack. The earlier we get treatment for a heart attack, the greater the chance that it can be interrupted, and we can salvage the bulk of the heart muscle supplied by the culprit artery. Remember, the loosely clumped platelet plug is readily broken up, while the fibrin network is tougher. This fibrin network is time-dependent and becomes more and more mature, remodeling busily, as though clot formation is in your best interest. The longer these stunned but courageous cells are starved for oxygen and nutrients, the greater the population of cells that will ultimately perish. The term "Time is Muscle" has become the mantra of the cardiologist.

The heart muscle can scream for oxygen only so long before it is killed off. There is significant individual variation in the susceptibility of heart muscle cells to oxygen deprivation. There is a point, however, after oxygen deprivation is initiated due to complete coronary blockage, when the muscle cells simply start to die off. The ones at the epicenter of the heart attack zone die off first. As the distance from the epicenter increases, more cells are merely stunned, can potentially recover, and then can eventually be reclaimed as a vital part of the heart pump once again. The longer these stunned but courageous cells are starved for oxygen and nutrients, the more they will ultimately perish. The greater the population of cell death, the greater the future compromise of the individual's life, both in quality and duration. *Time is muscle!*

Time is Muscle *and* Life

There is a more immediate reason to obtain early attention for a heart attack. When a coronary artery closes, there is a significant risk of a fatal disruption of the normal rhythm of the heart. This chaotic electrical storm, triggered by oxygen-deprivation to the heart muscle cells, is called *ventricular tachycardia,* and this frequently deteriorates into *ventricular fibrillation.* These are very rapid, ineffectual heart rhythms which are incapable of producing an adequate blood pressure. If this happens outside the hospital or, more appropriately these days, outside of an environment where a defibrillator is on hand, death ensues. Therefore, the mantra should perhaps be "Time is muscle *and* life." The story of my former secretary underscores this point quite dramatically.

Symptoms of a Heart Attack

What exactly are the symptoms of a heart attack? In the most classic form, they consist of a squeezing, vice-like pain in the middle of the chest, perhaps with radiation to the arms or jaws, associated with sweating and perhaps nausea just like we learned in medical school. Here's the catch. The symptoms aren't always classic. In fact, they frequently aren't. The longer I practice medicine, the more patients I see with atypical discomfort. I may be getting cynical because, when someone gives me a list of symptoms that are classic for a heart attack, I start worrying that something else, perhaps more exotic, is happening.

There is a reason for this variation and seeming paradox—or at least for some of it. I'm not sure it explains the gender difference but it does explain some of the individual variation. The location of heart pain is related to how you developed as an embryo within your mother's womb. When the heart tube that will eventually become the formed heart is developing within the embryo, nerve structure is also being developed. The primitive jelly that will become the heart begins in roughly the throat area. As the heart forms, folds, and develops recognizable structures, it moves downward within the chest to the area where it resides thereafter. If the nerve structures develop rapidly, for example, they invest the heart (while it is still in the throat region) with the same system of pain receptors that serve the jaw and throat. If the development and migration of the heart tube progresses in advance of its investment with nerves, these may be the same nerve structures that serve the shoulder girdle and arms, while yet a later development might predominantly involve the nerves that supply the chest wall. Therefore, pain that develops when oxygen is shut off to the heart muscle may vary all the way from pain in the jaws to isolated pain in the mid-chest or to discomfort as low as the upper abdomen, especially in women. This embryonic developmental nuance determines your symptoms 50 or 60 years later.

Additionally, we've all seen an individual who has a so-called high pain tolerance. This may not always be a good thing. Diabetics notoriously have heart attacks without much pain due to generalized neuropathy—a decrease in their quality of sensation, including pain—due to diabetic obliteration of the nerve fibers. Others without obvious neuropathy can also have a heart attack with very little pain in any location. Individuals who have inadequate oxygen delivery to heart tissue but do not sense it as pain, are said to have *silent ischemia.* We know, for example, if we run a continuous 24-hour electromagnetic tape recording of such a person's heart, we will see variations in the electrocardiogram that show evidence of ischemia but without symptoms. This can be dangerous, as such individuals can go right on exercising without knowing they are in danger. Their warning mechanism is faulty. Just about everyone with a full-blown heart attack will have some pain or at least significant symptoms of some sort. However, silent ischemia is fairly common in the general population. This is one of the reasons why detection is so difficult but also so very important.

Symptoms separate from pain almost always occur during a heart attack. These are generally related to something going terribly wrong in the body. They include nausea and sweating. Also, a sizable percentage will have shortness of breath. This is likely related more or less to an increase of water within the air spaces of the lungs due to impaired pumping action of the heart.

Other problems may develop in an artery-specific fashion. For example, an acute occlusion of the right coronary artery is much more apt to result in development of complete heart block, a total blockage in transmission of electrical impulses from the upper chambers to the lower. However, it is much less apt to result in ventricular fibrillation, a fatal electrical disturbance in the rhythm of the heart. On the other hand, occlusion of the large artery down the front of the heart, the left anterior descending, is much more likely to cause ventricular fibrillation, but is unlikely to cause heart block.

Diagnosis of a Heart Attack

It should be clear by now that heart attacks don't always start with a boom. One usually has pain and other symptoms as the artery begins to close. These symptoms may resolve partially or even completely as blood under pressure is forced through the loosely formed clot to provide blood and oxygen to the muscle past the partial obstruction. Then as the clot becomes more mature and chokes off blood flow even more completely, the pain may recur with a vengeance.

It should now be apparent that the earlier this process can be interrupted, the more likely you are to achieve a great result with less muscle loss and, subsequently, less trouble down the road. However, even the most educated people rarely make it to the ER within the first hour. It shouldn't take long for you to determine if you're having a medical emergency. If, for example, your "indigestion" doesn't promptly respond to antacids, it probably isn't indigestion after all. It is likely something much more serious, especially if accompanied by nausea or sweating. What if it is something else like, perhaps, a gallstone? It still needs attention. If you get to the emergency room right away with chest pain, you will become a high-priority patient and will receive an immediate electrocardiogram (ECG). If it's a false alarm, great! The doctors will then get on with the business of determining just what caused you all of this distress.

On the other hand, if it is a heart attack, you are now in a safe environment so that if you develop a fatal arrhythmia, you can promptly be defibrillated just like the treatment the young lady received at the airport. Additionally, you can immediately get started on a fast track to restoring wide-open blood flow to the artery supplying the threatened heart muscle.

The actual diagnosis of an acute myocardial infarction should really take no longer than it takes to obtain an ECG in most people. Sometimes heart attacks are not obvious on electrocardiograms, especially if the arterial occlusion is on the back surface of the heart. However, at least 98% are obvious.

Treatment of a Heart Attack

Since the initial blockage of the coronary artery is primarily resulting from a clump of platelets adhering to the ruptured plaque, and since we know that this clump is poorly formed and readily dispersible, the quicker you can get something to tear down this obstructive clump, the better. A readily available poison for platelets is aspirin. I tell my patients, "If you think you're having a heart attack, grab a couple of aspirin and chew them." They may just open this emerging latticework of clot in the coronary. Every little bit helps!

Once the diagnosis of a heart attack is made, within 5–10 minutes, what are your therapeutic options? This depends entirely on where you are located geographically. If in a remote area in a hospital that does not have a catheterization laboratory, you should receive a powerful thrombolytic/fibrinolytic drug (the clot is *thrombus*, the emerging network of clots is *fibrin*) known as a *clot-buster* unless there is some significant contraindication. Such a contraindication would be any process that would make you more apt to bleed inappropriately, such as recent blunt trauma especially to the head, recent surgery or stroke and, as a softer contraindication, advanced age. These drugs are engineered to lyse and disperse the thrombus (clot) that has formed in the coronary artery, thus the term *thrombolytic* drugs. Again, it is worth emphasizing that the earlier they are administered, the more likely clot dissolution will occur.

These thrombolytic drugs will not work on a totally occluded artery and make it look totally normal. They will, in a substantial percentage of patients, dissolve the clot so that blood flow can be restored enough to stop heart damage from proceeding. Plans should then be made for immediate transfer to a facility with a catheterization lab even if you're completely stable. Why? Because about one-third of all patients won't achieve an opening in the coronary artery with the use of this drug. Remember: *Time is muscle.* You don't want to sit around in pain, waiting and waiting to see if this drug has done what it is supposed to do, all the while enduring more heart muscle damage. If your artery doesn't open, you want to be on your way to a hospital that has a busy 24-hour-a-day catheterization lab so they can get you right in and open your artery with a stent.

Let's say the vessel *does* open in response to the thrombolytic drug. The story is still not over. Once the vessel is opened with the drug, depending on the thrombus burden (the amount of clot) involved, there is a variable potential for acute re-occlusion. Heart muscle that survived the first insult might well give up the ghost upon repeated insult. All patients who have received thrombolytic therapy for a heart attack, whether or not the artery opens right away, should be referred without delay to a tertiary care center where a heart catheterization laboratory is located. If the artery opened in response to the drug, they will be in an environment where they can immediately be taken to the laboratory in the event the artery closes again. It can be stented without delay or, if the coronary artery anatomy is compelling, coronary artery bypass surgery can be performed whenever the effects of the thrombolytic therapy wears off. Patients who remain stable should still receive angiography prior to being dismissed and, if there is significant residual material within the coronary artery, and there almost always is, the artery should be stented prior to discharge. A stent is a metal mesh-like device, frequently impregnated with a drug to prevent tissue growth within it. It can be deployed with a balloon under high pressure in order to restore a normal opening in the coronary artery.

If someone with a heart attack initially lands in a hospital that has a cardiac catheterization laboratory, this is even better. The best approach with this scenario is to give aspirin and also Heparin, an anticoagulant to prevent further clot formation, and hope for some clot dissolution as a bonus. This is given immediately while preparations are made to go directly to the laboratory for an angiographic determination of the process, and acute intervention.

With this approach, once we find the area of coronary occlusion, we thread a horse hair-like wire across the occlusion and deploy (insert) a coronary stent. This is a stainless steel structure that is crimped onto a balloon. We deploy this, properly sized to the culprit artery, at high pressure. This serves two purposes: It immediately disperses the clot that has formed on the ruptured plaque system and it seals off the plaque rupture. (Figure 10a)

There are potential hazards with this. However, the results are usually much better if you can get immediately into the catheterization lab rather than waiting for thrombolytic therapy to work. Additionally, with thrombolytic therapy, the ugly-looking ulcerated

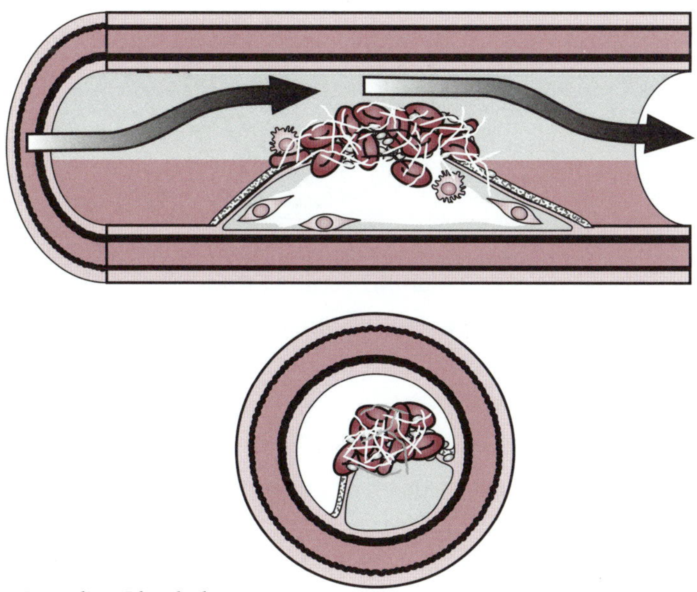

Figure 10a Clot Impeding Blood Flow

plaque is still just as it was originally, its jagged contents protruding into the coronary artery. This presents a source for more clot proliferation.

Not only that, but the thrombolytic drug carries with it the tendency for a bleeding complication to occur—and the older the patient, the more likely a bleed. This risk is relatively low, and unless the patient has a predisposition to bleed, such as recent trauma or stroke, it is worth the potential benefit. By the same token, why take the risk if you don't have to? The risk of a calamitous bleed, such as an intra-cranial hemorrhage (bleeding into the substance of the brain), is much higher in the elderly. This is also the age-defined population that suffers the preponderance of heart attacks. We reduce the dosage of the thromobolytics in the elderly for that reason.

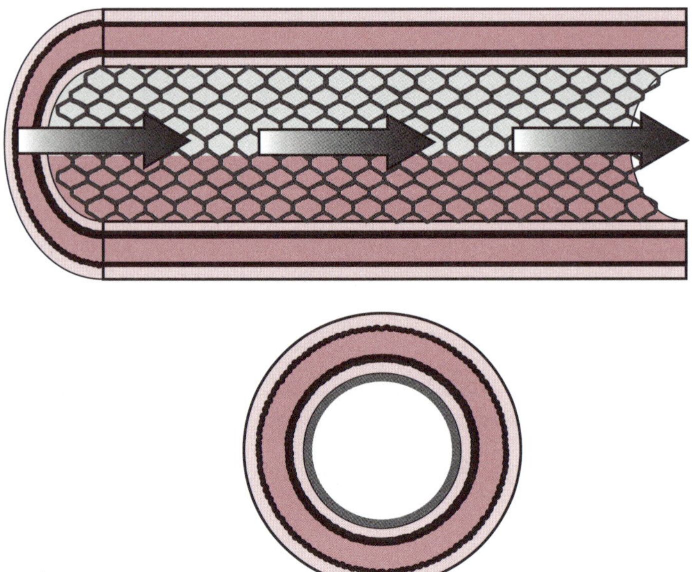

Figure 10b Stented Artery

The use of a strong platelet-active drug called Plavix is given at different times in the course of treatment depending upon which avenue of treatment the individual takes. For example, if the person suffers a heart attack while in a remote area, Plavix should be given immediately, as it will aid in thrombus dissolution. If the heart attack occurs in a more urban environment and the individual is taken to a large hospital where the doctor is going to try to open this artery directly with a stent, (Figure 10b) Plavix should be withheld until the doctor determines the coronary anatomy, usually within 30 minutes. Why? Because in a busy invasive cardiology practice, about one out of every 30–40 patients with heart attacks needs to go right on to the operating room for coronary artery bypass surgery due to the anatomy that the angiogram displayed. If Plavix is on board, the incidence of post-operative bleeding is very high and this raises the morbidity (incidence of associated complications) and the mortality rate. It has been reported that former President Bill Clinton recently received Plavix in the emergency room for a threatened heart attack, only to have to wait the requisite three days while new platelets were formed before he could undergo a safer coronary bypass operation. Fortunately, he was stable during those three days. Things might well have turned out very differently if he had threatened closure of a coronary artery, prompting emergency surgery while the platelets were still poisoned.

The same consideration is true regarding the use of a group of intravenous agents that enjoy the reputation as the strongest platelet-inhibitors known, the so-called IIb/IIIa glycoprotein receptor-inhibitors. These drugs should be started immediately when a catheterization lab isn't available, especially if the coronary artery shows no signs of opening right away with the thrombolytic drug. However, in a hospital with a catheterization lab, these drugs should be withheld until the coronary anatomy is known. If for some compelling anatomic reason, such as major blockage in the left main coronary artery with a totally occluded right coronary artery, the patient would be best served by going to the operating room for immediate coronary bypass surgery. These drugs would impose a very high risk of life-threatening bleeding following the operation, dramatic testimony that they do, indeed, work in their intended purpose.

The firmer the clot, a time-dependent process, the more difficult it is to break up. And by now you know the mantra, *Time is muscle!* For this reason, the patient with a heart attack should either be directed toward a catheterization lab for immediate intervention, or drugs should be started immediately in order to try to open the artery. Doing nothing for any period of time is not acceptable.

Frequently, we are presented with an individual who has waited too long for intervention or whose artery would not open with thrombolytic therapy given in a rural environment, and he or she now has a large heart attack. Sometimes such a patient even shows up with a complication of the muscle damage, such as congestive heart failure, evidence of water damming up in the lungs due to inadequate pump function. We go ahead and open these arteries because the evidence is overwhelming that these patients ultimately fare better with a wide-open coronary artery. Then we frequently place a temporary intra-aortic balloon pump to aid the heart in pumping blood and to unload the heart. In other words, this reduces the work load of the heart by displacing a portion of the blood the heart has to pump. The theory behind this therapy is that borderline-stunned heart muscle cells might turn around and survive if they do not have to struggle to pump blood. Remember, this is virtually the only organ in the body that has to mend on the run. We can put everything else to rest for a while. Not the heart. It has to keep doing its work even though it is badly wounded. No wonder the term "brave heart" was coined.

At the same time we're working on the acutely blocked artery, we may well recognize another coronary artery that is in precarious trouble with perhaps a 90% occlusion. We almost never meddle with this other artery, restricting our efforts to the heart attack culprit artery. In such a situation, we often hear the comment, "Well, gosh (or worse), why didn't you just finish the job while you were in there?" I live in Texas and people live large here. All Texans like to think that they are risk-takers by virtue of heritage. However, I'm sure they hear the same thing in New York and Baltimore, just with a different accent. The reason we avoid the non-culprit artery is that, if it were to clot off, it might well be fatal. One zone of muscle has already been insulted, some cells stunned, others destroyed. We would like to give these stunned cells some time to recoup. Many times, we could probably open the non-culprit vessel promptly and without incident; however, if it were to block off even for a little while, it might be the straw to break the camel's back in that this additional insult might wipe out the patient's blood pressure. Even one death out of a thousand from a reckless move is one too many. We simply want to get some time under our belt, let the offended heart muscle recover as best it can, then go back on a more elective basis and open the other one. However, we don't want to just piddle around until it closes too, and if the individual is truly having trouble, we'll go ahead and open it.

Treatment Following a Heart Attack

Treatment following a heart attack and intervention is especially important. There are many aspects to treatment and, unfortunately, such patients usually leave the hospital with a sizable number of expensive drugs. They clearly should be on both aspirin and Plavix to prevent further platelet aggregation that might result in coronary artery and stent occlusion. They should usually be on a low dosage of a beta-blocker to decrease the heart rate and initial phase of muscle contraction, the determinants of myocardial oxygen consumption. This allows for as much salvage of stunned muscle as possible, and also helps prevent arrhythmias (disruption in the electrical running of the heart) emanating from the damaged muscle zone. This beta-blocker should be Coreg due to its unique properties that are especially beneficial in patients with muscle damage and wall motion abnormalities. An angiotensin-converting enzyme-inhibitor

(ACE-I) should usually be given to relieve the workload on the heart and to reverse the dysfunction that exists within the inner layer of the blood vessel, the endothelium. Finally, the patient should be started on a statin drug to drop the LDL-cholesterol to approximately 70, as this is the level where progression of arteriosclerosis is interrupted.

This statin drug is very important. It not only drops the bad cholesterol, it helps to stabilize and reinforce the integrity of fibrous caps covering multiple plaques that are almost always scattered about. This is similar to the cockroach theory, "If you see one, there are others." The heart attack-producing plaque is seldom the only one in the arteries; there are usually many more in there. They don't even have to be very obvious, maybe just appearing as little flat indentations in the lumen of the coronary artery. You stent one and, unfortunately, there are frequently many more remaining (some perhaps of the vulnerable variety ready to pop). Hopefully, this protective function of the statin drug will preserve the integrity of the remaining plaque systems. As we have discussed, we know that *inflammation* drives arteriosclerosis and, specifically, converts an inactive process to an active and very dangerous one. Since the discovery that the statin drugs also partially reverse this Machiavellian inflammatory component, we feel much better after treating aggressively with these drugs.

We believe they have three currently recognized benefits:

1. They drop the LDL-cholesterol fraction.
2. They reinforce the integrity and toughness of the fibrous cap.
3. They reduce inflammation.

The end result of their use in this situation has been a sharp reduction in secondary events, such as *recurrent* heart attack and stroke, following a heart attack or intervention for an acute coronary syndrome. The incidence of congestive heart failure following heart attack has probably gone down as well. We know that the inflammatory cytokine level is high in many people with congestive heart failure. It appears that aspirin, ACE-I drugs, and statins all work toward reducing the effective cytokine level. In doing so, they likely suppress this culprit inflammatory component that is so detrimental. The role of the cytokines may actually run deeper than we had even wildly imagined. For example, we know that depressed people are more apt to have heart attacks than non-depressed individuals. We also know that cytokine levels are frequently elevated in depressed people. Is this the culprit? I don't know, but they are very important in producing heart attacks.

I always tell patients that we can probably wean them off of some of these drugs; however, there is proven value for each of them following a heart attack, and there is just no way around that fact. In some parts of Great Britain and Europe, you can purchase capsules with several of these drugs mixed together. This seems sensible. Instead of having six bottles containing individual drugs, you'd only have one bottle. This would be much more efficient and it would seem to make it less likely that a drug would be left off. Plus, it is less costly. We must do something sensible about this problem or we will break the bank with health care costs.

REMINDERS

1. *Time is muscle.* The earlier you get to a hospital with a heart attack, the earlier the artery can be opened with less loss of heart muscle. Every muscle cell counts and influences your quality of life.
2. If you're not in a hospital containing a catheterization lab, get transferred to one as soon as your treatment begins. It's very important that the artery be opened as soon as possible in case the "clot-buster" thrombolytic drug fails to open it. If it does open the artery, you still need to be in a protective environment in the event of re-occlusion of the artery.
3. The symptoms of a coronary occlusion are variable and unique to each individual. Women are most apt to have atypical pain, frequently in the area just below the sternum. They are more likely to have alternative sets of symptoms consisting of sweating and nausea.
4. I tell my patients to chew a couple of aspirin as soon as they think they may be experiencing a heart attack. This will help "poison" the platelets (the first responders in building a clot to close off the artery).
5. If "heartburn" doesn't go away after chewing a couple of Maalox or taking a proton pump-inhibitor such as Prevacid, it is likely *real* heart-burn—a burning discomfort resulting from accumulation of lactic acid as the heart muscle valiantly keeps on trying to work even though part of its arterial blood source has been blocked. Get medical help immediately!

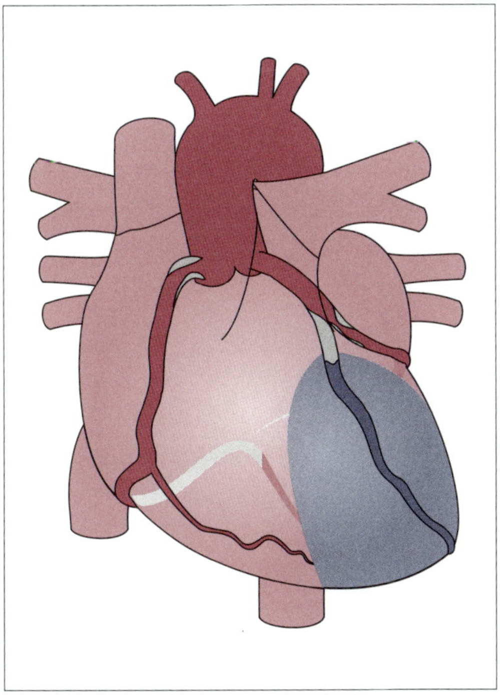

EMOTIONS AND HEART DISEASE

Your Thoughts Run Your Life

FOR MANY YEARS WE HAVE RECOGNIZED that people's emotional status and how they approach their disease has a lot to do with their happiness and with the outcome of their disease. Attitudes are exceptionally important, not only in life in general, but especially after you are stricken with a disease.

Patients who become clinically depressed following a heart attack, for example, have a much higher incidence of complications and death. I have always believed this to be a major reason why women, in general, do worse than men following a heart attack. It has been shown that women under age 60 have a 40% chance of developing major depression following a heart attack. Since the incidence of death in the six months following a heart attack is three to five times higher in significantly depressed people, this assumes massive importance. The same is true for bypass surgery. It is such a strong predictor that we will not operate on a clinically depressed patient unless it is an emergency. It has also been well shown that the immune system very abruptly changes for the worse following development of depression or great sadness. In short, your thoughts run your life, not the other way around.

Not only does your emotional state influence the way you handle your disease, in some instances, it also may have contributed to the development of your disease. For example, epidemiologic studies have shown that clinical depression is an independent risk factor in causing coronary artery disease, even when other risk factors are excluded. It is felt that the inside of the arteries, the endothelium, becomes dysfunctional in depressed people. This poses an adverse influence, presumably due to the increased blood levels of cortisol that many profoundly depressed individuals seem to carry around. Also, it has been well shown that depressed people frequently possess excess levels of cytokines that seem to trigger the inflammatory action leading to a full-blown heart attack.

I have talked with patients now for 35 years, advising them to take a positive, optimistic approach to life and to illness. I hope that I have never failed to offer encouragement when needed and have never appeared cocky or arrogant. When I began writing this book, I was a healthy 60-year-old cardiologist with over 30 years of clinical experience under my belt. I performed over 1,000 invasive procedures each year.

And then I got sick. *Very* sick. This resulted in a diffuse polyneuropathy, a painful and disabling loss of myelin insulation around my nerve fibers from which I am slowly recovering. I learned a lot in the last several months, not only about myself, but about doctors in general. Since I had worked in health care for 12 to 16 hours a day for 30 years, I knew something about the strengths of the system. During the last several months, I also learned of the weaknesses.

First, the diagnosis that something is wrong with our body is a great trauma. All at once, we are past influenza and the common cold. Now there is something *really* wrong. In my case, it was in the nervous system, something I knew little about. The threat of just what might happen, and how far it might go, was devastating. I went from spending 80 hours a week taking care of others to full-time trying to take care of myself. I went to the Internet to read about what my doctors said I had and scared myself half to death. The Internet is great but it has no soul, no heart, and no compassion. When I was afraid, it didn't put its arms around me to comfort me.

From the Internet I did learn a plethora of possible outcomes. I did not, however, learn anything about how to watch my disease or how to become comfortable with the fate that had gripped and taken control of my life. I couldn't figure out why this had happened to me. I was a nervous wreck. I have always been known to keep my cool under pressure. Well, this was a different kind of pressure. This was me.

I also came into contact with the mind-numbing beaurocracy of the medical world. Endless communication with insurance companies, discussions with the disability panel, and prior approval for treatment became my life. Unfortunately, these came at a time when I was at my very worst to cope with them. But cope I did, because I had to.

I had two insurance policies. This was more complicated than one because no matter which one I used, they said the other was liable, even though they both had been issued by the same company! I soon learned not to indicate on the form that I had a second policy. That's when it dawned on me how confusing the medical community is! I already knew this. I was just too preoccupied with my work to think about it much.

Another fact struck me hard and actually led to writing this book. I had a great neurologist and he had a great nurse practitioner, but there was no way he or she could give me enough face time. I had an unusual disease I didn't understand (I didn't know it existed until I got it) and a huge, ever-expanding list of questions, some I thought of in the middle of the night. They answered my first six or so calls promptly. Then I wore them out and their answers were less forthcoming. It wasn't their fault. I wasn't their only patient.

Eventually I settled down and realized I had to take my own advice that I had been delivering to my patients for years. I had to work on my attitude daily. I had to learn to be positive even in the face of what seemed the most negative of diseases. "I can still walk," I told myself. "I can still talk and think and enjoy my family." However, frequently I couldn't. I was unable to capably button my shirt so I switched to sweaters. I was ashamed of my situation and worried that someone would find out about it. I became sequestered within my own sensory-deprived microcosm. On my worst days, my hands would shake and I'd spill my morning coffee onto my sweater or I was unable to turn the pages of my book.

I felt extremely isolated and very sorry for myself. I'd pray all day to get better and that my problem would heal. After waking up 50 or 60 times a night, I would then pray that I would die in my sleep. Enough sleep deprivation will truly make you crazy! This was a hopeless, helpless dichotomy of passions. I finally began to realize that my disease was running my life and that I had to conquer it. Only then, I realized, would I overcome my fears.

During this terrible time of uncertainty, I kept a little book constantly at my side. Appropriately enough, it is called *Secrets of Serenity*. One of my favorite sayings in the book is, "I am I plus my circumstances," a quote from the Spanish philosopher

José Ortega y Gasset. Another was one by Hugh Downs: "A happy person is not a person in a certain set of circumstances but rather a person with a certain set of attitudes." Well known around the hospital for being up-beat and positive, I had a horrible time keeping my attitude adjusted.

I have always quoted Gandhi, especially to my Indian friends when they seemed to be turning negative: "Your thoughts control your life." What Gandhi really said was "Happiness is when what you think, what you say, and what you do are in harmony." Obviously, I was not in harmony. I was too tied up with my disease and what it had done to my career and to my life. I began reading the Dalai Lama to try to find some peace in his wisdom. I read everything. I read scriptures. I had several prayer groups trying to help me. My wife, my sister, and my daughter were all trying to help.

One person in particular helped me a great deal and, as is often the case in matters of this sort, he is unaware of it. Dr. Larry Dossey was an accomplished internist in Dallas, Texas for a long period of time. During the course of his practice, he began to notice that some patients who should do badly, actually did quite well. He studied the effects of mood, music, family support, and prayer on healing. Some of his books are *Healing Beyond the Body: Medicine and the Infinite Reach of the Mind, Recovering the Soul,* and *Be Careful What You Pray For...You Just Might Get It.* I heartily recommend them all.

I began to seek out quotations by famous people who had experienced trouble. Out of the thousands I found, one here and there would stand out. For example, Franklin Delano Roosevelt, though a product of a privileged upbringing, had his share of challenges. He purportedly refused to believe that he was paralyzed throughout life and started what became the March of Dimes. One of his quotes was, "When you get to the end of your rope, tie a knot and hang on."

These books, and other inspirational efforts, slowly began to change my attitude. But let me tell you, it took a lot of work. It's the emotional equivalent of turning the Titanic. You can't just sit back and think that someone else will take care of you. You have to take an active role in your own care. God bless him, my internist Jose Beceiro, a good friend and contemporary, called me every day when he knew that I was so sleep-deprived I was having a hard time holding on. All of this led me to take full charge of my thoughts.

That is the main function of this book. I want you to understand enough about your disease so that you become empowered to participate in your care. You will need to *know* your disease. I used to wake up in agony and would actually talk to my disease. And let me assure you that it was not always in the nicest tone!

I've been privileged to work with some of the greatest cardiologists in the world and to interact with some of the greatest doctors in every discipline. I've also had to work with some of the worst. I would not trade that experience, for I learned a great deal from the greatest, and perhaps even more from the worst. They were of all races, religions, and beliefs. Along with their obvious medical skills, the greatest attribute the really top-notch physicians had to offer was their ability to reassure the patient that there was something to do, that they would not leave them in this mess, and that they were going to be okay.

Nonetheless, we must all die. As the Bible tells us, it is a part of living, completing the cycle. In fact, some think that it is the most important part.

In 1996 I came across the eulogy that the renowned heart surgeon Dr. Denton A. Cooley had written about Dr. Robert Leachman, a wonderful cardiologist and teacher to us all. He quoted a stanza from a poem by Edmund Vance Cooke. I kept it.

And though you be done to death, what then?
If you battled the best you could;
If you played your part in the world of men,
Why, the Critic will call it good.
Death comes with a crawl, or comes with a pounce,
And whether he's slow or spry,
It isn't the fact that you're dead that counts,
But only, how did you die?

He ended by saying, "Bob Leachman counted in the world of men, and I will miss him."

It's beautiful. It gives us a format for living our lives. It gives us a sense of courage in dealing with our infirmities. It gives us finality, a pride in "fighting the good fight."

Take comfort that the healer, now the sick, has to make a solid effort to remain positive, just as you do. To quote Proverbs 23:7, "As he thinketh in his heart, so is he." I think about building myelin over my nerves. You may want to think about whizzing through your bypass surgery and zipping back to a fully active life. Picture a positive outcome in your mind, over and over again. Take great solace in knowing that we are all in this together. As the saying goes, "Open your heart and all the world will help." Make sure you have at least two people who will call you each day to make sure you're doing okay.

Our emotional status and our attitude have everything in the world to do with how we cope with our disease and with healing. I don't think any of us truly understands it. However, there is absolutely no doubt that people's attitudes dictate, in large measure, their course in life and that includes their hospital course. It has to be a true belief from within, from inside your soul. When it comes from the soul, we don't have to understand it.

To underscore this point, a reputable medical center recently carried out a study involving a large number of patients who were undergoing coronary bypass surgery. One third were told that other people would be praying for them; one third were told that others would not be asked to pray for them; and one third didn't know. Many were dismayed to learn that the group who had been prayed for by various prayer groups did the worst. I wasn't dismayed. I think it's great if you have people praying for you when you're ill. However, a positive attitude, an "I can do it" attitude, has to come from within. It is your disease, your soul, your anxiety, your surgery, and your life. You have to summon the strength from within yourself (and we all have it!) to construct an image of improvement, recovery, happiness, and contentment.

Dr. Richard Bergland, a prominent neurosurgeon and the author of the brilliant book *The Fabric of Mind* was an early and strong proponent of the influence of brain hormones—chemical molecules produced by the brain—on thoughts and function, including satisfaction, sadness or happiness, pleasure and, ultimately, healing. As he eloquently explains, tears produced in response to sadness or tragedy have a distinctly different chemical composition from those produced in response to sudden happiness. He goes on to tell us that "Powerful healing forces can flow from your brain to your body or vice versa." I strongly believe that our concentrated and repetitive thoughts, driven by positive influences, can significantly alter our response to illness—and to healing.

REMINDERS

1. **Your life follows your thoughts, not the other way around.**
2. **Attitude is not only genetically endowed and chemically powered, it is learned.**
3. **Anyone can build a positive attitude.**
4. **Your attitude can change your life. Insist on optimism!**
5. **Always remember, "I am I, plus my circumstances."**

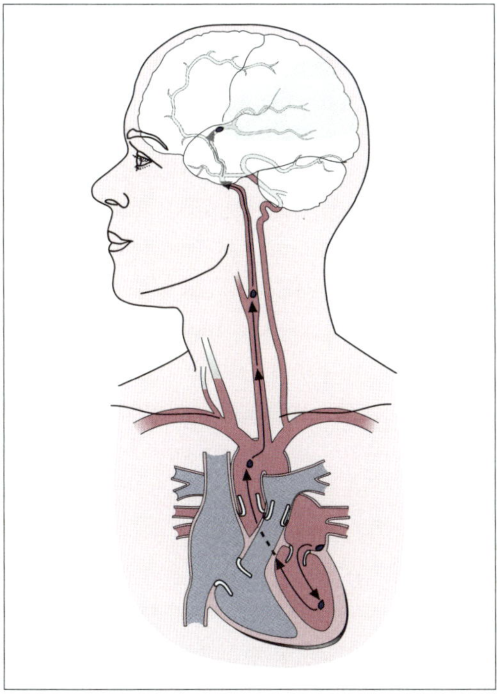

5 STROKE

Trouble in the Command Center

AS WE GET PAST 50 YEARS OF AGE, the one thing we all fear is stroke or some other neurological process that renders us unable to care for ourselves and robs us of our ability to be happy. I remember many comments from patients throughout the years, "Please, death before stroke." We don't always get to choose, but recognizing the warning signs can help. Some strokes, such as some intra-cerebral bleeds, are frequently unavoidable. Many others are avoidable.

Many of us yearn for the simpler times of yesteryear. However, while living may have been simpler then, so was medicine. We are now living in an age of markedly enhanced understanding of *transient cerebral ischemic attacks* (TIAs) and *cerebrovascular accidents* (stroke or CVA). With that understanding comes dramatic new forms of therapy. Though we can't live in a simpler time, we do have access to sophisticated treatment.

Arterial Circulation to the Brain

Everyone's brain is supplied by four arterial blood vessels. The common carotid artery on either side of the neck branches into external and internal carotid arteries. We are not particularly interested in the external carotids which supply blood to the face and can close off without consequence because the face has rich, over-lapping blood supplies. We are interested in them only because, in the event of internal carotid artery occlusion, they can send a few collateral vessels up to aid in blood supply to the afflicted zone. Conversely, we are very interested in the internal carotid arteries because they are the conduits that supply the cerebral cortex of the brain on either side. This is the part of the brain that controls motor movements, thinking, and speech. These fibers, on their way to the spinal cord carrying orders from the brain, cross over in the mid-brain in a process called *decussation*. Therefore, the left side of the brain controls arm and leg function on the right and, of course, vice versa.

The dominant side of the brain has largely to do with being either right- or left-handed. If you are right-handed, the left cerebral motor strip is your dominant side. If a stroke involves that side, speech will likely be affected as well. Therefore, dominant hemispheric strokes are usually much more significant. Their significance affects surveillance and treatment.

Since the internal carotid arteries go straight up toward the brain, any debris or clot that is formed in the heart usually goes north to the brain rather than taking the acute curve in the aorta to travel south toward the belly and feet. Occasionally we see someone with an irregular heart rhythm, usually *atrial fibrillation,* who has formed a blood clot in the left atrial appendage. When it subsequently dislodges, it may travel to one of the leg arteries. We talk about how lucky this person is. Had the embolus (a clot that travels) gone the more usual non-circuitous route to the brain, it would have been life-changing or life-ending. But luck is relative because in many instances we still have to retrieve the embolus from the leg artery to prevent loss of viability.

The other two arterial blood vessels that carry blood to the brain are the vertebral arteries. These vessels are usually right or left dominant as well, but only with regard to each vessel's relative size. The vertebral arteries are actually branches of the arteries supplying the arms—the subclavian arteries. These vertebral arteries supply the cerebellum, the specialized back portion of the brain. This part of the brain controls equilibrium and proprioception, which lets you know where you are in relation to other objects. Dizziness is one symptom of oxygen deprivation of the cerebellum;

difficulty with balance is another. If someone has a history of severe dizziness, careening into structures that they normally could easily walk around, we suspect a problem with the cerebellum.

So there you have it—four arteries to the brain, one internal carotid and one vertebral on each side. Problems with these arteries result in totally different symptoms and disease processes. Let's explore what can go wrong, how to prevent it, and what to do about it if it starts to happen.

Completely Reversible Neurologic Deficit (TIA)

A *transient cerebral ischemic attack* is a short-lived event resulting in a neurologic deficit that is completely reversible. It is caused by a brief interruption of adequate oxygen delivery to a portion of the brain. This implies that something has gotten loose either from a heart chamber, a heart valve, the aorta, or from the wall of the carotid artery and has lodged in a small arterial branch in the brain. This obstruction causes temporary cessation of activity of that particular afflicted area of the brain until the debris is broken up and cleared from the circulation.

A TIA is very different from a stroke (a cerebrovascular accident or CVA). They both have the same initial symptoms due to inadequate blood flow to part of the brain. However, while adequate circulation is restored in time to prevent irreversible loss of brain function in the case of a TIA, a persistent insult (unrelenting oxygen deficiency of the brain tissue) can last long enough to render permanent loss of brain cells and become a stroke. A stroke can be limited or massive, depending on the situation. It is determined by how large the branch is that is obstructed, how long it is closed, and whether or not there is any cross circulation to that area. The distinction between a TIA and a full-blown stroke is very important. Think of a TIA as a warning of something much worse to come if you do not get treatment to head it off.

For example, if you are right-handed and the debris lands in a branch of your left cerebral artery, you might transiently be unable to use your right hand and leg or you might develop slurred speech or become unable to speak at all for awhile. Remember, this speech problem usually goes along with a temporary blockage of blood flow to the dominant side of the brain. As soon as this debris is broken up and cleared to the extent that blood can get through to the brain tissue, there is a prompt return of function. If this same debris was to make a turn and go to the left retinal artery instead of the cerebral cortex, you would temporarily lose vision in the left eye, a condition called *amaurosis fugax*. This is a transient ischemic attack of the eye.

Causes of a TIA

A TIA is always caused by a tiny clump of debris. The debris has to be loosely organized to the extent that blood flow pounding against it is able to disrupt it quickly.

Just as in the coronary artery to the heart, one of these much larger carotid arteries might well develop a deposit of cholesterol, debris, and calcium to make up a typical arteriosclerotic plaque covered by a protective covering known as a fibrous cap. This fibrous cap is protective because it keeps the material within the plaque from opening up or rupturing its contents into the lumen of the carotid artery where the blood is circulating. When a plaque ruptures as a result of a thinning out of the fibrous cap, it doesn't release its material into the blood stream, it merely opens the plaque within the inside of the artery. The plaque is the consistency of Monterey Jack cheese that has been left in the refrigerator too long, has hardened, and subsequently cracked open. When this happens, this material that has been accumulating over the years splits open and the body defense mechanisms recognize this as an injury. The first responders in the blood stream are the platelets, which initiate thrombus (clot) formation.

Imagine a jagged, ulcerated plaque split open within the wall of the carotid artery. (Figure 11a) As platelets hold hands in the formation of the early beginnings of a clot, they form an aggregate, a little clump of platelets loosely bound to one another. Blood is whizzing past this complex (but still totally silent) lesion—the clump attached to the wall of the blood vessel—at a substantial velocity. Each time blood goes past, it tries to sweep the platelet clump off its attachment. The platelet aggregate continues to grow and as the blood whooshes past, it is swept forward like seaweed in the current. Finally, as the platelet clump becomes larger and larger, it absorbs enough force from the passing blood to be washed free of its mooring to the carotid wall. Now it's within the carotid circulation, totally subject to the whims of bloodstream turbulence as it goes hither and yon on its way to its ultimate landing zone. This landing zone is most commonly the middle cerebral arterial branch, as it is the straightest. However, the clot may careen against a vessel wall and choose the retinal artery, for example, as an alternative landing zone.

In the first case, the individual will temporarily lose motor function of the other side of the body (remember, the fibers cross over in the mid-brain). If it lands within the dominant side, the individual will also suffer transient speech disturbance. If it is on the non-dominant side, the speech will usually be spared. If the clot lands in the retinal artery, the individual will develop temporary blindness in that eye. Again, the important

Figure 11a Transient Ischemic Attack (TIA)

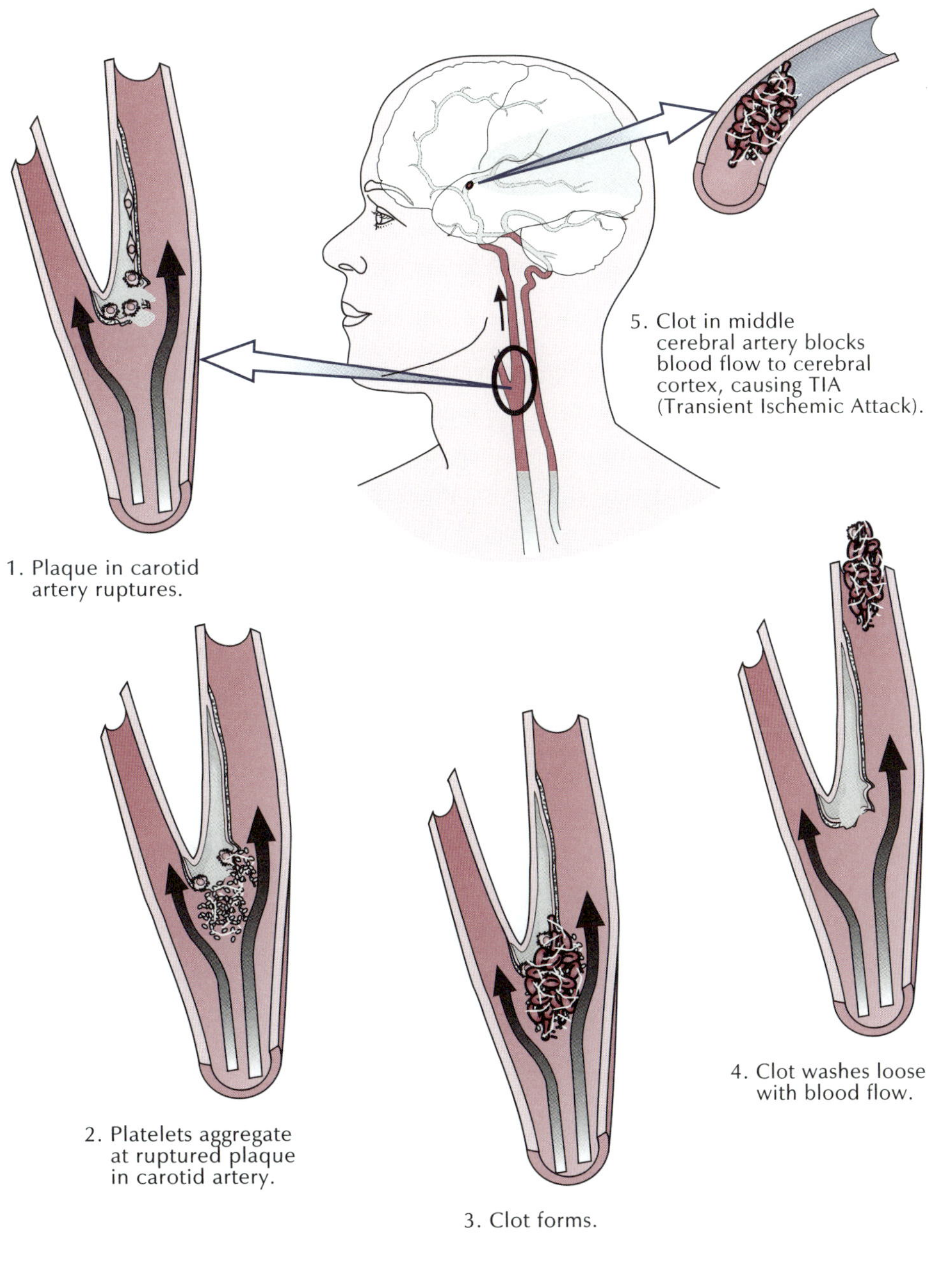

Figure 11b Resolution of TIA

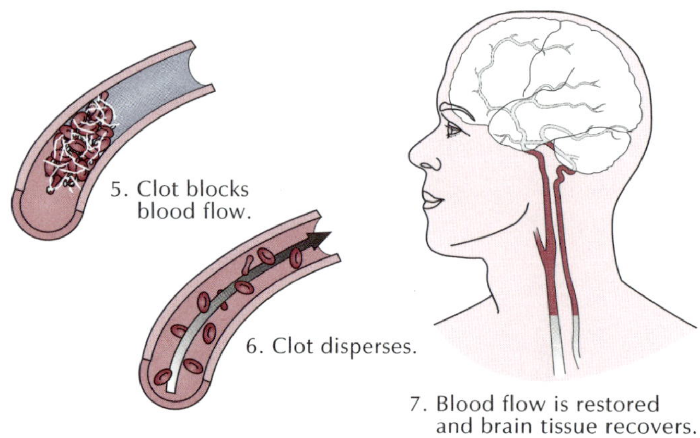

aspect is that, with a TIA, these changes will completely reverse. After the obstruction has been cleared and function promptly returns to normal, you'll breathe a sigh of relief. This has been a huge warning light in your life and needs to be heeded. (Figure 11b)

A clot to the brain could also have originated from a previous heart attack zone in the left ventricle. All of the muscle in the left ventricle should work in concert to pump blood into the aorta during systole, the phase during which the muscle cells shorten. If a heart attack has previously occurred, there will frequently be a zone in the ventricle that no longer contracts, especially if it is at the apex of the heart and particularly if it causes aneurysm formation (an out-pouching in the wall like a small bag). It may serve as a stagnant area where a clot can form.

Material tends to adhere to any stagnant area within the heart and blood vessels. The ventricle shrugs off any potentially adherent debris during contraction. However, a non-functioning zone of the heart wall can allow clot formation. When that accumulation gets large enough, it might be washed off and begin its rapid journey to the brain.

Paroxysmal atrial fibrillation is another potential and fairly frequent cause of a TIA or even a stroke. This is an irregular rhythm within the upper heart chambers. There is an evolutionary vestige, called a left atrial appendage, a pouch of the left atrium. If a person develops this type of irregular heart beat, the atria, including this appendage, cease to squeeze aggressively and a clot may form within this little appendage. When the clot ultimately loses its attachment to the deep recesses of the appendage, it enters the aorta as an embolus. The most convenient place for it to land is the cerebral circulation. Again, it could potentially travel to the retinal artery or it could even turn the curve in the aorta, careening off the aorta wall, and could wind up traveling to one of the gut vessels, a renal artery, or to the leg vessels. The leg vessel is by far the best place for it to land. It is, however, much more likely to go to one of the brain vessels because, as I mentioned earlier, it is a straight shot.

Because this irregular heart beat starts abruptly, lasts a while, then reverts back to normal rhythm, it is sometimes difficult to detect. For example, we have seen multiple individuals with a TIA where the cause was obscure, as they were in normal sinus rhythm when they made their way to the ER. Sometimes they said they felt that their heart was "out of rhythm." Occasionally we find nothing else to blame for the TIA so we anticoagulate the patient (tie up the clotting factors in the blood with a drug) to prevent further recurrences only to discover later that paroxysmal atrial fibrillation recurred. That's okay because we had the situation appropriately treated, just in case. It's important to treat these individuals in a preventive fashion because the next clot from the heart might be larger and might be life-changing.

This same scenario occurs in *fixed* atrial fibrillation. The cause is more obscure if the arrhythmia occurs on a paroxysmal (intermittent) basis. Our greatest fear in any individual with atrial fibrillation is stroke. The back and forth atrial fibrillation, called *paroxysmal*, is the most dangerous. In this situation, the arrhythmia will go on for perhaps a week, long enough for clot material to form in the atrial appendage and then convert back to sinus rhythm. When this occurs, the clot formed in the little appendage may break loose into the arterial circulation where it can be swept away to the brain. Unfortunately, it may be well-formed and therefore resistant to fragmentation by blood pounding against it. It all depends on how long the clot had been in the left atrial appendage because the clot is remodeled and becomes more rigid as it matures.

This debris might be a tiny clot that formed in the leg veins and traveled to the right heart, crossing a *patent foramen ovale* to the left heart, and then entered the aorta on its way to the left carotid artery. A patent foramen ovale is a small hole that is present in embryonic life and in some of us doesn't completely close over when we are born. It can serve as a communication (an opening) through which a clot may pass. When a clot in a vein gets loose, travels first through the venous circulation, then crosses over to the arterial circulation, it creates a situation we refer to as a *paradoxical embolus*. See Chapter 35 on *Patent Foramen Ovale* for details.

Some TIAs come from plaque systems in the aortic arch. Most of these go to the left side of the brain. However, these are large, dense plaques and any release of material from them is usually large enough to cause a stroke. Sometimes, a TIA is a harbinger of something worse to come from this zone.

There is an important distinction. When a loosely formed platelet clump breaks up from blood pounding against it, then through it, as a tiny channel is formed, brain or eye function will return. However, if the clot is so tightly formed and compacted—an older, more mature clot—that it can't be broken up completely, a stroke, or CVA, will result. Sometimes, not infrequently, the patient is left with something in between—a very small or intermediate, persistent defect, something we might refer to simply as an incomplete stroke.

So now you have the complete picture:

1. TIA—Blockage of a vessel with early resolution and complete recovery of brain function.
2. Limited stroke—An intermediate problem with a variable amount of damage to brain tissue.
3. Completed stroke—Severe damage to brain tissue from persistent blockage of an artery.

Vertebral Disease

Interestingly, embolic material almost never enters the vertebral circulation. This is because these arteries are relatively inaccessible to loose material within the aorta due to their acute take-off from their parent artery. Also, while we may frequently see high-grade arteriosclerotic plaque within the mouth of the vertebral artery, these arteries seldom close off completely unless they were tiny to start with. It's a good thing because large strokes from vertebral occlusion are frequently devastating. These individuals can be plagued by vertigo and dizziness, as well as gait disturbances, for the rest of their lives.

Urgency of Evaluation of a TIA

As you can probably understand, finding the source and the cause of thrombus formation and why and how the clot will embolize to a particular area is of some urgency. During the last 30 years, I have seen many patients come in very frightened with this problem, and understandably so. They have just experienced a situation that they understood right away could change their life forever, and then it cleared up completely in many instances. It must seem like a miracle.

When a frightened individual comes into the hospital or our office relating symptoms and yet is totally normal on examination, it is tempting to think that we have all the time in the world to evaluate it. We may not. We never know when the next one is going to strike and we don't know whether or not the next event may, indeed, be life-changing, because it may not be a TIA but a large stroke. Presentation with a TIA should be regarded with the utmost urgency and the cause should be fairly well known within a few hours.

Emergency Evaluation and Treatment

Investigation of the source of the embolic clot is fairly clear-cut and can frequently be performed in about an hour or two. The very first step when someone presents with a TIA to the physician or the emergency department is to be absolutely sure that a bleed has not occurred within brain tissue. We can do this with a quick CT scan or MRI. The results can be available within minutes. If there is no bleed, and there usually isn't, the physician should initiate treatment without further delay. If the patient is in atrial fibrillation, he should be anticoagulated with Heparin or Lovenox immediately. This is to prevent even more clot formation in the left atrial appendage, as this has to be considered the source of the embolic material until proven otherwise.

If the patient is in normal sinus rhythm, we must assume that the clot was from one of the other sources discussed and since platelet aggregation is the first step in the clotbuilding process, a strong platelet-inhibitor should be given. The strongest and most effective is Plavix. The patient should receive between 300 and 600 milligrams as a loading dose, followed by a daily dose of 75 milligrams. This should be given along with the age-old platelet-inhibitor—aspirin. Anticoagulation should also be started in this situation so clot formation can be stopped in its tracks. We can then begin our investigation.

Finding the Source of the Problem

An Echo/Doppler examination is the mainstay of evaluation. I order an immediate echocardiogram and carotid Doppler exam. The first will tell me if there is an abnormal heart valve or if a flat spot or outpouching exists in the left ventricle. It will tell me if there is an infectious process, called *endocarditis*, on a valve. A small particle of such a process can break off and escape into the cerebral circulation. It will not always tell me if this little communication between the upper heart chambers, a patent foramen ovale, is present, though it sometimes does. The second test, the carotid study, will tell me if there is significant carotid artery plaque. It will quantify the severity of the plaque and will sometimes tell me whether or not the plaque is ruptured.

The most common cause of a TIA is a cholesterol deposit in the wall of the carotid artery. The second most likely cause is atrial fibrillation. These two causes constitute over 50% of all possible etiologies. Less likely are left ventricular, valvular, aortic arch, and patent foramen ovale sources.

If the evaluation obtained from the two quick and non-invasive studies using the Echo/Doppler machine is clean, we still have no obvious explanation. At this point, we have not yet identified a source and have no idea how aggressive to be in treatment. This is where we may begin to suspect that there is a more unusual explanation for the TIA.

The next step in evaluation is a *transesophageal echocardiogram*. In performing this procedure, the patient is sedated and a small echo probe is passed down the esophagus to a point just behind the heart. Because we are in close proximity to the heart, we can obtain great pictures of the heart structures. Not only do we obtain a better view of the heart valves and chambers, we get to examine a part of the heart that can escape detection by other means like the elusive patent foramen ovale, the small corridor sometimes connecting the upper chambers of the heart. If we inject agitated normal saline (a syringe of sterile salt water shaken vigorously) into the I.V. in a peripheral vein and have the patient strain down (or if too sedated, we apply pressure on the upper abdomen to simulate this maneuver), we may see tiny bubbles pass from the right atrium, where they should be, over to the left atrium, where they shouldn't be. With this straining maneuver, called a *Valsalva*, we have raised the pressure in the right atrium which, in turn, lifts the flap covering the hole on the left atrial side. This allows passage of tiny air bubbles across the septum. If this can occur with small air bubbles, it can also occur with small clots. Within a ten-minute period, we have made the diagnosis of a patent foramen ovale. In absence of a more compelling explanation for the TIA, especially if the heart and carotid arteries are completely clean, this is likely the source for the embolus. Because it began in the venous circulation and then crossed over into the arterial circulation, it is a *paradoxical embolus*.

Because we have determined that the clot had to come from somewhere in the venous circulation, that "somewhere" is almost always the deep venous system draining blue blood from the legs. So we ask the technician to haul out the trusty old echo machine again and this time, do a thorough survey of the venous drainage. We want to determine if there is, indeed, a clot present and, if so, how extensive it is. If it is not in the leg system, the clot probably originated within the pelvis.

An individual who has experienced a TIA, is found to have a patent foramen ovale, and is subsequently found to have a lower-extremity deep venous system chock-full of clot is in a very high-risk situation. I would likely recommend prompt closure of the communication (opening in the septum between the two upper chambers) and then try to find the cause of the extensive thrombotic process. I would also recommend the deployment of an inferior vena cava filter. This is a stainless steel mesh "trap" deployed in the inferior vena cava which carries all blue blood draining from the legs and pelvis back to the heart. We do this through a needle stick puncture in the groin which can be performed within 20 minutes. Its purpose is to trap any clot that gets loose from its attachment to the leg or pelvic vein wall. In placing this, we are attempting to prevent a catastrophe should a large amount of the adherent clot break loose. In the event this occurred while the patent foramen is still wide open, it could cause a huge stroke. After the hole between the upper chambers is closed, it could still cause a disaster; this one would be from a huge embolus of clot to the lung artery, a pulmonary embolus. Both can be prevented by the inferior vena cava filter.

Treatment of a TIA

There are basically two situations in which treatment of a TIA mandates the use of anticoagulation. We first use Heparin, an intravenous drug, to prevent more clot formation and to help disperse some of the previously formed clot. It is followed by Coumadin, an orally-administered drug that ties up clotting factors in prevention of clot formation. One situation that calls for such an approach is atrial fibrillation, which we have already discussed. The other is a paradoxical embolus, presumably from the legs or pelvis. In this instance, unless the individual has had recent trauma or surgery that can cause inappropriate clot formation, we still don't have a full explanation for what precipitated the formation of a clot. Perhaps the individual took a 12- to 15-hour international flight a few days prior. Perhaps he drove cross-country with very few stops. We know that most people tend to drink inadequate quantities of water when they travel, as they don't want to spend all of their time stopping to go to the bathroom. Maybe the dehydration, coupled with the dependent position of the legs, resulted in a tiny clot in a leg vein.

If these explanations don't apply, the patient should be checked for an *occult neoplasm*, a malignant tumor not obvious to the patient or the doctor. To explore this possibility, he or she should have an abdominal and pelvis CT scan, a mammogram if female, and a prostate specific antigen if male. These tests, coupled with the initial CT of the head and a chest x-ray, pick up almost all hidden cancers that have been incriminated in causing accelerated clot formation.

If these tests are negative, I recommend blood tests to be sure the patient doesn't have a *thrombophilic disorder*. This is a disorder, frequently inherited, that causes inappropriate clot formation. A test can be done with one blood drawing looking for Protein C and S, Antithrombin III, Leiden Factor V, Antiphospholipid Antibody, and Lupus Anticoagulant. I know these are complex medical terms and they likely won't stick as you read this. *However, if you have a loved one with this problem, use a yellow marker to outline this area and ask your doctor if these tests have been drawn.*

This process can be stopped at any step along the way as soon as the cause for the TIA has been found. It is not enough to take Plavix and aspirin and wait to see if it recurs. This individual has suffered transient loss of motor function and perhaps the ability for speech formation. He barely dodged the bullet! What we want is to *prevent* devastating illness or loss.

There are new tools on the horizon that may make the work-up simpler and even more streamlined. A magnetic resonance image (MRI) angiogram can identify the cause of 95% of all TIAs and strokes. Just as "Time is Muscle" refers to the need for emergency opening of the artery in the case of coronary artery occlusion, the mantra in the stroke world should be "Time is Memory" or "Time is Function."

Causes of Stroke

Stroke can usually be considered the result of one of five different causes:

1. Lacunar Stroke

Probably the most common, and the mildest, is what we refer to as a *lacunar* stroke. It is almost always a result of hypertension and happens when a small intra-cerebral artery (one within brain tissue) simply closes off. This is treated with blood pressure control and platelet-active drugs such as Plavix and aspirin. Folks almost always recover completely, or at least markedly, from such strokes.

2. Intra-Cerebral Hemorrhage

Frequently the most devastating cause of stroke is an *intra-cerebral hemorrhage*, a bleed within the brain tissue. Fortunately, this is also the rarest, caused either from rupture of a small aneurysm within the arterial circulation of the brain, sometimes called a *Berry aneurysm*, or from an intra-cerebral bleed due to uncontrolled hypertension.

3. Embolic Stroke

The third variety is caused by an embolus, a large or well-formed clot formed elsewhere that broke off and traveled to one of the branches of the internal carotid artery distribution. This may be due to disease within the carotid artery, an arteriosclerotic plaque, with ultimate plaque rupture and platelet aggregation.

Earlier I demonstrated how a TIA can result from a loosely formed platelet clump washing off and lodging in the cerebral circulation. The circulation is restored as the clump breaks up. A more ominous situation develops when a large, mature (firm) clot breaks away from its moorings, either from a lesion in the carotid artery or from a more distant source.

These sources are the same ones discussed as causes for TIA; the clot is just more mature and firmer. As the clot breaks away, it results in a large stroke that is difficult to interrupt because the clot is mature and rigid. For example, it is not unusual to find diffuse, dense, thick plaques in the transverse aorta (the portion giving off the head vessels) of an arteriosclerotic 80-year-old person. We can detect these by transesophageal echocardiography. These plaques sometimes rupture spontaneously, shedding this debris usually into the left cerebral circulation and causing a dense stroke. Similarly, the clots from a heart attack zone in the left ventricle, a chronically fibrillating left atrial appendage (Figure 12), or a clot from a leg vein that has crossed a patent foramen ovale, are frequently rigid clots capable of lodging in a cerebral arterial branch with a resultant large stroke.

Figure 12 Stroke

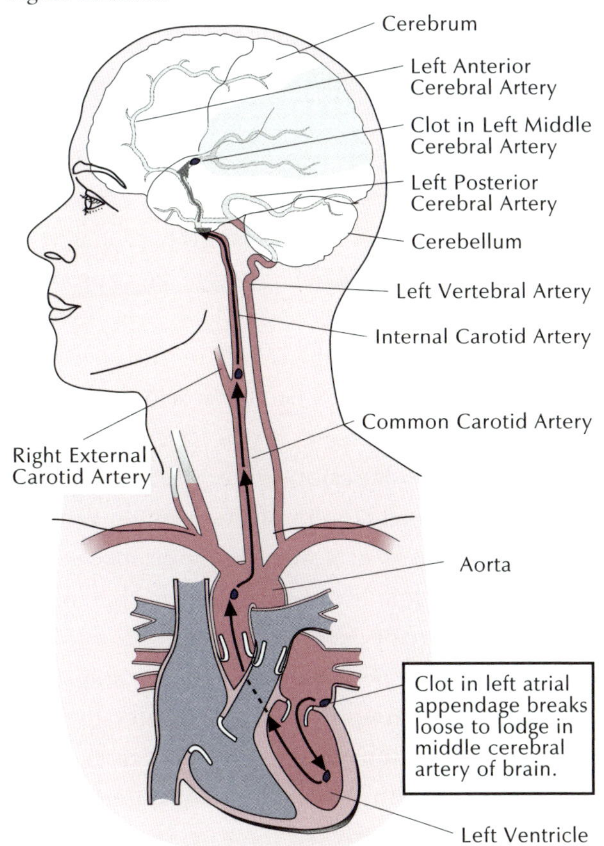

4. Complete Occlusion of an Internal Carotid Artery by Thrombosis

This fourth variety can result in a huge stroke. This is when the internal carotid in the neck clots off completely. This usually occurs when a carotid plaque has silently become more and more obstructive until it now is 90% or more occlusive. If plaque rupture occurs in this setting, the carotid artery is almost completely blocked off by the shift of this complex, unstable plaque system. A clot that forms on this ulcerated lesion doesn't always break away. Instead, it may completely plug the carotid artery at the site of the previous plaque, as very little clot is needed to take a 98% blockage to total occlusion. At the point when this occurs, brain tissue in the distribution of the internal carotid may well start to suffer from profound oxygen deprivation. This is a stroke in progress and usually a rather large one at that, as the entire internal carotid, supplying half the memory/motor system of the brain, is obstructed. While a total occlusion of a middle cerebral artery within the cranium (the head) causes a very large stroke, occlusion of its parent artery, the internal carotid within the neck causes a much larger one. Every branch coming off this large parent artery is suddenly carrying no blood at all and a large amount of brain tissue may well start to suffer, starving for oxygen-rich arterial blood.

The brain tissue *may* begin to suffer. There are exceptions. We all are born with a right and a left internal carotid artery carrying red, oxygen-enriched blood to the right and left sides of the brain. There is potential for communication between these two sides at the base of the brain through an anatomic variant known as the Circle of Willis (named after Dr. Thomas Willis, who extensively studied various patterns of the circulation of the brain). If you are fortunate enough to have a well-developed Circle of Willis, you might well be able to close off one carotid artery and never even know it!

On the other hand, if you have no communication through the Circle of Willis, a complete internal carotid artery occlusion can spell disaster unless quickly treated. A partially formed communication might result in a limited stroke. Needless to say, this vascular circle is of immense importance. Unfortunately, you don't get to choose this attractive option. If you have it, offer up a toast to your parents for their considerate gift of this important genome.

With complete blockage of the internal carotid artery in a setting with little communication via the Circle of Willis, there is no mistaking the diagnosis. The entire opposite side (remember, the fibers cross over) will become flaccid and functionless. If this involves the dominant hemisphere, the speech will be totally lost. This is clearly a medical emergency. In the past, since we had little to offer, timely treatment was less urgent. Now, we have much to offer in treatment. Again, *time is brain function*. Get your loved one to a good hospital which has a stroke team as soon as possible. They may well be able to open the artery and save brain tissue from destruction.

5. Cryptogenic

To complete the causes of stroke, there is a fifth category: *cryptogenic*. This is Latin for "obscure cause." We used to see a lot of cryptogenic strokes before we figured out that plaques in the transverse aorta could cause strokes, and before we had a good tool to use in detection of a patent foramen ovale. The tool in each of these evaluations is the transesophageal echocardiogram. Now it is rare to call a stroke "cryptogenic." When we have to use it, we still figure that an embolic cause was somehow the most likely scenario and treat accordingly. Before we use this fall-back term, we should make sure that we have done everything possible, within reason, to identify the exact source.

Therapy for Stroke

What is the therapy for a stroke? Just as in a TIA, the very first step is to be absolutely sure that an intracerebral bleed has not developed. We certainly don't want to be giving a drug to break up a clot if the cause of the stroke was actually a bleed. A bleed can act the same way as an occlusion from a clot. When the individual is sent to the CT scanner, the Doppler technician should be called to come to the ER as soon as possible. If the CT scan shows no bleed, a five-minute exam with the Doppler should confirm or rule out the diagnosis of a total internal carotid blockage due to a clot. If not, a CT angiogram should tell us if there is a clot in the middle cerebral artery supplying the motor strip.

If this is confirmed and there is no particular contraindication such as recent surgery or significant trauma, especially to the head, *thrombolytic* ("clot-buster") therapy should be initiated without further ado. As its name suggests, this is a very strong medication that has affinity for the thrombus, tearing it apart. In many instances, this drug will open the thin shelf of clot blocking the artery and the resurgence of arterial blood flow will allow for cessation of the stroke in progress. (Figure 13, page 76) The return of function is sometimes nothing short of sensational.

Well after we have treated a TIA or a stroke due to a carotid lesion, we will need to make a decision about any intervention. Some of these carotid lesions are not occlusive and will seal off with no more TIAs. Others are occlusive, 75% or greater

Figure 13a Before Clot-buster, Thrombolytic Therapy

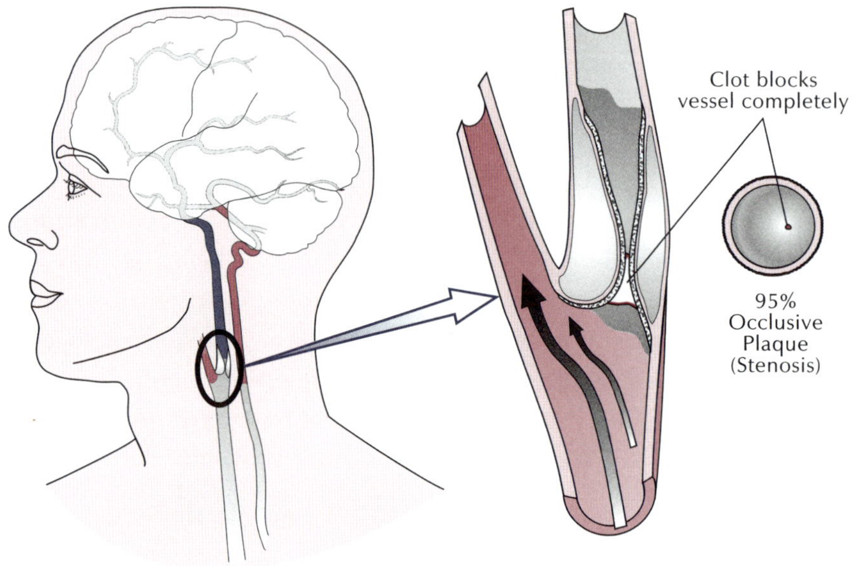

Figure 13b After Clot-buster, Thrombolytic Therapy

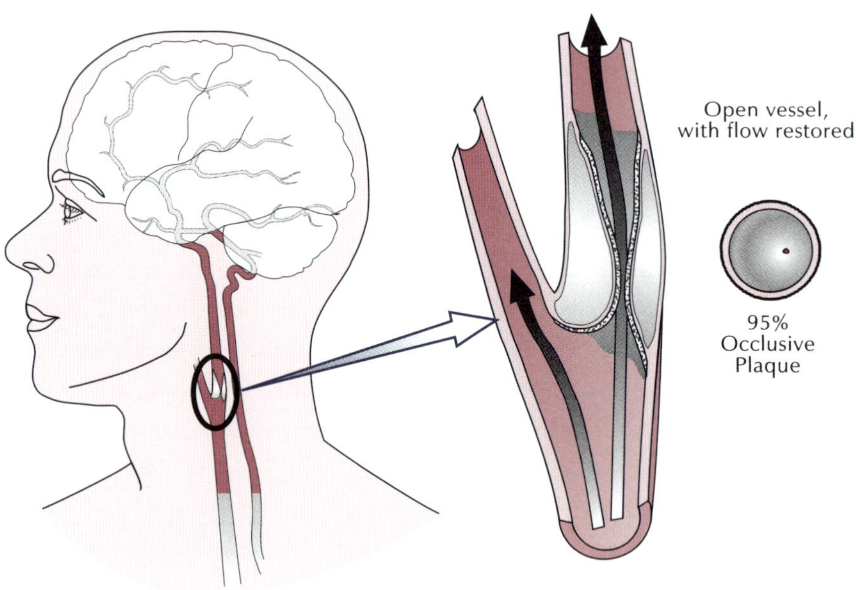

in severity. When the person has been treated for awhile, these should be addressed with carotid *endarterectomy*, where the artery is "apple-cored," removing the plaque along with the inside of the artery, or by stent deployment if the plaque is now completely clean. I still send these complex carotid plaque systems for surgery because the surgeons that I use have a less-than-3% incidence of peri-operative stroke. Also, I'm never sure that the debris, the partially formed clot, is cleared out completely and I wouldn't want it released during stent deployment. I believe all of these carotid lesions that are high-grade and have resulted in a previous TIA or limited CVA should be managed surgically.

Similarly, if someone has had a TIA due to a non-obstructive carotid plaque and they have subsequent events while on anti-platelet therapy, I refer them straightaway for carotid surgery. Again, I feel that the recurrent nature of this TIA is trying to tell us something. What it's usually trying to tell us is that there is a possibility of calamity if we don't address the problem.

Prevention of Stroke

Some forms of treatment are logical. The main treatment of a stroke is to control atherosclerotic risk factors such as high blood pressure, diabetes, elevated cholesterol, smoking, and obesity. We now know that a plaque in the carotid can remain stable for years, slowly accumulating bulk, only to become unstable and rupture under the influence of inflammatory molecules. This situation can be treated with a statin drug, an angiotensin, converting enzyme-inhibitor, and aspirin. However, when this newer generation of treatment began, we had no idea that the statin might sharply mitigate the incidence of stroke. Interestingly, a statin, when used in patients with Type 2 diabetes, coupled with one or more known risk factors, decreases the incidence of stroke by almost 50%. This is astounding data that I believe is due largely to plaque stabilization, reversal of the inflammatory trigger and, to a lesser degree, plaque regression.

The statin is one of the few drugs we have to at least partially treat the effects of inflammation. We now know that inflammatory molecules, called cytokines, are released by a particular cell, triggering clotting and erosion of the fibrous caps that cover plaques. These effects set the stage for development of what is known as a vulnerable plaque, one ripe for rupture and clot formation. This can happen, not only in the coronary circulation of the heart, but also in the carotid circulation to the brain. Indeed, it is not unusual for one to find an ulcerated plaque in a carotid in a heart-attack victim, evidence that "plaques travel in packs." In other words, this triggering event, leading to vulnerable plaques, seems to be a generalized phenomenon. The statin drug will, in large measure, block this inflammation triggering process. *If it is found that you have plaque formation in your carotid arteries, you should typically be on platelet-active drugs to prevent clot formation. These drugs are aspirin and Plavix.* This is a very important part of your care in the prevention of a potentially devastating stroke.

REMINDERS

1. A thorough search has to be carried out for the cause of a TIA or stroke. A reason can be found in more than 95% of cases.
2. If no explanation is discovered, a transesophageal echo should be performed to rule out a patent foramen ovale.
3. Platelet anti-clumping drugs, such as Plavix, may prevent recurrent TIA or stroke. The "loading dose" should be 300 to 600 milligrams, depending on the size of the individual.
4. *Time is brain function.* Prompt treatment by a stroke team may save brain function in the event of a total internal carotid artery occlusion or a middle cerebral artery blockage. Thrombolytic drugs should be given early, increasing the likelihood the clot will be dispersed and blood flow restored.
5. With a completely formed Circle of Willis connecting the right and left arterial circulations in the brain, a total occlusion of an internal carotid artery can occur without resultant stroke.
6. A statin offers a great protection against stroke.

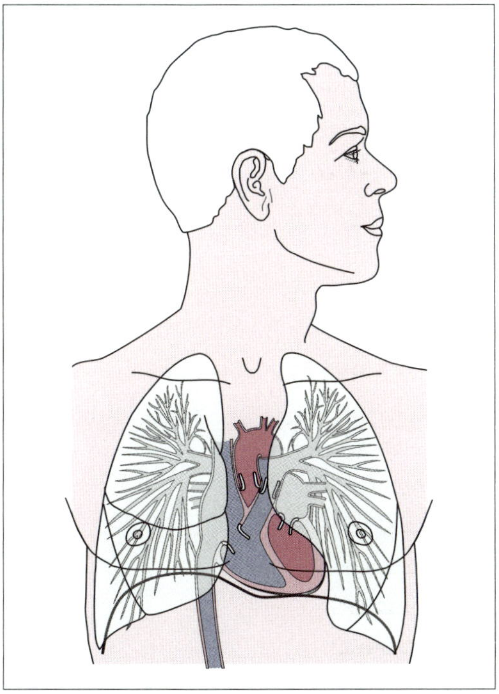

6 EMERGENCY TACTICS

How to Handle Cardiac Emergencies in the Home

THIS BOOK IS ABOUT EMPOWERING you to interact proactively in your care. Our medical staff will soon be stretched beyond belief so you must be educated about problems you may face. In the case of an emergency at home and with no medical personnel available, you are on your own. If you perform any of the procedures detailed here, please realize that, unless done properly, they can damage someone. Even if done properly, they can still damage someone. However, if you understand them and why you are doing them, they are very helpful procedures to know and just may save the life of someone you love. Otherwise, you're going to be in the same spot the guys in the ad on television are in: They see their friend choking next to them at the dinner table, comment on it, discuss it amongst themselves and agree he's surely choking, but continue eating their meal without doing anything and then watch as another guy walks over and effectively performs a Heimlich maneuver on him.

This chapter will help you recognize at-home cardiac emergencies. The material has to be used in a common-sense manner. Before you're faced with an emergency at home, check it out with your medical professional. If he or she agrees, this will serve as an excellent day-to-day resource so that you can be prepared if the need arises. **If your doctor doesn't agree with it—and endorse it—don't use it.**

Resuscitation or Not: Write It Down and Sign It!

Family members of a cardiac patient frequently ask, "What on earth do I do if he or she falls over at home?" There is no easy answer. A lot of what should be done depends on what the individual in question has expressed about quality of life, expectations, and wishes. It's important that each person considers establishing a directive about what he or she wants done near the end of life; not a pleasant subject for any of us. While I don't want anyone to dwell on it, I do feel that we have lagged behind medicine's innovations and advances in expressing our determination about how we will deal with death. It is the responsibility of each of us to make a decision about how we want people to respond to potential life-ending events. Let our family members know beyond a shadow of doubt, write it down, and sign it.

The most heartbreaking and emotionally devastating example of how the best intentions can go awry is illustrated by the following true story: An elderly man with severe heart and lung disease needed an abdominal operation. I had taken care of his heart for many years and he had specifically turned down an offer to implant an Automatic Implantable Cardiac Defibrillator (AICD), a device that is frequently implanted in sick hearts that are particularly prone to develop a fatal arrhythmia. We had discussed this on several occasions and his response was, "Doctor, when my time comes, I want to go be with the Lord." I advised him to get his wishes written down, recorded, and signed. I also advised him to share his decision with his family. He shared it with his wife but not with his daughter, a woman in her 40s who lived 200 miles away.

After careful consideration, the gentleman decided to go for the abdominal operation. He was miserable and needed to have his problem repaired. The major question was how he would fare during and following the operation. He called me over to his bed and made me promise that we would abide by his wishes that he not be intubated (have a breathing tube placed in his trachea) or have closed chest massage performed, if he were to arrest following the operation. He initially did well after the operation, and then started to decline. We continued doing our best with his management but made sure the nurses all knew he was DNR (do not resuscitate) status. He was very ill for two weeks, clearly dying, and I had several discussions with his wife. The daughter was not to be seen.

I received a frantic call from the nurse taking care of him. He had deteriorated sharply and I questioned why they were calling me in such a state. The nurse replied that his daughter was there demanding that something be done. I was only a couple of minutes away. When I arrived, the patient was dying. I quickly talked with his wife, who nodded in her grief. Right then, his daughter ran down the hall screaming, "If you don't do everything you can to keep my daddy alive, I'm going to sue you for every ★★#__★★ cent you have. I'll see that you never practice medicine again. I'll ★★#__★★ sue you for manslaughter." She was beyond reason. I intubated the patient, did closed chest massage, administered the proper drugs, all to no avail. Everything I did ran counter to what he had wanted. I did it, not because I was frightened of what this grief-crazed and probably guilt-ridden woman threatened, but because the man's wife stepped in and calmly asked me to please resuscitate her husband if possible. I felt then, and now, as though we violated the gentleman's carefully thought-out requests and told her so. I did this gently to the man's wife, less so to his daughter. It was a ridiculous, disturbing situation and most doctors have found themselves in similar circumstances.

In my view, every person over 21 years of age should be required to carry a notarized card stating personal wishes regarding efforts to be expended in the event of a life-ending accident or illness. This would save time, money, frustration, and bitterness. One of the most distasteful situations that occurs is to have a person brought into the emergency room arrested, to work on him aggressively for some time, only to have a family member arrive and summarily announce, as though we all should know, "Oh, don't do that, he has lung cancer and doesn't want to have anything like this done."

The tragic case of Terri Schiavo focused the national spotlight on the problem of what can be done or not done if you have not written it down. Tragedy knows no age. If you are mature, you need to fill out an "advanced medical directive." You can do this through the Internet for about $15. You can download a form, fill it out to reflect your personal wishes regarding resuscitation, intubation, and artificial feeding, have it witnessed by two people who have nothing to gain from your death, and get it notarized. Make a copy for your spouse, friend, or parent and you are covered. It will come into play only if you are mentally incompetent and unable to make medical decisions on your own. A power of attorney gives someone you trust the legal authority to act on your behalf, making these same decisions only after the fact, hopefully tailoring decisions appropriately for your unique circumstances.

Everyone should have one or both. Most people put off doing it. Young people think they're not vulnerable and they'll do it someday; middle-aged people are too busy; older people are put off by it, thinking they have to visit an attorney, the fee will be huge, and they'll do it when they receive a bad diagnosis. Do it now!

Sudden Collapse: What to Do

What do you do if your 50-year-old wife suddenly collapses? Most people don't have a clue. Sometimes a very simple maneuver can save her life. However, you don't have a lot of time. You have to assume that she has inadequate oxygen delivery to her brain. In this circumstance, *time is brain function*. You must do something to restore at least some oxygen delivery to her brain within about three minutes if she is to avoid brain damage. If you think you can call about it, read about it, or even think much about it, forget it! This is like driving on an icy road. You have to have considered it beforehand. How you react has a lot to do with the situation at hand. Below are two examples. They are exactly the way we physicians work through such problems.

A. Café Coronary

If she is eating, suddenly has trouble speaking, and turns blue, it is likely that a piece of food is stuck in her throat, the so-called *café coronary*. It is thought most commonly to occur in steak houses, frequently involving a chunk of beef that was a too large and unyielding. More often than not, it occurs in someone who has been consuming alcohol. Most of these occur at home, usually in someone elderly. The back of the throat, the oropharynx, is where this piece of food gets lodged. It blocks off the airway. Because the afflicted individual can't get air, she can't cough, she panics and reflexively fights to bring in needed air. By sharply drawing in air, she lodges the foreign object into her throat more solidly. Soon, it's impossible to either exhale or inhale. It's not a pretty sight.

You must quickly go through the following steps of the famous Heimlich maneuver (named after the doctor who discovered its utility for those who are choking):

1. Open her mouth and see if there is something that can be readily removed. If there isn't, don't dig deeply with your finger or you'll push whatever is lodged even more firmly against the back of her throat, further blocking the airway.

2. Stand behind her, she can be sitting or standing, and wrap your arms around her. Make a double fist with your interlocked hands just below her sternum and ribs but above the waist, and suddenly pull your fists toward you violently—a sudden and violent bear-hug. The purpose is to suddenly transmit air and energy upward, hopefully expelling the lodged piece of food through the mouth, relieving the tracheal airway obstruction.

3. If this doesn't work, do it again, then again, and again, using a sharp, aggressive squeeze each time.

4. Because this is always the most common cause of sudden collapse while eating, stop only after several repeated efforts have failed to eliminate the lodged material. It is hard to do, especially if it is your loved one, but you must repeat this maneuver several times, sometimes even after the victim has completely lost consciousness. As the brain becomes starved for oxygen, the muscles of the trachea and the back of the throat will often relax and a persistent effort may finally dislodge the bolus of food.

5. If the Heimlich has clearly failed, lay her down on the floor and start cardiopulmonary resuscitation. (I'll explain how to do it later in this chapter).

6. Call 911. This is the universal number to call when you need emergency help.

Fatal arrhythmias look exactly the same as the café coronary. However, a café coronary still has to be considered the most likely cause of a collapse at the dinner table, especially if the person is eating solid food, such as steak. We have to start with the most likely maneuver to yield success. It is not a rare occurrence and as we get older, our swallowing mechanism is less effective.

A café coronary can also happen in the young. One of our cath lab personnel had a café coronary in the break room. He had little time to eat, as he was needed to run part of the equipment. In the midst of a bite, he turned blue as a squid and was making wild gestures with his hands, unable to breath or cough. A cardiologist who was present promptly performed a Heimlich. A huge chunk of donut hit the wall at warp speed. The man coughed, said thanks, and sheepishly went back to work. The only thing between disaster and another 40 years of living was that maneuver.

B. Sudden Collapse While Not Eating

If the 50-year-old woman collapsed while reading, talking, or performing a routine household task, the circumstances are much different and so is your response. In that event, you need to have the ABCs of resuscitation in mind. Again, you have to "pre-learn" these. If the woman is clearly unresponsive, you must assume that her heart has developed a fatal arrhythmia (ventricular tachycardia or fibrillation) or has developed cardiac standstill (no electrical activity). Since the sooner you intervene, the more likely a favorable result, you must act quickly. First, ball up your fist and strike her very forcefully and sharply in the center of the sternum, the flat, bony plate right in the front and center of the chest. The energy expended to the chest wall is transmitted to the heart. This will sometimes convert an arrhythmia or restart the heart beat. They have to be strong efforts. A couple of these are adequate. This is difficult to do if you are overwhelmed with grief and concern for your loved one. It's the ultimate expression of "tough love."

If this doesn't work, move on quickly to the ABCs of resuscitation. They are:

A. Airway. Sweep your curved finger through the mouth, making sure there is nothing to obstruct the airway. Remove any foreign material, including dentures. If the woman has vomited, turn her to allow the vomit to drain.

B. Breathing. Cover her mouth with yours and give her a couple of good breaths with her chin tilted upward to open the airway.

C. Circulation. Start closed chest massage. With the heel of your dominant hand over the center of the sternum, place your other hand on top of it, and then sharply push the sternum inward. This is not gentle but is forceful and thrusting. You are compressing the heart between the sternum beneath your hand and her backbone, pushing blood through arteries to the vital organs—the brain, heart, and kidneys. A good compressor can generate a good strong pulse at about 80 compressions a minute. If you are alone, stop after about ten compressions to give her another large breath by mouth-to-mouth. If others are present, have them give the victim a breath every half-dozen compressions. If you do this for a couple of minutes with no response, call 911. If possible, do it with a cell phone so you can continue your endeavors. After a couple of minutes, stop to check if the woman is breathing or if she has a palpable pulse over a large vessel, such as the carotid in the neck.

During this time of attempted resuscitation, if you possess an in-home external cardiac defibrillator, go ahead and discharge it. In fact, do this as the first maneuver on a pulseless, unconscious person. *Remember: The earlier someone is shocked after they develop a fatal arrhythmia, the more effective it will be.* Still, don't forget the other procedures, especially clearing the airway. Additionally, if the heart is stopped, a couple of minutes of closed massage may bring back an effective heart beat.

911

I am often asked, "Wouldn't it be better to call 911 first?" No one who has ever had to call 911 bothers to ask this. Don't get me wrong. I love the 911 system. The operators are committed and work quickly and efficiently under great pressure. However, they have to get your information, they are frequently inundated (sometimes by crank calls), and the processing takes time. As my dad used to say, they have to separate the wheat from the chaff, and that's hard to do over the phone. The operator gives you instructions but meanwhile, your loved one is without help, quiet, and the brain is receiving no oxygen. Any effort directed toward restoration of air flow, heartbeat, and blood flow is more apt to be successful if instituted early. I think it is best to offer someone who is completely unresponsive at least two or three minutes of full, aggressive resuscitation effort, and start it as soon as possible. Of course, emergency procedures are most effective if another person is available to call 911 at the same time.

All of the procedures mentioned can cause bodily injury. Talk to your doctor about them before the need arises or take emergency medical courses offered within your community. In performing the Heimlich maneuver, there have been instances of broken ribs, rupture of the stomach, and other problems. With the thump version (using a blow to the chest) and with closed chest massage, there have been many instances of separation of the ribs from the sternum. I know from first-hand experience what it's like to cause trauma to one you love. I thought my father hung the moon every night and then got up early to remove it again. When he arrested in the small-town hospital close to our home, I traveled there to be with him. He suffered a cardiac arrest shortly after I arrived and, unfortunately, I was the only one around who could hope to resuscitate him. I put down his endotracheal tube and performed closed chest massage. By the time I stopped, his ribs had partially separated from his sternum. However, I did what I had to do to try to save his life.

Do not use the maneuvers I've just outlined unless someone is clearly in trouble and looks as though they are going to die if you sit idly by. If you choose to respond to a medical emergency, be sure you have thoroughly studied these tactics first and feel confident you can do them. If you have to perform closed chest massage, start out gently for the first two or three thrusts. If the person is old or thin, it doesn't take too much to squeeze the heart. If they are large, it takes more energy. If you have to perform a Heimlich, be sure you get below the ribs so you won't break them.

It would, of course, be better if a doctor happened to be having dinner in the same restaurant when someone loses consciousness. But you can't count on it. The measures I have outlined will help you in the event you are isolated or alone when someone you love collapses.

I believe that we will only improve the world if we are willing to help others. There is a Good Samaritan law in effect in the United States and Canada, as well as in many countries in Europe. This law protects from blame those who choose to aid others who are injured or ill. In some countries, knowledge of first aid is a prerequisite to receiving a driver's license. In the United States, no one is required to offer first aid to a victim unless that person is involved in a caretaker relationship with them. Some people have failed to help because they were worried about infection or legal implications. Medical professionals are not protected by Good Samaritan laws when performing aid in conjunction with their employment; they are protected if they won't be receiving remuneration for it.

Whether or not you provide assistance is an individual decision. If you learn the procedures well and do your best, you can feel proud of your efforts even if the end result is not altered.

Partial Collapse

If someone has slumped over, seems in distress, but is still able to respond and speak, don't institute the Heimlich or closed chest massage. We see this all the time. Oxygen delivery to the brain has become diminished by either a drop in blood pressure or heart rate or by some process that doesn't allow for adequate uptake of oxygen by the red blood cells.

Help her to the floor. By getting her flat, you are allowing the blood to be pumped on a level, rather than uphill to the brain, and you're preventing a potential fall resulting in injury. If she is blue, suggesting inadequate oxygen delivery, or if she is having severe shortness of breath or chest pain, call 911 without delay. If she is not blue or struggling for air but has a pulse that is regular but weak, gently take both legs, keep them straight, and elevate them above the level of the heart. When you elevate her legs, you are dumping blood that has pooled in the legs back into the central circulation. The person will frequently come back around. If you do a Heimlich or closed chest massage on such a person, she's going to be angry when she gets better. I've heard a few really bad words uttered from a wife to her husband over this type of situation.

External Defibrillators

External defibrillators are appearing in more and more public places, like schools and airports. They'll soon be in many homes. First, be sure that your loved one wants to be resuscitated in the event of an emergency. Practice finding a major pulse, such as the carotid artery in the neck, if you are going to have a defibrillator in your home. You wouldn't want to shock someone if you can readily feel a pulse beating strong and regular at a reasonable rate. When a situation occurs, make sure the person is unresponsive, not just drunk or sleeping. I have personally seen one person shocked from a deep slumber. He said almost exactly the same words uttered by the woman mentioned earlier when her husband did the unnecessary chest massage

It is not pleasant to be shocked when alert. While working on an arrested fireman when I was an exhausted new intern, I bent over to perform a blood gas analysis and then sat back on the bed. I couldn't have positioned myself better on the paddles if I had tried. The paddles discharged, delivering 360 Joules of energy to my derrière, blowing me against the wall. Trust me: **Do not shock someone unless the person is clearly unconscious.**

Viagra Problems

If we are ever going to come out of the closet on this one, this is the time and place. The very person who needs a drug like Viagra is the same person who is at some risk from using it.

An erection is maintained by a reservoir of blood entrapped within the penis. There are multiple reasons why a man may have difficulty obtaining and maintaining an erection. The most common in the over-50 crowd is that of partial compromise of blood supply to the penis as a manifestation of arteriosclerosis. This is frequently coupled with a neuropathic process (altered nerve function) in conditions such as diabetes. If you can't get adequate blood to the penis to become entrapped or if you have inadequate nerve reflexes, an erection is improbable. This is where Viagra comes into action—by relaxing the small arterioles so enough blood can enter to allow for an erection.

It works. Most people are happy with this drug. However, it is not without risks. I've spent many hours educating patients about the safe use of these drugs. For the most part, men who ask for this drug do it almost furtively, as though it's illegal, immoral or, at the very least, naughty.

The most important thing to remember is that all of the drugs engineered to treat erectile dysfunction can drop your blood pressure. The very people who need this drug frequently have large prostates and are taking medications like Flomax to bring about better urinary flow. However, Flomax can also drop your blood pressure. Therefore, Viagra and Flomax should not be taken together. The warning is on the instructions you receive with your Viagra. The drug company is covered. You, the person who is taking the drug, have to be the one to heed the instructions. Nitroglycerin and the long-acting forms, such as Isordil, will drop your blood pressure. If you are taking nitroglycerin compounds, you should never ever use Viagra.

As they say, boys will be boys. Therefore, we often see men take Viagra when they are taking Flomax or a similar drug. We see men who take both of these and are also secretly using nitroglycerin! These are the men who are apt to get into trouble with hypotension (low blood pressure) and suffer a serious problem.

The other folks at risk are those with carotid artery blockage. If you suddenly drop your systolic blood pressure from 140 down to 80 mmHg, you will not pass out if you have wide open arteries supplying the brain. However, if you have a 75% blockage in your dominant carotid artery and 50% blockage in the other, you could be in serious trouble when your blood pressure falls.

A third group of individuals at risk are the ones who need Viagra the most—diabetics. They frequently have diffuse arteriosclerotic disease, sometimes involving the smaller arteries, such as the retinal artery. They frequently have faulty nerve-driven automatic reflexes. If someone with normal reflexes has a drop in blood pressure, his heart rate will automatically increase in a desperate effort of the circulatory system to meet the perfusion (blood delivery) requirements of the brain. If these reflexes are faulty and his blood pressure falls, perfusion of the head with oxygen-carrying blood may be dramatically decreased. These men are at risk of developing visual problems, including unilateral blindness.

Since anyone can get into trouble with Viagra, keep this in mind: If you develop severe dizziness, lightheadness, or chest pain, don't try to stand or walk, the normal response to a panic situation. Instead, assume that your blood pressure has fallen dramatically. In response, move over until you can get your legs way up on the wall or the bed frame. If you are unable to do this on your own, get some help. Don't try to be macho! You are dumping the pooled blood in your legs back into the central circulation so that the brain and eyeballs can be properly supplied with blood. You will likely recover quickly. Don't even try to move until you have equilibrated for several minutes. Since many people walk around dehydrated, have your wife or friend get you a large amount of water to drink. If you continue to feel bad, take your pulse. If it is irregular, very rapid, or you continue to feel terrible, call 911 and get some help. But lie there until they come!

In addition to avoiding other drugs that drop the blood pressure when using Viagra, drink alcohol in moderation. It dehydrates you. Stay well hydrated with water. And don't have sex using Viagra after consuming a heavy meal. These suggestions will help you have a pleasant experience rather than a life-threatening one.

Rapid Regular Palpitations

Most people who have a rapid, regular heart rhythm, known as *paroxysmal supraventricular tachycardia (PSVT)*, have made at least one trip to the doctor's office or, more likely, to the emergency room. Though it is alarming, most of these spells are not dangerous, just a menace. With the first spell, you should be seen by a doctor so that you can be sure you don't have one of the unusual anomalous fiber tracts that render your situation more dangerous. Many people have an electrical fiber tract that causes them to conduct electrical impulses abnormally. Usually, these are just nuisances. Some can result in very rapid rhythms. Many people elect to have such a nuisance fiber tract burned with radiofrequency ablation to rid them of this problem. Then they can eliminate their drugs for it. Others just have a spell only every four years or so.

If you have a spell and are away from home or it occurs in the middle of the night or when guests are present, and if you know that you have a tendency to develop this arrhythmia, the following maneuver will stop it in about 75% of instances. Fill a basin with ice-cube cold water, take a deep breath, grab your nose between finger and thumb, and submerse your face in the water for a minute or two. This triggers a diving reflex, which slows our heart rate when we dive deeply into colder water (the same reflex the dolphins have). This simple measure may well snap you out of the PSVT and eliminate the need to visit an ER.

The other rapid, regular arrhythmia, much more dangerous and usually unresponsive to the diving reflex, is ventricular tachycardia. Most people know they have something dreadfully wrong when this occurs. See Chapter 14 on *Palpitations* for a better understanding of this worrisome arrhythmia.

Congestive Heart Failure with Pulmonary Edema

If you know you have congestive heart failure and you awake suddenly, acutely short of breath, you are likely having what we refer to as pulmonary edema. You can accumulate a great amount of water in your body without knowing it. It distributes within the abdomen and the legs and can be fairly unnoticeable, especially if you feel well and don't tax yourself physically. If you have congestive heart failure, you should weigh yourself every day so this water weight gain doesn't slip up on you. When you lie down, this water redistributes, but it takes two to four hours for this to occur. When it re-enters the central circulation, you suddenly have way too much water within your bloodstream. Water is pushed across the pulmonary capillary-alveolar membrane, that interface where the blood cells take on oxygen and drop off carbon dioxide. You wake up smothering for air as your air pockets are filled with water. This is known as pulmonary edema.

Though I educate my patients regarding this potential, they still have to go to the emergency room. I tell them how to ease their plight while they are preparing to go. I ask them to place a nitroglycerin pill under their tongue even if they have no chest pain. Nitroglycerin works by dilating the veins as well as the arteries in the body. In doing so, it dramatically reduces the amount of work the heart has to perform. There is less blood returned to the right heart, the huge maze of veins in the body are relaxed, and the blood pressure drops slightly reducing the burden of the left ventricle.

I ask them to take a "bail-out" pill, a strong diuretic called Zaroxolyn, when they become water-logged. It works in a different part of the kidney than your usual diuretic and will sometimes start the process of dumping water. Frequently, when my patients with this problem get to the ER, they are already much better. They are certainly appreciative that they didn't have to starve for oxygen during the transfer to the hospital. I have also had many of them do this on cruises and other travel where they didn't have access to their usual medical care personnel. It made a difference. I've had very good results with this precaution.

Go over this information with your doctor and make sure he or she is okay with it. They may disagree because of a difference in your particular situation.

Stroke vs. Too Much to Drink or Sleepiness

During the last 30 years, I've seen several individuals who had suffered a neurologic event and were put to bed because they were "sleepy" or "drunk." As we age, we are unable to process alcohol as well as a few years ago. It's easy to assume that someone has had one too many glasses of wine. It occurs at dinner parties, watching television, and during other events where you might logically make a judgment that your loved one was merely experiencing a "lapse" of some sort.

Here is how to quickly check to determine if someone is having a neurologic process: Ask him to squeeze your second and third fingers with both hands. His hand grasps should be equal. Ask him to speak. Even a sleepy or inebriated person should be able to form a word. Ask him to stick his tongue out. It should be in the middle. If one hand is weak, he can't form a word or the tongue deviates to one side, he may well have experienced some sort of neurologic insult, a clot to an artery in the brain or a bleed into the brain. He needs urgent attention.

A caveat is in order here. You may have heard the term "brain attack," in which the brain doesn't receive enough oxygen, compared to a "heart attack," in which the heart muscle doesn't get enough oxygen. You may have heard the recommendation to take a couple of aspirin for a heart attack. You might logically make the assumption that this should be done for a "brain attack" as well. Don't! When the heart hurts, it can only be caused by a blockage. When the brain tissue isn't working properly, it can be caused by either a blockage of an artery or a bleed. Aspirin would be great treatment for a blockage due to a fresh clot but would be terrible if a small bleed has occurred. You can't tell the difference. Let the doctor in the ER decide after conducting a scan to determine which it is, a clot or a bleed.

REMINDERS

1. If someone turns blue and collapses at the dinner table, he most likely has experienced a café coronary, an obstruction of the airway due to a large chunk of food lodged in the oropharynx. The Heimlich maneuver may save his life.
2. When food is not obstructing the airway, a sudden and complete collapse may mean the person has experienced a life-threatening arrhythmia or cardiovascular standstill. Make sure his airway is clear, then give him one or two sharp whacks in the center of the sternum. This will sometimes restart the heart.
3. CPR should immediately be started if clearing the throat and the sharp whacks aren't effective. Pay attention to the ABCs of resuscitation: A-Airway, B-Breathing, and C-Circulation.
4. Don't perform a chest thump or CPR when the individual is still responsive and speaking.

6\. If you are concerned that your loved one has had a stroke, check his hand grasp, his ability to form a word, and his tongue protrusion. If abnormal, it might be a stroke. Have him evaluated by a professional.

5\. Understand how to perform these maneuvers before you do them. Check with your doctor or your community's emergency procedures program. You can induce injury if wrongly performed.

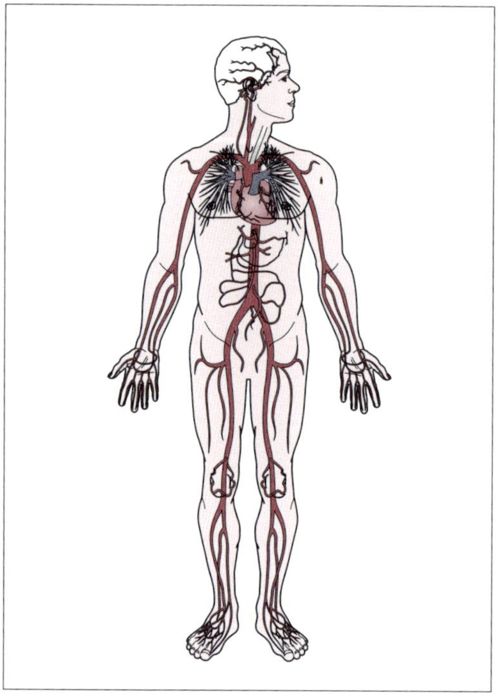

7 HIGH BLOOD PRESSURE

Hypertension

HIGH BLOOD PRESSURE, THE CHRONICALLY ELEVATED pressure measured with an arm cuff, is also called arterial or systemic hypertension and is common worldwide. It's difficult to get a true reading of the population with this disorder but it is estimated at over 30 million in the U.S. alone. Even though high blood pressure is not a disease of the heart, it is a frequent cause of heart disease. It is rarely due to blood vessel disease, but it can lead to or contributes to blood vessel disease. Most people are interested in hypertension and, specifically, how to prevent it and treat it.

Hypertension is called the "silent killer" for good reason. But it doesn't have to be a killer; it can be tamed. It is silent because it usually shows no symptoms whatsoever until it has caused organ damage. It is so silent that many people feel better with an elevated blood pressure. It gives them a "zing" similar to caffeine. Some people who have had chronic hypertension for years say they feel terrible when their blood pressure is well controlled. This is particularly common in those who seem to have a genetic tendency for high blood pressure to develop. It's as though their pressure gauge was incorrectly set by Mother Nature.

Left uncontrolled, high blood pressure will lead to renal (kidney) failure in a substantial number of patients. Renal specialists tell me that we baby boomers are about to experience an epidemic of end-stage renal disease, primarily due to high blood pressure and diabetes. We need to learn how to control our blood pressure before it causes damage to the "end" organs commonly affected by excessive driving or pounding pressure—the brain, kidneys, and heart.

High blood pressure will also lead to arteriosclerosis ("hardening" of the arteries due to cholesterol deposits), especially of the coronary arteries. There is absolutely no question that the stress exerted on the wall of the arteries is a strong contributor to formation and propagation of arterial disease. Additionally, the very factors that may well have influenced the development of high blood pressure in the first place—obesity, sedentary lifestyle, Type 2 diabetes, smoking, stress, excess alcohol consumption, and noise pollution—also cause coronary artery disease.

High blood pressure is also a leading contributor to the ever-growing population of individuals with congestive heart failure. This is especially true for African-Americans with high blood pressure. There are currently close to five million Americans with congestive heart failure caused by a stiff heart from hypertension, diabetes, coronary artery disease, and age. An estimated 750,000 of these are African-Americans. This is too many. When African-Americans develop high blood pressure, they are more apt to ultimately develop heart failure. In my experience, high blood pressure is more difficult to treat in this population. It tends to be more severe, requiring more drugs, and associated with more end-organ damage than in the non-black population. I mention it only because it points out the need for more aggressive efforts at blood pressure control in this group, especially the middle-aged. This is the time when you are developing the early architectural changes in the heart muscle that ultimately result in congestive heart failure, the beginning damage to the kidneys, and possibly the forerunner of changes that will affect your brain.

In terms of human suffering and mortality, the price paid for this silent disease to run its course undetected or untreated is too great. For example, hypertension is one of the most common causes of stroke, either a bland stroke due to the closure of a tiny vessel supplying the brain or a hemorrhagic stroke, the more devastating variety brought about by bleeding into the brain tissue. While we see stroke in individuals with normal blood pressure, the incidence goes up several-fold in the hypertensive population. This is usually related to the damage incurred to the small arterial blood vessels in the brain by the pounding of excess blood pressure. It finally results in enough damage that a small vessel closes off causing the so-called lacunar stroke. However, high blood pressure also causes damage to the inside of the carotid arteries, the large arteries in the neck providing arterial blood to the entire brain. They are more apt to develop cholesterol plaque within their walls, potentially leading to a larger stroke than we see when a small vessel within the brain tissue closes off. See Chapter 5 on *Stroke*.

This brain end-organ damage story keeps getting worse: The cognitive decline may be an unanticipated effect of hypertension. In other words, the longer you have high blood pressure and the worse it is, left uncontrolled, the more apt you are to lose skills in thinking, formulating answers to problems, remembering where you left your keys, your neighbor's name, etc. This is certainly not the complete answer to the increasing question of what causes dementia, but it is part of it.

For years I've thought that a lot of these effects had to do with the pounding the brain tissue gets when exposed to unremitting high blood pressure. Consider, for example, a very high blood pressure for 20 years. We know that this type of pressure will damage kidneys, making them small and shrunken, a condition we refer to as *nephrosclerosis*. It is known that the excess pressure causes multiple small scars to develop within the kidney tissue and as a consequence, they shrink. Why can't this happen to brain tissue as well? It's a straight shot to the brain. I believe that's precisely what happens: The brain develops tiny scars throughout its mass and it shrinks. It doesn't shrink a lot, just a bit, but each tiny punctuate scar may represent thousands of brain cells replaced by scar tissue. Scar tissue doesn't remember where you left your house keys. I believe that brain damage, in the form of either cognitive disruption or stroke, represents the most important reason for aggressive handling of high blood pressure. And I don't believe it has received nearly enough attention. The other end-organ insults and injuries are, of course, important. However, there is no greater life-changing event than that incurred by damage to the brain.

Definition of Hypertension

Hypertension is defined as a *persistent* abnormal elevation in systemic, or arterial, blood pressure. This is the blood pressure measured in the arm with a blood pressure cuff. A single abnormal reading does not make the diagnosis unless it is significantly high. Multiple readings in the elevated category do make the diagnosis. This is the reason it is so important to perform multiple blood pressure checks under a variety of situations in order to "trend" your blood pressure.

What constitutes an abnormal reading? Normally we consider a systolic pressure (the "top" number) of over 140 mmHg (millimeters of mercury, what every cuff measures) or a diastolic pressure (the "bottom" number) of greater than 90mmHg as an abnormal reading. If you routinely exceed these numbers, you have hypertension. However, we now know that even chronic systolic pressures over 120 mmHg but under 140 cause typical hypertension-related insults to the end organs and probably should be treated. In other words, just like cholesterol numbers, the blood pressure numbers that define the upper end of normal keep coming down as we accumulate more data.

I'm frequently told, "But doctor, I have 'white coat syndrome.' I always have a high blood pressure in the doctor's office but it's absolutely normal at home." That may be the case. However, if coming to the doctor's office causes the blood pressure to become elevated, other stressors in life probably cause the same reaction. Therefore, these are usually true readings in that person under stress. This is one of the reasons that a trend is important in making the diagnosis and is equally important in following therapy.

Causes of Hypertension

There is a strong familial tendency to develop high blood pressure. Blood pressure is dramatically altered by the volume status within the body at any given time. In other words, if you ingest a large amount of sodium chloride, plain old table salt, you will hold onto an equivalent amount of water. In many young people, this is of no consequence. But as we get older, the "pipes" (arteries) are stiffer and have less give, so salt and water loading is apt to drive up the blood pressure.

Again, this development is greatly influenced by your genetics. This genetic tendency toward high blood pressure cannot be overstated. You simply can't give some people high blood pressure, no matter how much salt they ingest. Others can carefully restrict the amount of sodium they ingest and still carry around an astounding level of hypertension. It has been shown that somewhere around 60–70% of individuals with high blood pressure are able to influence the level of their blood pressure with variation in salt intake. This is very important!

There are actually only a few mechanical or chemical explanations for elevated blood pressure. One of these mechanical processes actually leads to a chemical cause as well. This is *renal artery stenosis*, a primary disease of blood vessels, caused almost always by arteriosclerosis. The mechanical process, a blockage in the mouth of the renal artery supplying the kidney caused by cholesterol deposit, leads to the chemical cause for elevated blood pressure. The chemicals released are renin, angiotensin, and aldosterone, all poured out because the kidney is not receiving enough blood to satisfy its needs due to the blockage in the artery. Angiotensin causes the small muscular arteries throughout the body to become smaller, increasing the pressure the heart has to pump against. Aldosterone causes the kidneys to hold onto salt and water, also driving up the pressure. These chemicals are produced in response to the kidney's self-preservation "clarion call" demands to increase its own unique blood supply. In the course of doing this, the overall blood pressure is elevated, sometimes dramatically. This activation of the *Renin-Angiotensin-Aldosterone System* (RAAS) is not unique to renal arterial stenosis; it is activated in heart failure also. Certainly, they are interrelated events. We would expect this system to become activated when the blood pressure drops, as with a hemorrhage somewhere, and it is. Otherwise, it becomes an inappropriate reflex, elaborate in its form, damaging in its action. In this case, the kidney hormone, renin, tells the adrenal gland to produce another hormone, aldosterone, which exerts its action back on both kidneys, making them conserve salt and water. You can see that activation of this system will cause you to hold onto salt and water, sometimes in dangerous levels, and then causes vasoconstriction of millions of small arteries, resulting in elevated blood pressure.

Another mechanical cause is *coarctation* of the aorta, a congenital process whereby the descending aorta is narrowed from the time of birth. This problem requires surgical or stent repair. Its detection rarely escapes the teenage years.

Yet another mechanical cause is *fibromuscular dysplasia* or hyperplasia. This is the "string of beads" narrowing of a renal artery—usually only one, though both may be affected—almost always found in young women. These are tough to treat, as the narrowed segments frequently are repeated right down to the kidney.

Pure chemical causes are limited as well. The more common is caused by a tumor of the adrenal gland. It is usually benign in cell type but not in symptoms. This tumor, called a pheochromocytoma, produces large quantities of the "fight or flight" chemicals, epinephrine and norepinephrine. These are actually neurotransmitter-type hormones, exerting their influence widely throughout the body. These patients look, feel, and act like speed junkies due to the endogenous "speed" they are manufacturing. They are jumpy, have a rapid heart rate and a markedly elevated blood pressure, frequently have lost weight and are skinny, and sometimes have diarrhea. By measuring urinary metanephrines, the end product of the metabolism of these chemicals, we can detect this tumor. As the saying goes, "You won't find it unless you look for it." We have to perform about 200 such tests on various individuals with high blood pressure before we find a positive result. However, it is imperative to detect it so it can be effectively treated. The symptom complex sounds as though this tumor should be obvious. It's not. In fact, there are only about two or three diseases that have consistently made a monkey of me in my career and this is one of them.

Another chemical cause of high blood pressure is an elevated blood level of calcium, frequently due to a tumor within the parathyroid gland. Other causes exist, but this one is the most common. This is a very rare cause of hypertension.

These mechanical and chemical causes of hypertension constitute far less than 1% of all cases of hypertension. The rest are due to a combination of genetics and habits such as salt-loading, obesity, smoking, lack of exercise, alcohol, caffeine, and stress. I'm sure we'll discover other sources as research continues.

I'm often asked, "Doctor, what part does stress play in this high blood pressure problem?" I believe it plays a major role in quite a few people. We know, for example, that the stress hormone cortisol is poured out in greater quantities in people who handle stress poorly. We also know that its level rises drastically in the early morning hours, between 4 and 6 a.m., faithfully following our 24-hour cyclical response to light. It is no accident that this is also the time of peak occurrence of heart attack, stroke, and sudden death. Constant exposure to a high level of ambient noise has been shown to cause hypertension, probably similar to constant sensory bombardment of any type. I don't think "happily stressed" people, those whose jobs entail some stress but who love their work, necessarily have a sharply increased incidence of hypertension. However, I believe that chronically unhappy people, who frequently hate their jobs that involve multi-tasking and stress, have a significantly increased incidence of hypertension.

The Special Role of High Blood Pressure in Producing Heart Failure

For decades, we have known that untreated high blood pressure would ultimately bring about congestive heart failure in some people. We were puzzled by why some folks with a chronic, very high systolic pressure of 180 mmHg would go along seemingly unfazed by this tremendous burden, while others with a similar pressure would develop dramatic thickening of the wall of the left ventricle, and some would even go on to develop significant enlargement of the left ventricle, as well as loss of contractility. We used to call this "burned-out" hypertensive heart failure. We also knew that African-Americans were more predisposed to have heart failure from uncontrolled high blood pressure. There are many variables and much more of an explanation to come explaining this unusual, apparently random selection process. Now, however, we seem to have at least a couple more pieces of the puzzle put together.

We have, for example, discovered that aldosterone, the end product of an elaborate chemical pathway activated by the kidney, can damage the heart, causing muscle cells to drop out, replaced by scar tissue instead. As we discussed previously, this renin-angiotensin-aldosterone system acts as one of the monitors of the body, helping decide how much salt and water to hold onto, how much to eliminate, and how much to tighten the small blood vessels regulating blood flow to all tissues in the body. One of the chemicals produced is a strong vasoconstrictor, causing increased tone in the small muscular arterioles throughout the body. Instead of just water-logging us, excess aldosterone also damages the heart muscle. Therefore, anything that activates this renin-angiotensin-aldosterone system can cause a world of trouble. This system is very frequently activated in congestive heart failure, causing more hypertension, then more heart failure—an endless loop that, unless interrupted, will wreak havoc in all of the end organs.

Fortunately, we now have drugs that block the development of these vasoconstrictors and also drugs that block their effects at the tissue level. For many years, we had a drug to counteract the actions of aldosterone. We just didn't know how important it was to block it until recently. Now we know that blocking the end-organ effects of aldosterone is extremely important in the treatment of congestive heart failure.

The Natural Way of Prevention and Treatment

Too many people have taken the view that medicine has advanced to the degree that it can bail them out of almost any situation. The attitude seems to be, *I'll do as I want; medicine will fix it.*

The very best way to treat hypertension is by taking a natural approach. For example, if I could take over the habits of each patient with hypertension, I could cure about 75% of all cases. If I could control how that person exercises, eats, thinks, and reacts to life stressors, I could eliminate hypertension in that individual. There will, of course, continue to be a substantial number of people who have such a familial tendency for hypertension that it can't be corrected with simple measures.

My first advice is to throw away the salt shaker. Stop buying salty chips and other salt-laden food products, and stay clear of monosodium glutamate (MSG), a common ingredient in restaurants. Quiz the servers and inform them you are not to receive any MSG under any circumstances. It is a taste enhancer and should not have to be used to make food palatable. Poor chefs will use it liberally. It is a very potent salt product. Specifically, it is a sodium salt of glutamic acid. When you ingest it, it breaks down into sodium, the harmful ion that elevates your blood pressure and holds onto water and glutamate. *Make sure it is not in your food.* Most servers are all too happy to help you out with this. They've been helpfully responding to my questions about it for years.

My second bit of advice is to eat small quantities of fruit at several intervals during the day. All of them, particularly bananas, are high in potassium. The kidneys are manufactured in a fashion such that sodium and potassium are handled in inverse proportions—the more potassium one ingests, the more sodium is excreted by the kidneys. When the sodium is excreted, water follows and the blood pressure falls.

Exercise is very important. I recommend daily walking. This goes a long way toward reducing hypertension. It is common for patients to drop their blood pressure by 10 or 20 points just from regularly walking two to three miles a day. It helps keep your weight down, relaxes you, and helps eliminate sodium through perspiration. Walking conditions your muscles and causes the blood vessels leading to these muscles to relax, or vasodilate. This is a good thing and will clearly drop the blood pressure.

Weight control is a key point. For each pound of fat, there is a mile of capillaries. If you are 20 pounds overweight, not uncommon in America, you possess 20 miles of unneeded capillaries. This is quite a maze of small pipes! The resistance against which the heart pumps is responsible for generating the blood pressure. We have already learned about the natural chemicals produced to regulate the small muscular arteries in the body and how the blood pressure goes crazy when too many of these chemicals are produced. However, if you have 20 miles of small pipes to pump blood through that you don't really need, your blood pressure will continue to be a problem as the resistance is increased simply due to the extra network of small arteries you have to feed. Keep your weight down.

Finally, we come to a critical key to controlling blood pressure. It is something that the bulk of Americans think is either malarkey or too time-consuming. It is called meditation. It is important to start off the day with meditation. Why? A mechanism is present in all of us that causes the release of the stress hormone cortisol, and the fight and flight hormones epinephrine and norepinephrine in the early morning hours. This mechanism, to which we are all captive, is called the Circadian rhythm. We are all hardwired to have this. It results in an outpouring of these hormones into the blood stream starting about 4 a.m. and lasting until about 8 a.m. We can't make it go away! It is an in-born part of all of us. These are all important hormones. They have vital functions and without them we would die. However, they are poured out abundantly in the early morning hours and there is a great deal of evidence that this peak is harmful to our blood pressure, our arteries, and our plaque systems within our arteries.

We can combat its effects. Instead of groaning your way into the kitchen to get a big cup of java when you awake, make a nice cup of green tea and go to your special place for meditation. This means something different to everyone. I read a little book called *The Daily Word* and then I think about my life and my day. I also read my little book called *Secrets of Serenity*. These are just short one- or two-sentence passages. They focus me, bring me down from my anxiety high (which I don't know I have until I get rid of it), and reaffirm to me what is important in life.

These simple measures are more important as we get older. They influence health, happiness, some measure of prosperity and, of course, love and care of family. In today's fast-paced world, it is too easy to start thinking that you have to get out there and slay the dragon. Well, let the dragon wait for awhile.

Everything else, including competition, should be secondary to our peace of mind. A lifetime of trying to get ahead of the pack is stressful and ultimately takes its toll on us one way or another. Competition is important because it pushes us to become all that we can be. However, meditating once or even several times a day resets our gauges and can be done at our desks as well as under a tree somewhere.

For some, the best form of meditation is prayer. For others, it is imaging something in nature, perhaps a mountain view or a waterfall. For others, it is reading poetry, the Bible, or the Koran. You'll need to find your own way of calming your soul. If it's closing the door and muttering a mantra, so be it. Do it your way, but do it—every day. It will do amazing things to your blood pressure!

You Need Your Own Blood Pressure Cuff!

If you have high blood pressure, purchase your own blood pressure cuff. Many times, your insurance carrier or Medicare will cover the expense if you have a prescription from your physician. There are many people out there who do have "White Coat Syndrome." Their blood pressure rises drastically when they come to a doctor's office. We suspect this when we put the person on a blood pressure regimen and they come back saying they've been dizzy or have blacked out. Their blood pressure may have gone back to a perfectly normal level the minute they walked out of my office. The medication was unneeded and taking it made them sick. Having your own blood pressure cuff is the most important component of good blood pressure treatment. Take it with you to your doctor's office so your manometer can be compared to the one in his or her office. You can follow your progress, you can learn your "triggers," you can see what your pressure is when you're dizzy, and you can even help us determine if you have lost your normal Circadian variation (blood pressure rises in the early morning hours when your stress hormones are peaking). For example, we know you frequently lose this variation with metabolic syndrome. Keep a diary.

24-Hour Blood Pressure Monitor

We can perform a 24-hour blood pressure monitor. These are especially helpful in cases of "refractory hypertension." Sometimes it is due to sleep apnea, a process in which you suspend breathing when asleep. Because we know that about half of all of those with congestive heart failure also have sleep apnea, and we know that their blood pressure rises drastically when pathologically apneic, the 24-hour blood pressure monitor is a helpful tool.

A Combination of Natural and Drug Treatment

If you do all of the above and still have high blood pressure, you need treatment with drugs. The traditional treatment has changed with time, as it should. Ideally, we would use a single drug when treating hypertension but we often find ourselves adding drug after drug for optimal blood pressure control. Because of this, it's so much better if you practice all of the "natural" methods of blood pressure control that I recommended. If you still have a persistently elevated blood pressure, a drug can be added to use in conjunction with your healthy practices. If your blood pressure is relatively refractory, we prefer to use smaller doses of multiple drugs rather than pushing a single drug until you get unpleasant side effects. But don't give up your natural methods just because you have to take a drug.

It's difficult for a physician to go over an entire list of natural treatment components in detail with each and every patient. Oftentimes, it's easier just to write out a prescription. Our problem as physicians is not having enough face-to-face time to explain it all. And even in a relaxed, conducive environment people retain only a fraction of what they are taught. In your doctor's office, with a million emotions colliding in your brain, it's a wonder you recall any of what is said.

As doctors, we're often surprised by how an intelligent person can have a disease that can cripple him with a stroke, heart attack, renal failure, or even end his life, and yet he forgets what we told him last week. To understand why a patient forgets, the doctor just needs to become a patient for awhile! It's difficult to learn it all and easy to forget some of it. Take notes and research your disease so you can ask your doctor about it on your next visit.

We have become a "drugged-up" society. Each medical issue seems to beg for a drug. The drug companies love it. It makes them rich. This is representative of a health care society run amok! You don't frequently see an advertisement on television telling you how to "naturally lower your blood pressure." The drug companies are trying to sell drugs and they're good at it. The typical person over age 65 takes an average of six drugs! As a common-sense approach, I try hard to control high blood pressure *without* a drug or I treat it with a drug while the patient does everything under his control to change harmful patterns—sedentary lifestyle, overeating, obesity, salt consumption, smoking, excess alcohol, and stress. As he gains control of these high blood pressure accentuating factors, we taper down and he discontinues the drug(s) as quickly as possible. This is ideal though it is the exception. I hope to change that for a variety of reasons. The most important is to prevent you from having so many *artificial* chemicals inside you. Another is the preservation of your hard-earned dollar. Even if you have medication insurance or Medicare, you are indirectly paying for the drug. A third reason is the self-satisfaction and feeling of triumph you will have when you "fix it on your own." There's nothing better for your health and nothing better for your soul.

Sir William Osler, a famous physician who taught and wrote prodigiously in the late 1800s was also famous for his quotes, some acerbic, some merely commentary. Two of them apply here:

1. "One of the first duties of the physician is to educate the masses not to take medicine."
2. "The desire to take medicine is perhaps the greatest feature which distinguishes man from animals."

If drug therapy is necessary for control of hypertension, I usually start with something that I customize for the patient. For example, if the patient's heart rate is very high, I may well start with a beta-blocker because the high rate, in absence of anemia or high thyroid levels, is an indicator of excess output of stress hormones. At the same time, I try to make sure this patient doesn't have a pheochromocytoma, one of the rare chemical causes for high blood pressure. It is a benign adrenal tumor that can pour out huge quantities of epinephrine.

On the other hand, if the individual comes in with a lot of edema fluid, I may just start with a simple diuretic in order to eliminate the water. If neither is the case, I may begin with either a calcium antagonist, such as Cardiazem, which is exceptionally well tolerated, or an ACE-I or ARB to block the complex renin-angiotensin-aldosterone system I outlined earlier. I almost always start off with a diuretic whether or not I find evidence of excess fluid. Water hides everywhere and the diuretic is inexpensive and well tolerated.

There are some truly exceptional drugs out there. There just aren't very many! There is a great drug for high blood pressure, an ACE-I, that has generated wonderful data. It's called Ramipril. The HOPE study, a large clinical trial, has demonstrated the qualities of this drug. As an ACE-I, it blocks the angiotensin-converting enzyme, a necessary part of normal physiology. But the end product of that metabolic conversion is manufactured in excess when the machinery is revved up because there is high blood pressure (the activated RAAS we have talked about). It turns out that this particular ACE-I has been shown to be especially valuable in patients over age 55 that have had a previous problem. We know, for example, there is a sharp rise in cardiovascular events after age 55. This is well documented by statistics from the American Heart Association. If you are over 55, with a history of coronary artery disease, stroke, or peripheral vascular disease, or if you have diabetes plus one other risk factor, Ramipril reduces the incidence of subsequent heart attack by 20% and stroke by 32%. It is certainly possible that the other ACE-I drugs will do the same. However, the data is in on this one and if the problem fits in this category, I want this drug.

Be aware that ACE-I drugs, by blocking this important enzyme gone ballistic, also allow for accumulation of bradykinin in the blood and tissues. Bradykinin is a "good" chemical, causing relaxation of blood vessels. It's broken down by the angiotensin-converting enzyme. If we block this enzyme, we block the breakdown of bradykinin too. This is part of the reason the drug works so well. Some never notice this increased level; others develop a dry cough. Rarely, few individuals taking the enzyme inhibitor ACE-I develop what is known as angioneurotic edema. This is a swelling of the throat and tissues, frequently associated with a blotchy appearance. If these occur, the drug needs to be stopped. It can be replaced by a drug that works only one metabolic step away, an angiotensin receptor-blocker, ARB for short. We don't have as much clinical data on this group of drugs, but they are the next best thing.

Also be aware that an ACE-I may cause birth defects if used in the first trimester of pregnancy. I've always told my young female hypertensive patients to, if possible, take nothing except a diuretic. For everyone else, the ACE-I is the drug of choice if you have to venture beyond a simple diuretic.

Another drug trial warrants mention because it is effective in serving as a possible treatment program for a problem that has been frustrating in the past: high blood pressure–related congestive heart failure. ALLHAT, another famous drug trial, showed that new-onset heart failure is significantly lower when the long-term drug treatment for high blood pressure is either a diuretic or an ACE-I rather than a calcium channel blocking drug. Since the African-American population is more prone to develop congestive heart failure in response to long-standing hypertension, the ACE-I would seem to be ideal. Unfortunately, they frequently respond poorly to this class of drugs. From the standpoint of heart failure, they do better on a combination of a long-acting vasodilator (like nitroglycerin) and an old-fashioned drug, Hydralazine. Both of these are vasodilators, implying that this subset of patients may have an inordinate degree of tone in the small muscular arteries that determines systemic vascular resistance. In other words, these vessels, called arterioles, always carry a certain amount of tone, usually determined by the nerves investing these vessels and influenced by chemicals within the bloodstream. This tone may be minor, so that the artery is relaxed, or very pronounced, so that the artery is constricted. This tone produces the resistance against which blood has to flow to reach the tissues. If we bleed, the vessel tone is increased so the blood pressure will remain in a reasonable range. In high blood pressure, the vessel tone is frequently too great. The fact that these two vasodilator drugs work so beautifully in the African-American population suggests that tone is an important factor. I don't think we know why they respond less to the ACE-I class of drugs that block vessel constriction. Nonetheless, this is badly needed information for this otherwise difficult-to-treat population.

Based on an amalgamation of good data, it is beneficial to start treatment of high blood pressure with a simple inexpensive diuretic, adding an ACE-I such as Ramipril if inadequate control is found after a month or two of doing everything right. In the African-American population, it makes sense to substitute the nitrate-Hydralazine combination when a drug needs to be added. Subsequent to these, the next likely drug would be a beta-blocking drug, such as Inderal or Lopressor.

Don't quit the simple lifestyle modifications I recommended just because you have to start on a drug. It doesn't have to be a case of one or the other. By necessity, it is frequently both. The simple lifestyle modifications I outlined may *limit* the number of drugs one has to take for good blood pressure control.

Surgical and Interventional Treatment of High Blood Pressure

There are basically only four surgical or interventional treatments for high blood pressure. If a coarctation of the aorta is found, it should be opened. It will not completely take care of the blood pressure problem. If a pheochromocytoma of the adrenal gland is found, it should be resected (surgically removed). This will frequently take care of the blood pressure problem unless kidney damage has occurred. If a tumor of the parathyroid gland is found to have significantly elevated the blood pressure, it should be resected.

This brings me to a treatment that has been controversial in the past: interventional opening of a blocked renal artery. The traditionalists will argue that opening a 75–90% blockage of a renal artery will not totally treat the blood pressure. That is certainly true. However, if that blockage is left alone, more and more renin will be poured into the blood stream, more angiotensin will be generated, and this will make it progressively more difficult to control the blood pressure. Not only that, but if we leave the tight blockage, the same thing that is causing the kidney to signal for greater production of these chemicals—starvation for blood and oxygen—will cause the kidney to lose tissue. We will ultimately wind up with a small, shrunken and useless kidney, now pouring out huge amounts of renin. To top it off, if we leave it alone, an unpredictable number will eventually close off the artery completely. This will result in what we call auto-infarction of the kidney: The kidney is lost completely due to a loss of its blood supply. In the past, when we had only a balloon to open the artery and we had to rely on this result, it was more controversial. Now, with good stents (stainless steel mesh-like devices that can be delivered in the artery, forcing the tight blockage into a wide-open configuration once again) it is no longer debatable. We can achieve good durable results in most of these arteries.

REMINDERS

1. The most common mechanical and/or chemical causes of hypertension are renal artery stenosis and pheochromocytoma. Look for them if your blood pressure is high or is difficult to regulate.
2. Though we don't know the cause for most cases of hypertension, we do know that genetics play a huge role.
3. Try to control moderately elevated blood pressure with natural measures first—lose weight, limit your intake of salt, and exercise.
4. Don't quit the natural measures if you go on an anti-hypertensive drug. It could mean the difference between taking one drug or three or four for blood pressure control.
5. Avoid ACE-I for high blood pressure if you're in the reproductive age group.
6. If you're African-American with high blood pressure, ask your doctor what drugs are most effective for you.

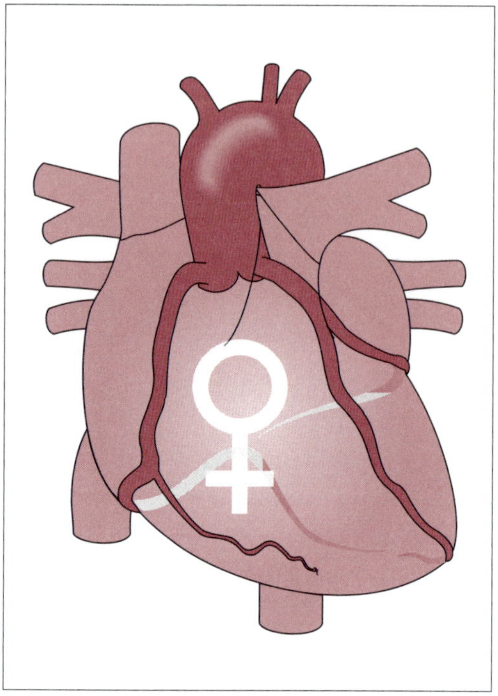

WOMEN AND HEART DISEASE

Women *Are* From Venus

THERE ARE NOTEWORTHY VARIATIONS IN HEART DISEASE seen predominantly in women. I think many of these important differences have been largely left out of traditional commentary regarding women and heart disease. I'll distinguish these features and show you when to get help and what type of help to get.

John Gray, in his 1992 book *Men Are from Mars, Women Are from Venus*, writes that women want their problems to be acknowledged. This chapter is an effort to do just that.

Coronary Artery Disease: The Problem is Detection

The problem, common to both sexes, is *detection* of the symptoms implicating a blocked coronary artery. Ever since William Heberden's initial classic description of angina, the pain that points to a blocked coronary artery, as a "vise-like" discomfort in the chest, this portrayal that has been passed down to each new crop of doctors. We have come to believe that a blocked artery announces its presence in the same persistent manner as *The Tell-Tale-Heart* written about by Edgar Allan Poe. I think we overlooked the complete description by Heberden. It is, "True angina, which is a rare disease, is characterized by paroxysms of agonizing pain in the region of the heart, extending into the arms and neck."

Other diseases were more likely to claim our ancestors when Heberden first made this pronouncement. "True angina" is certainly not the common symptom for a lot of people, especially women, with coronary artery disease causing heart attack. Detecting this mostly silent disease based on symptoms alone or even symptoms coupled with risk factors, is similar to interviewing 100 CEOs and determining which one is lying! The presence of this disease is often hidden because the symptoms of a blockage are as unique as fingerprints. *The mantra for the cardiac world has to be detection of the problem, especially in women, before it has a chance to wreak havoc.* We can't rely on symptoms to point out the population of women with this deadly disease. We must find it before it spells disaster for the women at risk.

Severity of the Problem in Women

First, I think the female population in America is just now becoming fully aware that heart and blood vessel disease is the number-one killer of women over age 25 in this country. At this time, heart and blood vessel disease is responsible for one of every 2.4 deaths in women in America. This means that if there are 240 women at a gathering, statistics tell us that 100 will die from cardiovascular disease. Since the emphasis on health care, prevention, and discovery should be meted out appropriate to the severity, frequency, and mortality of a particular disease process, we can see that we have sadly missed the mark with this one. If you go to any large city and run a survey of middle-aged women and ask about the most prevalent cause of death in their gender and age group, many would consider breast cancer to be their greatest threat. They would be wrong. Just the fact that this misconception exists is cause for concern that we have not done our job. **Coronary heart disease kills four times more women than breast cancer does.** This statistic is even worse for African-American women.

Women are naturally protected from arteriosclerosis, the deposit of cholesterol within the wall of blood vessels, until they reach menopause. The natural cycling of female hormones—estrogen and progesterone—confer a wonderful resistance to this disease. (Coronary heart disease can already be well established in many males by age 30.)

Women are becoming more prone to early coronary artery disease as the incidence of obesity and diabetes mellitus increases in women. The presence of diabetes essentially cancels out the protective benefit women have with hormonal influences. It has recently been shown that large numbers of women are diabetic or prediabetic and don't know it because the test for chronically elevated blood sugar levels is not routinely asked for nor performed. Additionally, the incidence of women smokers has not appreciatively decreased. An Italian study showed the significance of this by determining that women smokers have a higher risk of death from heart disease than male smokers; the difference is greatest for aggressive smokers.

These changes in habits and the gender differences have caused a demographic shift in the relative proportion of the population with coronary heart disease. While there is ongoing evidence that the incidence of cardiovascular death is diminishing in men, there is alarming evidence that the incidence in women is actually increasing, at least in the U.S. The latest data even suggests that more women than men have cardiovascular disease! We know that heart attacks are more apt to be fatal and recurrent in women than in men. Following a heart attack, women are more apt to die in the first year and for several years subsequent, than men and are more likely to have a second heart attack. This is no longer a "man's disease."

Coronary artery disease behaves somewhat differently in women. Generally, it is likely to occur about 10 to 15 years later than in men, largely due to the effects of hormones. It's also possibly influenced by differences in enzyme systems that drive metabolic pathways. It's well known that estrogen increases the good cholesterol (HDL-cholesterol) fraction. It has other protective benefits too. Yet it is still possible for pre-menopausal women to develop coronary artery disease or any form of arteriosclerosis.

Women who had low levels of estrogen prior to menopause have a greater-than-normal risk of developing early coronary artery disease. Additionally, there are plenty of women out there who have experienced surgical menopause secondary to removal of the ovaries. Many of them are too frightened of replacement hormone therapy to take it. Many others who have had a hysterectomy simply do not know whether or not the ovaries were also removed. Still, pre-menopausal structural coronary artery disease is usually seen in severe diabetics or those with a particularly heavy smoking history, frequently coupled with other highly weighted risk factors such as markedly elevated serum cholesterol. The combination of inflammation and a high LDL-cholesterol seems to be a particularly bad duo for women especially when in conjunction with other known risk factors. The most predictive of these risk factors is smoking. For the most part, in purely general terms, women are protected by menses.

At menopause, women catch up with men pretty quickly. When this occurs, an important gender difference emerges. Women tend to have smaller blood vessels than men, including those vessels that supply the heart muscle. This has a lot to do with the effects of testosterone in men. This difference in the size of arterial conduits is very important.

Symptoms of Coronary Artery Disease in Women

With the risk factors and given the strict admonition that detection of silent coronary disease is of utmost importance for women, we should consider the symptoms of *ischemia* (oxygen deprivation of the heart muscle, usually from a narrowed coronary artery) in women. What exactly are the warning signs of a blocked coronary artery in women, and are they different from those in men?

One of the first things I am struck with is that women with coronary artery disease are more likely than men to complain of fatigue. This is a very common occurrence in everyday life. However, it is more common in the female population that ultimately suffers from heart attack. Women complain of "overwhelming fatigue" or "I'm simply drained all the time." If a woman tells me this, my antennae perk up.

Many women do not complain of severe vise-like, squeezing chest pain. While this is the symptom we all learn about in medical school, it is not terribly common in women unless they are having an overt heart attack. Instead, they are more apt to complain of a barely detectable generalized discomfort in the front of the chest. I am also impressed that more women complain of "indigestion" in the epigastrium, the area just below the breastbone. It is usually associated with a bit of nausea, sweating, and they occasionally have difficulty catching their breath. These symptoms are frequently said by the patient to be "minor."

Women also complain of jaw, neck, or shoulder pain. In Chapter 3 on *Heart Attack*, I have discussed that the location of pain and discomfort has a lot to do with the region where the heart becomes invested by nerves that carry the messages of discomfort back to the brain. As a reminder, when the heart develops in the embryo, it starts out as a glob of gelatinous material in the region of the neck. As it descends to its ultimate position within the chest, it turns and folds. During this time of heart formation, other parts of the body are forming. For example, if nerve formation speeds ahead in one particular embryo, the nerves that invest the heart may be predominantly the ones that also supply the jaws or neck. As the heart descends, it may receive a reduced nerve supply from the nerves that also supply the chest. Those nerves may have already formed prior to the heart's positioning itself within the chest cavity. Therefore, the referral of discomfort perceived by the brain is exceptionally unique to each person. You may have received very few nerves to the heart at all during your formative adventure. Alternatively, you may have received a huge number of them. Your reaction 50 years later to the buildup of lactic acid in your struggling heart muscle—unhappy because it's not receiving enough oxygen-rich blood—is distinctly linked to this unique embryonic investment of the heart with nerve fibers. This is one reason why each person's symptoms are as unique as his or her fingerprints.

Our goal is to catch a heart problem in the making and do something about it on an elective basis, long before it causes a potential calamity.

Women, Read This Paragraph Carefully!

In Chapter 3, I related my former secretary's heart attack and sudden death episode while she was at the airport. Because of her job, she is familiar with the symptoms women commonly complain of when they have a coronary problem and could act accordingly. But how in the world can someone who is not involved in the medical world be expected to detect her symptoms? The short answer is: They frequently can't.

In a well-known study conducted in Framingham, Massachusetts, fully 63% of women who died *suddenly* of heart attacks had no warning. This is enough to scare the bejiggers out of any woman with significant coronary risk factors. It underscores an important point: *Education of potential warning signs and symptoms is only a small part of effective treatment! We have to recognize this disease before it causes a calamity and treat it aggressively before it kills. Detection of its presence in asymptomatic women is the key. We must have a well-utilized screening test for the detection of silent coronary artery disease in women.*

Detection of Silent Coronary Disease: Screening Tests (and Hazards)

One of the reasons women with coronary disease are identified later than men is that women's symptoms are sometimes so vague that physicians have trouble ferreting out the important from the mundane. This is coupled with the fact that we historically have had very poor tools for discovering hidden coronary disease. I don't think we are necessarily any more astute than we once were, but we are now better prepared because we have much better screening tools. By screening, I am referring to detection in the woman who has a variety of coronary risk factors but is *asymptomatic*. She is going along blithely in life, but she might be at significantly increased risk of a heart attack down the line.

When choosing a screening tool, it has to satisfy three criteria: inexpensive, safe, and reliable. We're all aware that no screening test is 100% reliable. However, if we are going to screen asymptomatic women with coronary risk factors, we absolutely have to offer complete safety. On the flip side, since 1 out of every 2.4 women is currently destined to die of a heart attack or some other atherosclerotic manifestation, we must have a screening test that is readily available to large numbers of women and that will detect this so-called vulnerable individual with some predictive accuracy.

There are over 75 million baby boomers turning 60. Fifty-one percent of these are women! We know from the incidence of cardiovascular disease that more than half need to be screened. These are dizzying numbers! Since we are going after this disease before it causes a calamity, we have to be sure the test is safe *and* reliable.

No test is perfect; however, some of the ones that have been traditionally used are very poor. Below is a current list of potential screening tools and the pros and cons of each so that you can have proactive input in your evaluation and care.

A. Coronary Calcium Score

By far the best test is the coronary calcium score. It detects and measures pixels of coronary artery calcium. As cholesterol plaques develop within the wall of an artery, we know that they calcify. This, too, occurs at an earlier age in men than in women. This test is effective for men over age 35 while a woman has to be at least 45 years of age for the test to be valid. This is the precise age when we should start screening women for the presence of beginning coronary artery disease. This test satisfies all of our criteria: It can be obtained without a physician's referral, costs only $100–$200, and takes less than 15 minutes to perform. It is safe, there is minimal radiation exposure (about one-sixth the amount each of us receives from sunshine each year), and requires no contrast agent, such as that used with an angiogram. You don't even need to have an intravenous started. It is reliable and tells you if you are at very low risk of having a cardiovascular event or if you need further testing.

We establish appropriate normal calcium amounts, called "scores," for each decade of life. In a woman, this score should be zero up to age 50, very low (less than 10 or 20) up to age 60, and then rises with each subsequent decade. If a 50-year-old woman, a couple of years shy of menopause and a smoker with elevated cholesterol is evaluated in such a manner, a zero calcium score is very reassuring. It is not 100%, but it is highly suggestive that she does not have high-grade structural coronary artery disease. On the other hand, if she has a score of 1,400, we quickly get moving with further investigation. Such a woman almost certainly has severe coronary artery disease.

Can a person, especially a woman, have significant coronary plaque without calcification? The answer is yes. Any screening tool will miss some. This test doesn't tell us whether or not a woman has a tight obstruction; it merely points out who is at low, intermediate, or high risk of having significant coronary artery disease. Obviously, if a woman, or a man for that matter, comes back with symptoms suggestive of a coronary blockage despite a wonderful coronary calcium score, we obtain an angiogram or some other test to make sure she is not suffering from coronary plaque that has not yet calcified.

The critics of this test like to point out that the soft *noncalcified* lipid-laden plaques with thinned-out fibrous caps are the ones that are the most likely to become eroded and fissured, thereby creating the substrate for coronary thrombosis and a heart attack. Their point is important, as it was the pathologists who pointed out such a plaque (the *vulnerable plaque* system) in arteries of those who had recently died of a heart attack. However, this criticism is not totally borne out statistically. One large trial of almost a thousand asymptomatic people—exactly the sort we are concerned with in our screening endeavor—were evaluated with calcium scores and also underwent coronary angiography. Those with zero coronary calcium had *no* cardiac events, such as heart attack, over the next three years. Those with coronary calcium had a substantial number.

Based on this study, we can feel fairly secure that a zero coronary calcium score portends a statistically excellent outlook. We are, after all, using this as a *screening* test. If someone, especially a woman, comes in with a zero coronary calcium score but has symptoms suggestive of a coronary artery problem, her doctor should be quick to remember this soft plaque concept, along with the fact that women calcify less and later than men. In order not to miss the soft plaque that may be threatening yet hasn't yet calcified, an angiogram should be ordered without delay in this circumstance.

What about those with positive scores? Again, we can look to a large clinical trial of asymptomatic people—almost 5,000 between 50 and 70 years of age and followed for 4.3 years. Over that time period, 119 people sustained at least one cardiovascular event, such as a heart attack. Almost all of them had a significantly elevated coronary calcium score. Fortunately, the incidence of a heart attack was only 0.1% a year in the group with a zero coronary calcium score! This is powerful data.

When 1,400 men and 500 women were compared using coronary calcium scores, the prevalence of calcium in women was about half that of men until age 60. In keeping with our earlier discussion about women following men by 10–15 years in developing coronary artery disease, the coronary calcium scores of 40- to 70-year-old men and 50- to 80-year-old women were largely identical.

Looking at the evidence from these large trials screening asymptomatic people, the utility of the coronary calcium score as an irreplaceable screening tool seems to stand up admirably. Will a few people with a zero coronary calcium score have a heart attack? Definitely. However, we can't think that millions of women should be subjected to a much larger radiation exposure, as well as contrast material, to be able to detect soft coronary plaques in an asymptomatic population! Reserve that for those who are at particularly high risk—those with very high LDL-cholesterol levels, a heavy smoking history, diabetes, or a high C-reactive protein (CRP) level indicative of inflammation, perhaps in combination or even coupled with symptoms suggestive of coronary blockage.

I don't have any doubt that the multi-slice cardiac CT angiogram detailed below is better and more reliable. However, it is usually much more expensive, carries a radiation exposure that is roughly ten times that of the calcium score, requires intravenous contrast material and, I believe, is not as suitable a screening tool for asymptomatic women. Keep in mind that we are dealing with at least 20 million women in the next few years! Keep in mind also that most are not interested in receiving any more radiation to their breasts than is absolutely necessary. Should the multi-slice scanner be used as a screening tool in women with symptoms? Absolutely. Should it be used to screen the general female population with coronary risk factors but no symptoms? Not at this time. We don't have the resources, for one. We do have the resources for a 15-minute coronary calcium score which delivers very little radiation to the breasts.

B. Multi-Slice CT Scanner

In the past, if we wanted to get an angiogram, a contrast study outlining the walls of the blood vessels, we had to introduce a catheter into the femoral artery in the groin and advance it up to the heart to inject an iodinated-based contrast material. Though relatively safe, there is always some risk (such as stroke or bleeding) with any invasive test, and the risk is high enough that we do not want to use it as a screening tool. If a person's coronary calcium score is high enough or, alternatively, if she continues to have chest discomfort or some other worrisome symptom, we obtain a multi-slice (currently 64-slice) CT angiogram. It will show us the coronary arteries and the arterial circulation throughout the body. This points out the presence or absence of coronary disease with reliable accuracy.

I think we are going to see more and more people, especially women with multiple risk factors, screened with the CT angiogram. I cannot over-emphasize the fact that women calcify coronary plaque less aggressively than men. I have made a great case for the use of the coronary calcium score as a screening tool, and I stick by it. However, we know that non-calcified plaques, especially in women, can be lipid-rich and may well be associated with an increased vulnerability for sudden plaque rupture which leads to acute coronary syndromes including heart attacks. This caveat regarding women bears repeating, as it is exceedingly important. This non-invasive angiogram is so important as a diagnostic tool that one should be in every large hospital emergency area. If you come in with chest pain but no evidence of a heart attack, you should have such a test before going home. If it is normal, you are predictably safe from the coronary standpoint. It should not be used as a general screening tool for coronary artery disease in my view, as the radiation exposure is not insignificant.

The way I envision the routine screening evaluation of the several million asymptomatic women with coronary risk factors is as follows:

1. Obtain a coronary calcium score: a 15-minute test, with no contrast agent used, a $100–$200 test that gives you about the same radiation exposure you get from sunshine during a cloudy summer. If your score is zero and you are not having symptoms suggestive of a blocked artery, go home with a smile on your face.
2. If your score is over 50 or you have had symptoms pointing to a blocked artery, they can start an I.V. on the spot and perform a multi-slice CT to determine if you have significant blockage.

This is a logical schematic to me. It allows for the screening of huge numbers of women with a multitude of risk factors, starting with the safest and least expensive method, and moving to the higher radiation, contrast exposure, and more expensive test when indicated.

C. Thallium Scan

This is a good place to illustrate what *not* to use as a screening tool. Traditionally, thallium imaging has been the best screening test available. Similar to a lung scan, it is a scan using a radioactive particle that is taken up by specific tissue, in this instance by the heart muscle. The radioactive tracer is thallous chloride. In the performance of the test, you are attached to an electrocardiogram, an I.V. is started, and you are given a provocative measure to cause the heart to demand more oxygenated blood. In some cases, this is a drug. In some, it is exercise. It is usually a combination. In this induced state of increased demand of the heart muscle for oxygen and nutrients, the thallium tracer is injected and your heart is scanned. The heart muscle loves potassium and removes it from the blood stream very efficiently. 95% of all potassium resides within the body's cells. Since the radioactive thallium is ionically identical to potassium, the heart muscle removes it equally efficiently; tucking it away within the cellular machinery. If you have wide open blood vessels to carry the oxygenated blood to the heart muscle and also have a normal heart muscle, which takes the tracer inside its cells, uptake by the thallium should be homogenous, with no holes and no defects. If you have a coronary blockage that is at least 75% in severity, we should see a defect with provocation that corrects after the stunned and oxygen-starved muscle cells have had a chance to recover. On the other hand, if you have already incurred muscle damage from coronary blockage, you should have an area that has been irreversibly injured and a persistent defect will show up.

This sounds great, doesn't it? What could be better? What's wrong with this? The answers are: "No, plenty, and lots!" For one thing, notice I mentioned a defect would appear if the artery were at least 75% blocked. It is pretty well known that women have a more dynamic element of coronary artery lumen size fluctuation than men. This is one of the important differences between women and men. For instance, they seem to intermittently vasoconstrict, or narrow the artery, especially in the zone contiguous to the plaque. This is due to contraction of the smooth muscle, triggered by some stimulus, within the wall of the artery. For example, take a woman who might have only a 50% blockage. She may be okay most of the time even if the fibrous cap containing and covering the plaque material has been breeched. The artery may be large enough, even with provocation, that the thallium scan is normal. But she may intermittently narrow the artery down to a 90% blockage due to a spasm of the muscle within the arterial wall. Even in the best of circumstances, it is not acceptable to just detect 75%+ obstructive arteries! I have seen many women who experienced spasm next to an ulcerated plaque system, with a perfectly normal thallium scan, yet had an unstable coronary problem. Almost all of these had some degree of coronary calcification.

Women with sizable amounts of breast tissue will notoriously show a defect in the region of the breast on the left side. Since this is in the exact region where an obstruction of the big left anterior descending coronary artery down the front of the heart would show up, we frequently find ourselves on the horns of a dilemma. Is this breast tissue attenuation (interference of detection of radioactive decay by breast tissue) or is it real due to a blocked artery? If you are overweight, the area of the heart that interfaces with the diaphragm, the bottom surface of the heart, may well show up as attenuated also. With this added bonus, it looks like you have not one but two defects. In reality, you may have none!

This is a fairly good test for determining if someone has a tightly blocked coronary artery. It is not a good test for detection of silent, sub-clinical coronary artery disease.

D. Screening for Coronary Risk Factors

We know that risk factors are additive, and the chances of a woman or a man having significant coronary artery disease increase with each risk factor. If a woman has a family history of coronary artery disease or elevated cholesterol, she should have a screening test for cholesterol and other blood lipid fractions every couple of years, starting at age 30. Any woman with symptoms that might represent a narrowed heart artery and any woman between the ages of 45 and 50, should receive a battery of screening tests to help determine her risk of having coronary artery disease. These tests should include a complete lipid profile including LDL and HDL fractions, triglycerides, and Lipoprotein (a); a homocysteine level, a measurement of the relative index of inflammation called a high-sensitivity C-reactive protein (hsCRP); and, at the very least, a blood test designed to determine the *chronic* blood sugar level—an A1 Hemoglobin level—should be drawn. This blood test will determine if someone is "borderline" diabetic. If any of these is abnormal or if there is a significant family history of coronary artery disease, a significant smoking history, a history of hypertension, or the patient is particularly obese, she should have a coronary calcium score.

If and when we identify risk factors, whether or not there is evidence of arteriosclerosis, we need to correct and modify those risk factors the best we can. It's not enough to see a woman who smokes and has a high LHL-cholesterol obtain a zero calcium score, and reassure her that she is lucky and has escaped. We need to council her to quit smoking and treat the high cholesterol so she can continue to be "lucky." She should be counseled regarding the importance of daily exercise, stopping smoking, and controlling her cholesterol, blood pressure, and stress levels.

Stress is a more significant influence in women than men. Methods of stress reduction, such as meditation, Pilates, yoga, and interaction in a warm, friendly environment need to be carried out. When you take the "RealAge" test, you'll see that social influences play a large role in your physiologic age. The RealAge test is a popular test that tells your physiologic age rather than your chronologic age. For example, a person who isolates herself is more likely to have a heart attack than one who is socially gregarious.

Tendency for Development of Peripheral Arteriosclerosis

There are a number of other unique features about heart disease in women as compared to men, most of which you don't read about. It has become obvious to me over the years that female smokers are at least as apt as men to develop more peripheral manifestations of arteriosclerosis in the leg, kidney, and arm vessels. Women sometimes develop blockages in the leg vessels and other vessels without forming equally tight blockages in the coronary arteries to the heart. By that I mean I have seen a large number of women, usually smokers, usually with hyperlipidemia and/or hypertension, who had an arteriosclerotic blockage in the subclavian artery (the artery leading to the arm), a renal artery (to the kidney), or the leg vessels. Sometimes there was blockage in all three and yet the coronary arteries may not have been affected. If a man has one of these, he almost always has severe coronary artery disease. I have also seen numerous women whose distal aorta, the giant blood tube carrying arterial blood to the legs, is completely blocked off without demonstrating much or any arteriosclerotic disease in the coronary arteries. This happens in men; it is just more likely to occur in a woman.

Why is it important to make this distinction? Men frequently come to our attention because of chest pain or some other indicator of a blockage in a coronary artery. In the process of evaluation, we notice that he has no pulses in his feet. We quiz him about pain in the calves of his legs when walking. Frequently the answer is no, since he is sedentary and may well be a smoker. An equally sedentary woman smoker may have a blockage of the same severity in the leg artery. However, if the heart circulation is spared, she may well not come to medical attention for months or even years. By that time, it is not uncommon to find that the thigh artery (the superficial femoral) has completely blocked off due to the arteriosclerosis. This creates a much more difficult problem, as we have limited resources to use in getting through this total blockage. If trouble develops in the downstream arteries to the foot, we sometimes have no option but to operate, usually on very small arteries that predict a high failure rate following the operation.

Silent atherosclerotic disease can spell a difficult course. This underscores the need for detection of this disease. While these women's coronary arteries may be spared in terms of blockage, they will also frequently have an elevated calcium score which alerts us to the possible presence of disease elsewhere. It points out the need for women with risk factors, particularly cigarette smoking, to have a good evaluation of their cardiovascular system every five years starting at age 30. It makes a strong plea for daily vigorous exercise. A good strong walk will clearly cause leg pain in someone who is narrowing down the main artery in her leg due to blockage and will point out the need for help.

The point should be made over and over and over in the literature read by women that **heart and blood vessel disease is the number one killer in women.** A woman who has no known coronary risk factors may relax a bit. Those with known risks of the traditional causes of arteriosclerosis should be aware that they should be exceptionally vigilant for the detection of this disease.

Coronary Artery Spasm

Women tend to have more exaggerated changes in the size of the arterial lumen, the central channel that carries blood, than men—especially in response to emotions or stress. All of us influence our coronary artery size by our actions and reactions. In response, the coronary artery becomes smaller or larger depending on conditions including our state of activity and emotional framework. This change in size can be extreme in women, frequently triggered by outside influences.

The role of the central nervous system in coronary artery size has been known since the early 17th century. The famous treatise *De Motu Cordis* written in 1628 by William Harvey, the father of cardiology, first recorded this: "Every affection of the mind that is attended with either pain or pleasure, hope or fear is the cause of an agitation whose influence extends to the heart." It can't be said better than that, even after almost 400 years of study.

Dr. William Osler, in his famous textbook of medicine written in 1892, also refers to the fact that vasomotion of the coronary arteries (great variation in size) is more common in women. He called it "pseudo-angina" and said that it was "never fatal." He also said, "Angina pectoris is a disease of middle life and occurs almost exclusively in men." He may have been trying to tell us that coronary artery disease is quieter in women than men. I suspect he was simply defining this a hundred years ago as a "man's disease." That has certainly changed! What all of these very astute statesmen in the field of cardiology were referring to is the tendency of the coronary artery to express profound changes in caliber size from moment to moment, many times influenced by stressors in life, some conscious and some not.

We now know that when a coronary artery plaque, the cholesterol deposit, becomes unstable, a contiguous segment of artery frequently develops a spasm. In other words, if the protective covering over this collection of cholesterol—the fibrous cap—ruptures, the situation immediately goes from being a stable process causing no symptoms to an unstable one that frequently leads to a complete blockage and a heart attack. In both men and women, the contiguous area of coronary artery may well develop spasm due to contraction of the muscle within the wall of the artery. But in my experience, coronary spasm is much more common in women than men.

Finally, women are more apt than men to demonstrate a phenomenon called *Prinzmetal*, or variant, angina. I believe this is the same syndrome referred to over a hundred years ago by Dr. Osler as "pseudo-angina." This is chest, jaw, or shoulder pain frequently associated with marked electrocardiographic (ECG) changes, usually occurring at night or at complete rest, often in the absence of any structural arteriosclerotic coronary artery disease whatsoever. Dr. Myron Prinzmetal, in 1959, determined it to be caused by "spasm" of the muscle within the wall of a normal coronary artery. It could be easily treated with nitroglycerin (NTG). The problem was that it might recur many times during the day or night, totally destroying normal life patterns.

It was not until the early 1970s that the etiology was established with certainty. At the University of Colorado, a young lady came in with recurrent pain associated with dramatic ECG changes, readily reversed with NTG. Since this would routinely occur during the very early morning hours, she was taken to the cauterization laboratory about midnight, a catheter was placed, angiography demonstrated normal coronary arteries, and a rather long wait began. Sometime after her usual hour of having a spell, perhaps because she had been sedated, she woke complaining of chest pain. Her ECG changed to a pattern suggesting a heart attack, and one of her coronary arteries had completely closed off. It opened up nicely when NTG was injected down the coronary artery. She was subsequently taken back to the laboratory another couple of times because the area showing trouble on the ECG was not always the same. Sure enough, it was not just one coronary artery that possessed this tendency to develop spasm, it was all three! This hallmark case showed us two things that are very important in Prinzmetal angina: First, as suspected by Dr. Prinzmetal, it is due to spasm of the muscle within the wall of the coronary artery and second, it can occur in several arteries within the same person. While it was not proven by this patient, the coronary arteries do not seem to all develop spasm at one time.

There is no doubt that this disease which is sometimes stubbornly resistant to treatment and very worrisome and life-changing to the patient, is more apt to occur in women. It is more apt to occur in smokers, and in those with a history of migraine. It is also more apt to occur in those who are entering menopause, notoriously a time of vasomotor instability.

Another subgroup that has intense spells of this phenomenon are cocaine users. The spasm in the wall of the coronary artery tends to be more intractable in these individuals and can easily be fatal. For example, we have seen a number of first-time cocaine users come in with a heart attack, cardiac arrhythmias, or death.

There is a fairly strong correlation between the migraine process and coronary spasm. We know that migraine is at least partially due to vasomotion within an arterial segment. Migraine sufferers (some studies suggest as many as 13% of the population) have been forced to sit by waiting while one explanation after another has been given as to the cause of their headaches. This is not due to lack of study. At this time, the most widely accepted theory is that there is a functional impairment of the trigeminal nerve, a major pain pathway in the nervous system, paired with a variation in the level of serotonin, the chemical which regulates pain messages. The first event may well be a drop in serotonin levels which in turn causes the trigeminal nerve to release compounds that cause blood vessels to dilate. This dilation brings about the severe headache that is characteristic of migraine. This is the result of "vasomotor instability." As mentioned above, these individuals are also much more prone than the non-migraine population to develop coronary spasm, also a demonstration of vasomotor instability.

The drug that is normally prescribed for migraine acts by exerting a strong vasoconstrictor effect, making the artery smaller again. An unwanted side effect may be the vasoconstriction of a susceptible segment of coronary artery, which is a drug-sensitive coronary zone.

Like coronary spasm, migraine seems to be most prevalent during a time of estrogen and progesterone hormonal fluctuations. Frequently, they become worse during the transition to menopause, just as the coronary spasm syndrome does. They are both frequently brought on by stress. Whatever the cause, they are inexplicably linked.

There is also an overlap between coronary spasm and a condition known as *Raynaud's Syndrome*. This is a tendency for spasm to develop within the digital arteries when the fingers and toes are exposed to cold. Such individuals develop cold white fingers when they get ice from the freezer. They develop white painful toes during the winter months, making them hate cold weather. Indeed, if you look at a pie wedge diagram, there is overlap amongst all three of these processes: coronary spasm,

Raynaud's, and migraine. This implies a "vaso-spastic" tendency within multiple arterial distributions.

Years ago, I was sent a young lady with absolutely no discernible coronary risk factors, but she had experienced a heart attack anyway. Angiography elsewhere showed a 90% blockage of a coronary artery, and she was sent to me for angioplasty with a balloon. Nitroglycerin had not been given during that angiogram to determine if this was perhaps coronary spasm. She was about 35 years of age, active, and had no evidence of anything that might lead to coronary spasm. She adamantly denied use of cocaine and her husband was a retired cop who informed me that if I asked the question again I would regret it. He smiled as he said it, but I got the point. We strongly suspected coronary spasm. Upon repeat angiography, we found she had normal arteries which lead to a diagnosis of intermittent coronary spasm.

The following day, she spontaneously developed severe chest pain, accompanied by ECG changes consistent with a heart attack. She was taken back to the laboratory where she was found to have complete occlusion of one of her coronary arteries, a different one than would have caused her first heart attack. It opened up when I injected NTG down the artery. I confirmed the diagnosis of coronary artery spasm without any doubt; however, I had no idea why she had it. She did not smoke and was nowhere near menopause.

As I was sitting in my study that same night, I read of a strange infiltrative process that had been found in a couple of hearts in very young women who had been taking L-Tryptophan for mood elevation. They had tragically died. At autopsy, these hearts were found to possess a scattering of eosinophils within the heart muscle. These are cells in the blood stream most commonly associated with allergic diseases and are almost never found in the heart under any circumstances. These two women had also experienced heart attacks but were nonsmokers and had none of the usual recognized coronary risk factors. I raced to my car, drove to the hospital, and breathlessly asked this young lady if she had been taking this drug which was sold without a prescription. She had! I was sure I had found the answer and formulated a test to prove it. I carefully explained it to her and her husband.

The next day, I carefully advanced a bioptome from its insertion in the groin vein up to the right side of the interventricular septum and took a couple of bites of heart muscle thinking that it would demonstrate eosinophils. It didn't. Dejected, since I had put her through some risk with the biopsy, I told her and her husband the bad news. They informed me that she hadn't taken any of the drug for the last week and asked if it was possible the cells had vanished, leaving behind some sort of substance that would continue to exert its deleterious influence on the coronary artery tone. I had just learned of the disease the night before. I didn't have a clue.

A great pathologist by the name of Andrew Horvath called me later that day and told me to send the slides to the National Institutes of Health. They could examine for the presence of a basic amino acid, the "footprint" of previous eosinophil infiltration. It turns out that this compound is the strongest vaso-active compound known to man. Her heart muscle tissue was chock-full of it! Subsequently, there was a large class-action lawsuit against the company that manufactured and distributed this over-the-counter medication. It was shown that the vehicle that carried the L-Tryptophan was perverted with a substance that caused an unusual allergic response, resulting in eosinophils moving into the heart muscle. I published an article on it and received far more requests for reprints of it than for any other article I had ever published, all from lawyers.

I have since seen one other young lady who had this same type of coronary artery spasm and was also taking a variety of over-the-counter compounds, including tree bark extract. It also was resolved with discontinuation of the medications. Both of these women eventually recovered from this tendency to develop spasm within the wall of their coronary arteries. It took about two months in the first example, only two weeks in the second. During that time, they both had to use frequent NTG in order to "break" a spasm. NTG is a strong relaxant of the arterial wall muscle, especially in the event of inappropriate vasoconstriction associated with this disorder. It works promptly. Nonetheless, both were immensely relieved when they no longer had to be constantly vigilant to the possible, sometimes violent, onset of this worrisome pain syndrome.

I've spent a lot of time on coronary spasm, including variant angina, because there is no doubt that it is more common in women than men. Women are more apt to have intense spasm in their coronary artery than men whether in otherwise normal arteries, variant angina, or ruptured plaque associated with arteriosclerosis. This susceptibility is due to a variety of influences. I suspect one of the greatest is that of endothelial dysfunction—the diseased function of the inside lining of the artery, with inflammatory molecules causing enhanced clotting and tendency to develop spasm. This is much more active in women than men. This angina of coronary spasm is treated with NTG for acute spells and, if recurrent, a long-acting calcium antagonist to keep the artery maximally dilated. The major thrust is to make sure it is not associated with structural coronary artery disease. Spasm is a major component of that clinical syndrome too, usually when a plaque has ruptured and the vessel is very unstable. To me, this vaso-reactivity is a significant difference between the coronary arteries of women and men. This concept is extremely important and has not received proper press and recognition.

Microvascular Coronary Syndrome: A Woman's Disease

For over 20 years I have heard the term "Syndrome X" refer to a woman with chest pain, frequently with signs of decreased blood flow to the heart tissues, associated with normal but small coronary arteries shown by contrast angiography. There is usually a tendency to have other vaso-spastic disorders such as migraine syndrome and Raynaud's phenomenon. It seems, however, to be different from Prinzmetal angina, since the ECG doesn't change in the same way when they have chest pain. Another distinction is that studies have shown reduced blood flow in the microvascular bed, the tiny blood vessels supplying the heart, even during periods of no pain.

Syndrome X is treated with nitroglycerin for acute spells and a calcium channel blocker as a prophylactic measure, exactly like Prinzmetal angina. Estrogen sometimes works also. This is something I discovered by accident when I cared for a woman who had a refractory case of Syndrome X and was placed on estrogen by another doctor. I do not recommend estrogen for these women, however, as I think most of them have structural coronary artery disease. I think it has something to do with "tone" in the smallest arteries (there is a point downstream when the small vessels lose their ability to constrict), probably in association with structural disease.

We have relatively new data from the Women's Ischemia Syndrome Study (WISE study) that seems to dovetail with Syndrome X. Women seem much more apt than men to deposit cholesterol plaque rather uniformly down the distal (farther down) coronary artery, in many instances extending into the smaller vessels. I think this is basically the same thing as Syndrome X. This may affect as many as two or three million American women and it frequently doesn't show up on an angiogram. Most of it might be uncovered by a coronary calcium scoring test with ultrafast CT, though I'm not aware that any study has been performed looking at this possibility. Many of these women are diabetic or prediabetic and many have metabolic syndrome (obesity, elevated LDL-cholesterol, insulin-resistant diabetes, evidence of coronary inflammation). This dramatically underscores the earlier proclamation that coronary risk factors have to be treated aggressively, especially in women and especially in women with chest pain, fatigue, or shortness of breath, and even those who have no evidence of discreet blockage of the coronary arteries by angiography. I fear that the multi-slice CT angiogram will miss this very important group of women, as the more illuminative selective coronary angiogram has already been shown to do.

Treatment of Coronary Artery Disease in Women

The treatment of arteriosclerotic coronary artery disease is the same for women as for men. It is just more difficult. Women are more apt to have significantly smaller vessels than men and they also become more diffusely diseased than those in men. This has made coronary bypass less effective, as the bypass grafts are more apt to close off in women. For the same reasons, it has traditionally made coronary stenting more difficult and less effective. Put simply, since the stent (a stainless steel mesh deployed within the coronary artery in order to open the blockage) imposes damage to the inside of the artery, some tissue proliferation occurs in response to this injury. This happens in men too. However, in men, with a larger artery, we might be able to deploy a stent that is very large—a 3.5 mm size. Some degree of re-stenosis (recurrent blockage with scar tissue) could be well tolerated since the artery is large and there is room to spare. In a more petite woman's artery, we might be stuck with using a 2 mm stent. The same amount of tissue growth that we saw in the man will almost totally block off this small artery. With the advent of drug-eluting stents, impregnated with a cancer drug to prevent tissue proliferation, we have seen an improvement of this end result. However, the smallest stents do not yet come in drug-eluting varieties, a deficit that must be rectified as soon as possible.

These features mean that we are more likely to have to treat women following intervention or surgery with drugs to reduce oxygen requirements by the heart muscle. These include a beta-blocker to slow the heart rate and the force of contractility and perhaps a calcium antagonist to enlarge the lumen of the vessel. This is sometimes disappointing in that most people who go through coronary bypass surgery want to throw away their angina medications. When preparing a woman with small to medium size coronary arteries for surgery, it is only fair that we mention that her complete treatment may well be a combination of the surgery and a medication. We are sometimes forced into this hybrid form of treatment in men as well; it is a more common necessity in women.

We make the point to smokers, especially women with petite arteries, that continued cigarette smoking might well induce coronary spasm. It will not only accelerate the arteriosclerotic problem, but will also increase the chances of bypass graft failure since cigarette smoke is a strong vasoconstricting agent. In the 1970s, we took a large group of male smokers, sedated them to keep them off cigarettes for several days, and then took coronary angiograms. After the angiogram, we allowed them to smoke a cigarette in the cath lab and then repeated the angiogram. It was not unusual for the lumen size of the coronary arteries to shrink to half the previous size following cigarette usage. If it shrinks the entire lumen of an artery due to its vasoconstrictor effect, what might it do to an area right next to plaque? It might induce intense vaso-spasm. Since we have discussed that women develop spasm in the artery more frequently and more aggressively than men, we must presume that cigarette smoking could cause such limited flow down a vessel that graft thrombosis could result.

The difficulty with intervention and bypass in women also makes aggressive treatment of coronary risks like hypertension, smoking, obesity, inactivity, and hyperlipidemia, all the more important. It drives home the message about early detection so we can alter the course of the disease before it reaches the stage of coronary bypass or intervention. **Discontinuation of cigarette smoking is an extremely important element in decreasing coronary risk factors in women.**

Controlling your diet is extremely important, also. Studies show that the Mediterranean diet can be a very effective method of *treating* arteriosclerosis. This study, sponsored by the Spanish Ministry and involving 800 men and women over four years, showed that the arteriosclerotic event rate, manifested by heart attack, stroke, need for intervention, and surgery, could be cut in half by strict adherence to this diet. There are many Mediterranean countries, all of which have their individual and legendary national foods. Common to all are abundant fruits, vegetables, nuts (especially walnuts), olive oil, some fish, little meat, and wine in moderation. Both nuts and olive oil possess monounsaturated fat that raises the good cholesterol. This diet also dramatically reduced the concentration of inflammatory molecules, those that we measure with the high sensitivity C-reactive protein, which seem to be a major problem in a fair number of women who have coronary artery disease and heart attacks.

While this diet is important for us all, it is probably especially important for women, as it is simply more difficult to guarantee them a great result with coronary bypass and stent deployment. Plus, we have repeatedly shown that women have a more difficult time detecting the presence of a blocked artery. I also aggressively treat women with coronary artery disease, or any other form of arteriosclerosis, with omega-3 fish oil and statins. It has been shown that the EPA and DHA in fish oil, the so-called omega-3 polyunsaturated fatty acids, help prevent coronary artery deposition of cholesterol, reduce the inflammation within the artery leading to clotting, and in the event of heart damage, help prevent a fatal arrhythmia. My goal with statins is to drop the LDL-cholesterol to a therapeutic level. Also because of the gender-dependent tendency towards more endothelial dysfunction (spasm due to reactivity of the innermost lining of the artery), I treat them with L-arginine. The arginine is used in the manufacture of nitric oxide within the endothelium. Nitric oxide is the strongest arterial relaxant we know. When I employ a statin, I am careful to use CoEnzyme Q10 as well. I also use an ACE-I, an angiotensin converting enzyme-inhibitor, known for its "soothing effect" on the inside of the blood vessel. Like L-arginine, it improves endothelial function and helps maintain the largest caliber possible. I use it in both men and women, but I am stronger in my language in incorporating it into the treatment program for women. Finally, if the coronary arteries are especially small and heavily diseased, I keep women on Plavix, a potent platelet-inhibitor, forever. We know that platelet aggregation is the first step in the formation of a clot within the coronary artery, and we must try to block this process should a plaque rupture despite our best efforts.

Non-Arteriosclerotic Heart Disease in Women: Possibly Enzyme Related

I am convinced that women also develop the other degenerative diseases of the heart at a later age than men. For example, women seem to show up about 10 to 15 years later with aortic stenosis than men. This is a degenerative, frequently calcific, disease of the aortic valve. It is initially called aortic sclerosis when it is not obstructive. Remember, this is the valve between the main pumping chamber, the left ventricle, and the aorta. The stresses on this valve are the same ones men have, if you consider only the blood pressure and heart rate. Something delays this age-dependent degeneration in women, postponing the laying down of calcium within cardiac structures and blood vessels. It may be entirely related to estrogen and progesterone and is just part of the overall process of arteriosclerosis. These valves do ultimately morph into a structure that looks like a large arteriosclerotic plaque.

I believe that women also develop apoptosis, the death of cells within the heart muscle called "programmed cell death," at a later age than men. I suspect this is one of many reasons why women live longer than men. I have no doubt that some of these phenomena, which have largely been attributed to hormonal influence, may be gender-specific and genetically programmed but in a different way than we presumed.

Prevention

Since we have just learned that women generally have smaller vessels than men; may have more diffuse involvement; possess a greater tendency for spasm; and have a less satisfying result from intervention than men suggests we should place an even greater emphasis on prevention of the problem. Prevention is important in men *and* women. We should be putting our best efforts toward preventing this problem from happening in the first place. I have made my reputation from working in the catheterization laboratory for 30 years. My favorite saying is, "I've made my living opening arteries, but I've gotten my greatest satisfaction preventing them from closing."

Much of what is good as prevention is also good as treatment. What we put between our lips and into our stomachs is the most important risk factor that we can alter. Think about it. Smoking accelerates arteriosclerotic coronary artery disease and induces coronary spasm. We can completely eliminate it as a risk factor! If we eliminate salt from our diets, the incidence of hypertension plummets. If we markedly decrease saturated fat in our diets, blood lipids will improve markedly. If we use monounsaturated fats, such as those obtained from walnuts and olive oil, HDL-cholesterol (the good stuff) will increase. Exercise will help even more, not to mention the additional benefit from weight control, blood pressure control, and proper sensitivity to insulin. Think about it. The only risk factor you can't modify, at least in part, is heredity. And you can't sue your parents for it!

The Lesson: Listen to the Man's Wife!

I had just performed a treadmill test on an elderly gentleman and he had almost died on the treadmill. He had dropped his blood pressure, had raised his ST segments on his ECG, a marker of a heart attack, and it took a lot of work to get him stabilized. These things suggest a left main coronary blockage, a life-threatening anatomic process. While I was talking to him, sandwiched between him and his wife after he had gotten stabilized and was dressed and comfortable, I was continuously interrupted by his wife. When he recited his symptoms, his wife would grab my elbow and enthusiastically comment in an excited, very loud whisper, "That's exactly what I have been having." It was annoying. After all, I was still rattled by the near death of the elderly gentleman on my left. The irritant, his wife on my right, was not formally my patient. I finally informed her, nicely but firmly, that she simply had to let me get on with my task at hand. I had to arrange for her husband to have an angiogram the next morning.

He had exactly what I expected and I was feeling pretty proud of myself. We took him right from the cath lab into the operating room and he received a very nice coronary bypass operation for a 95% blockage of his left main coronary with a totally blocked right coronary artery, certainly a life-threatening problem. As they wheeled him into the recovery room, doing fine, his wife suddenly hugged herself in pain, broke out in a deep sweat, and barely had time to whisper to her waiting room companion to call a doctor before she slumped to the floor with a very sizable heart attack, promptly going into complete heart block, necessitating the implantation of a temporary pacemaker. When I got her stabilized, her shock-level blood pressure barely acceptable on a large amount of intravenous medication, she took my hand in both of hers, smiled weakly, and said sweetly, "Honey, I kept trying to tell you I had the same symptoms as Herman." I was no longer cocky; I was ashamed and thoroughly embarrassed. I am fairly sure this nice lady had a structural blockage in her coronary artery and had effort-induced angina. Furthermore, I am strongly suspicious that she so intensely fretted about Herman, as he was having his operation, that she put her coronary artery into intense spasm. From that day in 1976 to the current time, whenever a wife tells me she is having the same symptoms as her spouse, I work her up until there is no doubt about the cause of the problem. I may have unwittingly ignored Herman's wife's not-so-muted plea for help; I haven't ignored one since. Whenever I see the surgeon who operated on her husband, he mimics the whole bedside disaster, making me go red even at age 60. Some things you just never live down, nor should you, or the past will become the future.

Hormone Replacement Therapy: A Continuing Controversy

No discussion of women and heart disease is complete without some attention to the perpetually controversial subject of hormone replacement therapy (HRT). We have studies that show that women who have low estrogen levels for several years prior to menopause are more likely to develop arteriosclerosis. In light of these results, it seemed a given that estrogen supplements would strongly *prevent* arteriosclerosis after menopause, especially since it was known to keep the skin younger, the bones stronger, the mood better—all the symptoms associated with making menopause manageable.

Estrogen combined with progesterone became known as HRT. Almost every post-menopausal woman took this therapy for years. Then articles began appearing regarding possible deleterious effects of HRT, especially with reference to those with established heart disease. Women shied away from it in droves, and for good reason. There were lawsuits. Confusion ran rampant. All at once, you couldn't force doctors to prescribe this drug, even for those with serious post-menopausal symptoms.

Here we are, several years later, and we still don't have concrete answers about how to prescribe HRT. This seems irresponsible and careless but it's more complex than that.

One large epidemiologic study suggests a harmful effect if HRT is administered to women who have known arteriosclerotic disease. I believe the answer for this group of women is in. They shouldn't take it. There has, on the other hand, been some data showing that HRT will actually help prevent arteriosclerosis, if administered to younger post-menopausal women with no evidence of established arteriosclerosis. Others have not corroborated this.

In summary, there is no good answer to the conundrum regarding HRT. But if a woman has particularly bothersome symptoms, aggressive bone density loss, mood swings, or any other markers of estrogen deficiency, I will order a coronary calcium score, take a good history, and look at coronary risk factors. If the compilation of this data looks acceptable, I allow her to take HRT under the direction of her internist or gynecologist. I do *not* want my known coronary patients taking it until this controversy is settled and the ratio of estrogen/progestin fine-tuned and individualized. Additionally, I do *not* think HRT should be used as a secondary prevention of arteriosclerosis. If someone comes to me on long-term HRT and has known coronary artery disease, I discuss continued HRT with her on a case-by-case basis. Some choose to continue. Their lives were too miserable without it.

I hope this helps you. You will need to accept your doctor's advice about it because each woman presents a different case for risk and preference.

REMINDERS

1. "Tone" within the wall of the artery creates significant differences in behavior of the coronary artery between women and men.

2. Women's arteries tend to be smaller than men's arteries making it more difficult to work on them with the same predicted results. This makes prevention more important.

3. Women are less likely than men to have severe, crushing chest pain as a manifestation of a coronary blockage. They are more apt to have a vague discomfort in the chest or just below the sternum.

4. Two risk factors that can be altered favorably are diet and exercise. Women should eat a healthy diet (such as the Mediterranean diet), stop smoking, and get on a routine exercise program.

5. HRT should be discussed with your doctor and determined on an individual basis.
6. If a woman smokes, has a family history of coronary artery disease or other risk factors, she should begin her cardiovascular surveillance program at age 30, with two-year incremental laboratory tests and ongoing efforts at risk factor modification.
7. A woman who has significant coronary risk factors should have a coronary calcium score test at age 45 or 50, which is the earliest age the test is valid in women.
8. If a woman has symptoms suggestive of coronary blockage, even with a low calcium score, she should have a CT angiogram to ensure she doesn't have major non-calcified coronary plaque.
9. Microvascular coronary disease and uniformly distributed plaque disease are present in a significant number of women with coronary artery disease.

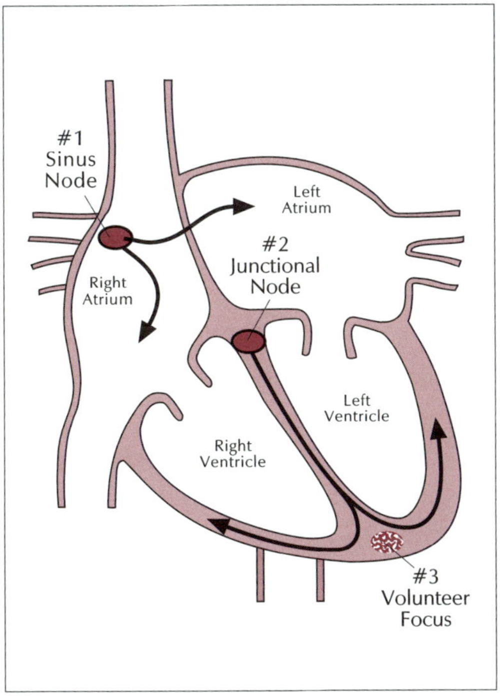

9 ATRIAL FIBRILLATION

The Most Common Rhythm Disturbance

ANY VARIATION FROM THE NORMAL SINUS RHYTHM of the heart is called an *arrhythmia. Atrial fibrillation*, a rapid chaotic heart beat, is the most common significant arrhythmia in the world. It is so common in the elderly population that it is unusual, in a group of a dozen friends over age 65, for someone *not* to know another person with this arrhythmia.

There are two or three caveats that are important to keep in mind to live comfortably and securely with the problem of atrial fibrillation. First and foremost is: This arrhythmia doesn't kill you, though it may seem as though it is going to when it first begins. Secondly: It is important to get effective treatment reasonably soon after onset. Thirdly: Many people who develop this arrhythmia do not have to remain in it forever.

Anatomy of the Normal Heart Beat

The normal electrical activity in the heart is so-called sinus rhythm. The heart muscle, both in the upper chambers, the atria, and in the lower chambers, the ventricles, has to be stimulated in order for it to perform. In response to a stimulus, in this case electrical, the muscle cells shorten, and contractility results. Contractility of the entire population of muscle cells, all at one time, causes that specific chamber to become smaller, pumping blood forward as it does so. The various heart valves open, then close, in response to this muscular pumping action of the heart. In order to initiate a single contraction of the heart, the heartbeat, a tiny electrical spark is emitted simultaneously from thousands of specialized cells located in the top part of the heart. It quickly spreads throughout the upper chambers, causing the pumping action of the atria. The current then travels to the border between the corners of the atria and the corners of the ventricles, an area called the atrio-ventricular node (AV node). The AV node conducts electricity much less rapidly than the other electrical conduits, effectively slowing transmission of the electrical impulse between the upper and lower chambers. Therefore, with any rapid activity of the heart in the upper chambers, it acts like an old-fashioned "governor" on the heart, allowing only a certain number of electrical impulses to reach the ventricles per time period. Most people my age know something about a governor. Back when I was young, it was not unusual for a father to put one on his car so his teenage son couldn't drive over a certain speed. This modulating effect by the AV node functions much the same way, slowing conduction so that a very rapid atrial rate of perhaps 300 beats per minute will be transmitted down into the ventricles at a rate of perhaps only 150.

When the electrical current makes its passage through the AV node, it goes through the ventricular conduction system and activates the ventricular muscle stimulating contraction of these pumping chambers, again by fiber shortening. The end result of this sophisticated electrical and mechanical interplay is a sinus beat with electrical spread throughout the heart, resulting in synchronized contraction of the upper chambers, then synchronized contraction of the lower chambers. The result is that blood is pumped from the atria into the ventricles and then pumped into the great vessels, all in one single electrical-mechanical event. The continuous repetition of this cycle is the rhythmic beating of the heart, the result of a miracle in design.

Anatomy of Atrial Fibrillation

People are always surprised when their heart goes "out of rhythm." Considering the complexity of the system and the conditions in which it has to function, I'm constantly surprised that it doesn't go out of rhythm much more commonly, especially as we get older. While there are many reasons for the development of atrial fibrillation, 90% of all cases are due to age and hypertension. This particular arrhythmia has gotten so common that it is unusual for a cardiologist not to see two or three new cases a week. It has become a virtual epidemic. By age 65, the incidence of atrial fibrillation is about 3% of that age group population. This climbs to about 5% by age 80. Currently, there are between one and two million Americans with atrial fibrillation. With aging of the baby boomers, this population is going to swell dramatically.

In atrial fibrillation, the top chambers are no longer activated by a synchronous electrical impulse originating in the sinus node. At a precise moment in time, the atrial muscle develops disorganized electrical activity. It *fibrillates*. If you were to go into an operating room and peer into an open chest of someone in atrial fibrillation who is about to undergo open-heart surgery, you would instantly be reminded of a ball of worms writhing about. Instead of pumping synchronously, the atrial muscle sort of quivers in a thoroughly disorganized manner.

The development of atrial fibrillation results in loss of meaningful contractile contribution by the atria. In other words, instead of blood being actively pumped from the atria into the main pumps (the ventricles), it passively flows by virtue only of pressure. Because of this, the atria do not completely empty. Not only that, but this writhing activity is very rapid, beating at a rate of 300 to 600 beats per minute. Were it not for the "governor" effect exerted by the AV node, slowing electrical passage, the ventricles would follow the atria and anyone who developed atrial fibrillation would promptly die from it.

Happily, this doesn't occur in the vast majority of folks. It takes a very unusual and extreme situation to allow for 1:1 transmission of electrical impulses through the AV node at rates of this magnitude. Up to a rate of around 180, a healthy heart will allow 1:1 conduction of electrical impulses. Not so with extremely rapid atrial rates. Instead, with atrial fibrillation, the AV node allows transmission of only about one out of three or four of the impulses reaching it, resulting in a ventricular rate of roughly 120 to 180 beats per minute in the majority of people who develop atrial fibrillation. While this is far superior to the much faster rate that would eventuate if there were no built-in modulator, it is still a pretty shocking thing for most people to go from a regular heart rate of 70 beats per minute up to a very chaotic and irregular heart rate of 160! Some people will have enough deterioration of the AV node cells from scar or cell dropout, that they will only conduct at a rate of 60 or so. A very small percentage of people will have a rate even slower in response to atrial fibrillation. Some of these individuals will actually pass out when they develop this arrhythmia if it is conducted at an extremely slow rate. Most, however, go along at a ventricular rate of 120 to180 beats a minute.

Causes of Atrial Fibrillation

What causes this very common arrhythmia that is so capable of disrupting your bridge game or waking you from sleep? The most common process is a gradual enlargement of the left atrium and, less commonly, the right atrium, resulting in disruption of the normal atrial electrical conduits. A frequent cause of this enlargement is hypertension, with thickening of the left ventricular wall and build-up of pressure within the left atrium. The simple process of old age will likely replace this etiology very soon. In this circumstance, the left atrium enlarges in response to nothing more than reduced elasticity of the left ventricle. Every elderly person, especially if the person develops a particularly stiff left ventricle, is *susceptible* to this rhythm disturbance. This is the reason it is so important to understand these mechanics. A thorough understanding of this ubiquitous problem will require a good bit of reading to serve as an adjunct to whatever your doctor has time to tell you.

If a person has hypertension, the left ventricular muscle thickens in response to this high pressure in a large percentage of individuals. There are a variety of very sophisticated and intricate mechanisms that are likely responsible for this wall-thickening process in some people but not in others. We call this increase in wall thickness in response to hypertension "remodeling" of the left ventricle. There can be remodeling in response to a variety of insults to the ventricle, such as that occurring in response to a heart attack with loss of muscle cells. The type that occurs in response to hypertension is simply an enlargement of healthy muscle fibers, comparable to those which develop in your arm and leg muscles when you lift weights.

The heart doesn't stop and rest. It does its thing—70 or so beats per minute—without a break. Therefore, if the pressure against which the heart is working is elevated, even part of the time, it is not unthinkable that enlargement, *hypertrophy*, of muscle fibers occurs. This occurs very aggressively in some, but is only moderate in others and doesn't occur at all in a few select individuals. For different reasons, this is akin to the variable extent that each of us bulks up in response to weight lifting.

When such enlargement of heart muscle fibers occurs, the muscle mass of the left ventricle relaxes less rapidly and also less completely. The valve between the left atrium and the left ventricle is the mitral valve. When the left ventricle is relaxed, this valve opens and blood pours from the holding chamber, the left atrium, into the left ventricle. If the left ventricular wall is thickened, stiff, and relaxes slowly, a greater pressure has to be generated within the left atrium in order to properly fill the ventricle. Over time, this will cause the left atrium to dilate (to enlarge). This, in turn, brings about stretch and distortion of the conduction system and perhaps even the laying down of scar tissue throughout the atria in response to this pressure phenomenon. This slowly brings about less-than-optimal synchronous electrical activity, eventually causing enough disruption in transmission of electrical impulses to result in atrial fibrillation.

I have no doubt that the simple process of enhanced longevity will eventually supplant hypertension as the major cause of atrial fibrillation. If you are over 50 and reach down and pull up a tent of skin on the back of your hand, you will notice that it takes a while for it to return to its normal form. Your skin may look pretty normal to you but if you ask a 15-year-old to do the same thing, you'll be dismayed to see their skin pops back into shape very quickly. A normal part of aging is the gradual loss of elastic fibers within our tissues. Billions of dollars have been made in the cosmetics industry selling products to halt or reverse this process. So far, the process goes on inevitably with each passing day after a certain age. A significant portion of this aging phenomenon is the result of free radical formation from cellular activity. Theoretically, this can be partially blocked by antioxidants. This is new information, however, and the process we see now reflects previous injury.

This same phenomenon involving loss of elasticity also occurs in the heart. After age 40, the filling pressure, which is the left atrial pressure necessary to adequately stretch the left ventricular muscle fibers and fill the tank, begins to increase. While we may be able cosmetically to hide the aging process in the skin, there is no proven way to prevent this gradual loss of elasticity of the ventricles, a process known as a *diastolic compliance dysfunction*. This is a mouthful that indicates the abnormal relaxation process of the ventricle in accepting blood from the atrium. *The ventricle becomes stiff!* The persistent and even progressive increase in left atrial pressure eventually stretches the left atrium, ultimately disrupting the normal electrical circuitry, and atrial fibrillation occurs.

There are other causes of atrial fibrillation. I have personally taken care of at least a half-dozen surgeons who developed atrial fibrillation during a stressful operation. This is not good! It means their stress is so internalized that they are pouring out tremendous amounts of epinephrine, the hormone that is responsible for the "fight and flight" reflex that we all possess. If this goes on in surgeons who are trained to deal with stress and to channel it into purposeful energy, it certainly happens in the remainder of the population. This may actually occur in fairly young individuals. There is now evidence that this *youthful* tendency may well be genetically ordained.

There are also individuals who, because of other co-morbid illnesses (other associated medical conditions), are primed to develop atrial fibrillation. These are individuals who might have underlying hypertension, coronary heart disease, obesity, lung disease, alcoholism, anemia, and a host of other possible problems. When such a person is suddenly thrust into a situation of great stress, he may consequently develop atrial fibrillation. That stressor may be variable: surgery for a fractured hip, high fever due to pneumonia or a urinary tract infection, or a motor vehicle accident with or without injury. It is also very common for a healthy 70-year-old person, with no known underlying health problems at all, to develop atrial fibrillation when faced with one of these stressful situations. Finally, we now know that sleep apnea (periods of suspended breathing during deep slumber), a condition usually found in a person with some degree of obesity and frequently with abundant "jowl" tissue, is commonly associated with atrial fibrillation.

Fully one-quarter of our post–coronary bypass patients develop atrial fibrillation. While this is doubtless partially caused by the stress of the surgery and some of the post-operative drugs that are used, it also seems that handling the heart is truly a unique stimulus for development of atrial fibrillation. In much this same category are those with an inflammation in the sac surrounding the heart, *pericarditis*. This is an example of an irritant of the heart bringing about this arrhythmia. Since many of our post-operative heart surgery patients develop a pericardial friction rub implying an inflammation in their heart sac, it may be that the atrial fibrillation develops primarily in response to this irritation.

Many individuals will develop atrial fibrillation secondary to a pressure or volume overload of one of the upper chambers. Undue stress imposed on either the right or the left atrium will trigger it. This is due to the fact that the electrical network is shared between the two atria. Therefore, stretch and distortion of the electrical circuitry in either atrium is capable of disrupting the normal activation of these upper chambers. In the case of mitral valve leakage, instead of having all of the blood that enters the left ventricle pushed out of the pump in a forward course, a variable amount leaks across a faulty mitral valve into the left atrium, thus enlarging the atrium and ultimately leading to atrial fibrillation. This is a classic example of volume overload. Similarly, people who have rheumatic mitral stenosis, scarring of the mitral valve in response to previous rheumatic fever, have a build-up of pressure within the left atrium because blood cannot be effectively pumped across the scarred valve. They are the most prone of all to develop atrial fibrillation. So here we have two examples of trouble with the mitral valve, one causing volume overload, the other causing pressure overload within the left atrium. It makes no difference. Either occurrence will bring about stretch and enlargement of the left atrium, disrupting the electrical fiber tracts, and eventually causing atrial fibrillation.

Any valvular leakage or obstruction can bring about atrial fibrillation. Similarly, any abnormal physiology that results in the heart having to handle the same blood repeatedly will bring it about. A great example is a shunt between the two upper chambers, an atrial septal defect. With each heartbeat, some of the blood escapes across the septum. It subsequently has to be pumped again and again. A good example of a pressure phenomenon is one that results from a blood clot to the lungs, what we call a pulmonary embolus. This is due to a clot that formed elsewhere, usually in the deep veins of the legs, and broke loose to travel to the lungs. This will frequently cause dramatic increases in the pulmonary artery pressure, which will secondarily put a burden on the right atrium and trigger atrial fibrillation.

A volume or pressure overload is not necessary for the development of atrial fibrillation, though it is the most prevalent cause in the general population. Yet another reason for atrial fibrillation is an endocrine disorder, such as a hyperactive thyroid gland. If too much thyroxin is pumped out, the heart will commonly develop atrial fibrillation. This can be corrected with suppression using a drug or removal of the over-active thyroid gland. Another endocrine disorder that is prone to cause atrial fibrillation is that of a benign tumor of the adrenal gland, a pheochromocytoma, pumping out excess quantities of epinephrine.

A new cause of atrial fibrillation may have been uncovered. This is cardiometabolic syndrome. This is closely linked to obesity as well as to insulin-resistance forms of diabetes, which are thought to be present in fully one-fourth of the adult population of America. It is also known to influence the development of atrial fibrillation, possibly as a function of one of its end-organ results, arteriosclerosis.

As you can see, there are many reasons why people develop this common condition. And the list is much longer than I have outlined. Those of you who are reading this chapter with particular interest because you have this condition can apply your own process to the anatomic/physiologic model I have portrayed, and you can determine why you, specifically, have developed this situation.

Importance of Ventricular Rate Control

We've learned that when the heart goes into atrial fibrillation, the rate is usually rapid and the rhythm is chaotic. In itself, this can precipitate heart failure or moisture in the lungs simply because the heart can't function properly. This is especially prone to occur if there is underlying blockage in the coronary arteries, or if the left ventricular wall is particularly thick and stiff. With a rapid rate, there is simply inadequate time for the left ventricle to properly fill. Plus, the left atrium may well enlarge even more with this inadequate emptying, which further increases the pressure in the left atrium. This pressure is transmitted into the veins draining the lungs (the pulmonary veins). This enhanced pressure, if high enough, will force water from the blood stream into the tiny air pockets, the alveoli. This condition is called congestive heart failure and it causes a sudden, severe shortness of breath. The most common complaint of someone with recent onset of atrial fibrillation with a rapid ventricular response is inability to get enough air or take a deep breath.

The very first thing that needs to be done in the majority of people who develop this problem is to get the ventricular response down to a reasonable rate, in the 70–100 beat per minute range. This can be done by administering a drug that influences the AV node in a suppressive manner, slowing the ventricular rate. An old-fashioned drug called Digoxin, given in increments until the proper response occurs, is effective. It can be done more quickly with an intravenous drip of a calcium-antagonist called Cardiazem. It, too, exerts an electrical slowing effect on the AV node, what we refer to as a negative chronotropic action. If the individual is in particular trouble, the most effective way to promptly improve the situation is to sedate the person and apply electrical shock, immediately restoring normal electrical activity in most instances.

Treatment to Prevent Stroke

Okay, so now we have the heart rate controlled. What next? Atrial fibrillation has been widely ignored in the past and has frequently even been treated with nonchalance, especially in the elderly. However, it is now well established that at least one-quarter of all strokes are caused by atrial fibrillation. Therefore, if there is no contraindication, the person who has just gone into atrial fibrillation should be anticoagulated promptly with Heparin or Lovenox, a Heparin fraction. This acute drug, used to stop proliferation of clots, should be given until a more durable drug can take its place. Such a drug is Coumadin, which works by tying up the clotting factors in the blood stream. You can't selectively tie up only those clotting factors that might work to form clots within the heart. Clotting everywhere in the body is affected. This is the reason this drug is difficult to use and its most common side effects are bleeding complications.

Why is clot-formation within the fibrillating left atrium such a problem? When the heart is in sinus rhythm, each beat of the heart acts to shrug off any material that would tend to adhere to the wall of the atrium or, even more likely, the left atrial appendage. For reasons we poorly understand, there is a small pouch attached to the left atrium, kind of like a watch pocket on a pair of jeans. I have pants that have watch pockets, though I have never carried a pocket watch and don't know anyone who does. Similarly, the left atrium has a little pocket over to the side. *Everyone* carries this atrial pocket, known as the left atrial appendage. But as far as we know, it has no useful function. At least my watch pocket doesn't cause me any trouble. This one, attached to the heart, can cause an ocean of trouble. When the heart is in normal sinus rhythm, the appendage contracts right along with the rest of the atrium. When the upper part of the heart is simply quivering with atrial fibrillation, blood can clot in that little stagnant pool. We can detect this clot material with transesophageal echocardiography, described later. (Figure 14) If it stays there, who cares? If it gets loose, it can't possibly go anywhere good, for it is now within the arterial circulation feeding the organs. And it usually goes north to the brain. In one second, a clot can be lobbed from the left atrial appendage into the left atrium, then the ventricle, out the aorta, into a carotid artery. It will travel as far as it can until it lodges in a blood vessel, clogging it, and stopping flow to the brain tissue serviced by that arterial branch. (Figure 12, page 73) In this instance, a stroke starts immediately. Since this is usually a well-formed clot that has been in the process of maturing for some time, it is firm and doesn't break up readily.

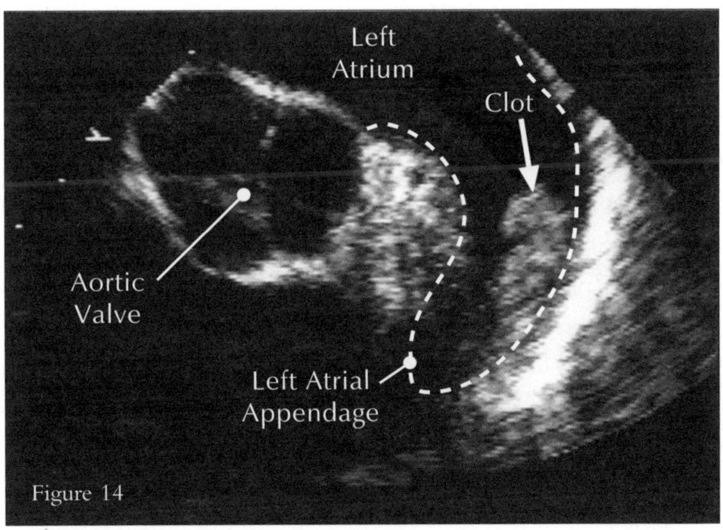

Figure 14

In other instances the clot may go south, landing eventually in an artery to the leg, or worse, the gut. Landing in the gut is usually catastrophe, especially if it results in dead bowel. In other words, if the clot lodges in a vital artery supplying the bowel wall, the bowel will turn blue and cramp terribly, as it is not getting enough oxygen-carrying red blood to satisfy its needs. Unless the clot breaks up, the bowel wall starts to die. We can seldom do anything surgically except remove the dead bowel. Fortunately, the clot that makes the turn around the aortic arch and heads south much more commonly enters one of the leg arteries. Usually we can retrieve such a clot from the leg artery and everything turns out just fine. However, a clot that results in a stroke or dead bowel frequently presents a bad situation. **This potentially life-changing event, clot embolization secondary to atrial fibrillation, must be prevented! This is by far the most important consideration in the care and management of atrial fibrillation.**

Why doesn't thrombus proliferation and embolization always occur in atrial fibrillation? I don't know. Theoretically it should, but it doesn't. All physicians who anticoagulate patients have had experience with people, recently diagnosed with atrial fibrillation, telling them that an uncle or friend or somebody they know, had atrial fibrillation for 20 years and never had a stroke. And they may well be right. There is no question that when we set out to anticoagulate everyone who has atrial fibrillation, we are treating all of these people with a dangerous drug, some of whom would never toss a clot from their left atrium if we simply left them alone. The questions is, who is and who isn't going to have an embolism with subsequent stroke or some other calamity? It is akin to high-risk behavior—some get by indefinitely with it; most do not. In order to prevent calamities in those who are prone to it, we must necessarily treat some who would not be.

We have, however, at least identified some low-risk people with atrial fibrillation. We know, for example, that very young people with normal hearts and normal blood pressure who occasionally go into atrial fibrillation are at very low risk of clot formation within the appendage. At the other end of the spectrum, we know that individuals who have had rheumatic fever and subsequent rheumatic mitral stenosis (a scarring of the mitral valve) are particularly prone to develop a clot in the left atrial appendage and embolize. All others are at variable intermediate risk. To some extent, the level of risk seems to be related to the size of the left atrium. However, this is not the singular consideration.

At this time, everyone except the very young with atrial fibrillation should be anticoagulated unless there is some pressing reason why they should not be. This is not a casual statement! Coumadin is the drug of choice for chronic anticoagulation. It ties up the clotting factors in the liver and has to be regulated very, very carefully. In my busy cardiology office, just collating the anticoagulation data and communicating with the patients in a timely fashion is an exhausting task. This alone requires over 50% of the time of two nurses!

Additionally, the populations we are usually dealing with regarding this condition are also in the age group where they are not only prone to this problem, but are at higher risk for others. For example, almost everyone over age 70 will occasionally develop severe joint pain. They are often given a non-steroidal anti-inflammatory drug, such as Ibuprofen. This drug makes the joint pain better but can cause irritation of the stomach lining. An inflamed stomach lining that might not bleed if the clotting elements had not been altered may bleed now since the person is taking Coumadin. Likewise, this elderly population is more prone to diverticulitis and polyps in the colon, both of which are easily made to bleed if Coumadin is being used. These older people are more apt to need emergency surgery, to have serious automobile accidents, and are more apt to fall—all situations that make them more apt to bleed on Coumadin therapy. Therefore, we are all constantly on the hunt for something to use that is less dangerous than Coumadin, but still possesses its protective features against catastrophic embolism from atrial fibrillation. While there are hints of a substitute, so far there is nothing else as effective in our armamentarium of approved drugs. We are, for example, frequently asked if platelet-active drugs, such as aspirin or Plavix, are effective against clot formation in the fibrillating left atrium for prevention of stroke. They are not.

Cardioversion from Atrial Fibrillation Back to Normal Sinus Rhythm

The majority of individuals who develop atrial fibrillation can be converted back to normal sinus rhythm. This not only markedly improves the hemodynamics (the presentation of red blood to vital organs and the prevention of moisture in the lungs), but also frequently allows safe temporary withdrawal of Coumadin in those who need surgery or have a bleeding problem.

I want to stress, before going on, that the decision as to whether you should be cardioverted from atrial fibrillation to normal sinus rhythm is something you have to work out with your cardiologist. Each person is unique, not only in our mannerisms, fingerprints, and appearance but also in the several features that figure into the equation about cardioversion. Only your physician, with your input, can make this decision.

I will try to present both sides: cardioversion from atrial fibrillation back to normal sinus rhythm versus leaving it alone. My view is based on my observations and experience. That doesn't mean that people are wrong if they disagree with it.

Your doctor may have a good reason not to try to get you back into normal sinus rhythm. Talk with your doctor about it.

There are several drugs that are exceptionally effective in maintaining sinus rhythm. Probably the best is Amiodarone. It is a powerful drug that initially had a bad reputation because, in the high doses first used, it caused an inflammatory change in the lungs. When used for atrial fibrillation, it usually doesn't take much of this drug to control the rhythm once the person is loaded with it. When combined with other drugs, it can frequently be given in exceptionally low doses, such as 200 milligrams only two or three days a week. When a patient comes to us with newly discovered atrial fibrillation, we first control the ventricular response so the person can enjoy a nice slow rate and avoid cardiac decompensation, with its resultant congestive heart failure. At the same time, we tie up clotting factors with Coumadin to prevent a clot from forming in the atrial appendage. After that, if the individual doesn't have severe lung disease, we load up with Amiodarone for a few weeks and then decrease the dosage to a very low amount, one that is not likely to cause problems. The major problem is that of pulmonary fibrosis, a scar-formation in the lungs. Therefore, we avoid using it in individuals with significant lung disease because they have no reserve in the event they develop this unusual side effect. While the pulmonary problem will reverse quickly if discovered early and treated with steroids, patients with lung disease may not have the reserve necessary to wait out the storm.

Any individual who is started on Amiodarone should be monitored every three to six months with a chest x-ray to rule out sensitivity to the drug. Occasionally, there are individuals who will develop pulmonary fibrosis with very low dosages of Amiodarone. There are other potential toxicity problems with it. One is abnormal thyroid function. Another less common side effect is a gait disturbance due to a neuropathy (nerve damage). Needless to say, the dosage should be kept at the bare minimum to do the job, and the patient should be well-versed as to what to look out for in the event of a side effect.

After the patient has been treated in this fashion for about a month to six weeks, long enough for any clot adherent to the left atrial appendage to have been eroded away, the person will be brought back into the hospital for a couple of hours in an effort at reclaiming a normal sinus rhythm. We sedate the patient, advance an echo probe down the esophagus behind the heart, and put echoes into the heart, much like sonar signals transmitted from a submarine. These bounce back and since different tissues possess different echo-absorption and deflection, we can determine if there is clot in the left atrial appendage. This is the transesophageal echocardiogram.

See Figure 14 on page 139 for a view of an appendage that *does* possess a clot—we would *not* want to cardiovert such a patient for fear of dislodging the clot.) If there is no clot found in the appendage, the patient is slightly more deeply sedated and shocked electrically through electrodes placed on the front and back of the chest, creating an electrical arc that momentarily stops electrical activity. The heart responds by coming back into sinus rhythm. This is called electrical cardioversion. Done under these circumstances by a skilled team, this is a safe procedure.

Once sinus rhythm is restored, the heart is happier. There is ample time for the left ventricle to fill, the rate is regular, and the atria are once again ultimately able to contribute to the total cardiac output. After a bit of time, the atrial appendage starts to contract normally again, thereby removing the threat of thrombus formation. Atrial contractility doesn't return overnight; it takes awhile, usually a few weeks.

Why isn't an effort made to convert almost everyone back to sinus rhythm? Beats me! But it isn't. The day before I wrote this chapter, I met a man in my office for the first time who had been cared for by a number of name-brand cardiologists in a large center well-publicized for cardiac care. He had been in atrial fibrillation ever since his coronary artery bypass six years prior. This is a sophisticated businessman who had a very thorough understanding of his clinical situation and came armed with reams of reports and lab values. He swore adamantly that no one had ever mentioned cardioversion to him. He has taken Coumadin for the last six years! This is particularly unfortunate because virtually everyone who develops this arrhythmia as a consequence of coronary bypass surgery can be converted back to sinus rhythm. Not only that, usually in about three months, once the effects of the surgery become mature with resolution of all inflammation, the patient can be removed from the drugs with very little incidence of recurrent atrial fibrillation.

There has been some literature stating that people do equally as well in atrial fibrillation as in sinus rhythm. In fact, a large clinical trial has just shown this. The trial took a large number of patients who had atrial fibrillation. Members of one group were allowed to remain in atrial fibrillation and were anticoagulated with Coumadin to prevent clot formation and stroke. The other group received intense efforts to reclaim and maintain the God-given normal sinus rhythm. They found no significant differences in survival and incidence of complication between the two groups.

I still believe that almost everyone deserves at least one effort to reclaim a normal sinus mechanism. An exception would be someone who has a giant left atrium; these will almost never remain in sinus rhythm even if the cardioversion is successful. Another is someone who has an artificial heart valve and will need to remain on

Coumadin indefinitely to protect against clot formation within the structure of the valve.

Since you still need to be anticoagulated with Coumadin once you have been converted from atrial fibrillation to sinus rhythm, the question is why we would ever try to convert anyone back to sinus rhythm. Why not just allow everyone who develops atrial fibrillation to continue in it, control their rate, anticoagulate them indefinitely, and leave well enough alone? I think there are several reasons. Discuss the pros and cons in your case with your physician and take the doctor's advice. I personally think there are several compelling reasons to try to reclaim and maintain sinus rhythm.

The first is due to the vastly superior hemodynamics that accrue to those in sinus rhythm as compared to atrial fibrillation. As the left ventricle becomes less effective as a pump—a fairly common situation with progressive age—the atrium contributes more and more to the total cardiac output, the amount of blood pumped each minute. No one knows when he or she may lose some pumping function, especially in older age. We *do* know that a condition known as programmed cell death (apoptosis) occurs frequently in advancing age. With loss of heart muscle cells, the left ventricular pump becomes less effective. In any circumstance, including heart attack, that reduces the efficiency of the pump, the atrium contributes more and more to take up the slack. I, for example, want to be in sinus rhythm so that my atrium can step up and help carry the burden if I lose muscle cells in my main heart pump. With a sick left ventricle, the left atrium can increase its contribution up to 35% of the total cardiac output instead of its usual 15%. One could say, "Well, wait on it. If I start losing left ventricular function because of some unforeseen problem, then I will get cardioverted." It isn't that easy. The longer one remains in atrial fibrillation, the harder it is to cardiovert to and hold a sinus mechanism.

There are other strong reasons to be cardioverted back to sinus rhythm. Not the least of these is the fact that one may be forced to discontinue Coumadin either temporarily or permanently, whether because of peptic ulcer disease with bleeding, the need for surgery, frequent falls, or dangerous hobbies. If this ever occurs, the one who is in sinus rhythm rather than atrial fibrillation can come off Coumadin without risk. If you remain in atrial fibrillation, you are at risk each time you stop Coumadin. It is the rare elderly individual who develops atrial fibrillation and makes it to a natural end of his life without being forced to quit Coumadin for awhile because of some compelling reason.

Yet another strong reason to try to get back into sinus rhythm is this: If you are in persistent atrial fibrillation, you must be fairly aggressively anticoagulated with Coumadin. An argument can be made that once you've had atrial fibrillation once, you are more likely to go back into it and, therefore, should be anticoagulated forever. However, the *level* of anticoagulation can be more relaxed in those shown to remain in sinus rhythm for a number of months. Therefore, their day-to-day risk of bleeding into the gastrointestinal tract is markedly reduced. In other words, if you remain in atrial fibrillation, you would have to maintain an INR (International Standard of Anticoagulation) of 2–2.5 (highly anticoagulated). This is compared to the level of 1.5–2 where you would need to be if in sinus rhythm. This may not seem like much; however, this value is logarithmically expressed, so this seemingly small increment can make a world of difference in bleeding tendency.

This decision has to be made through discussion between you and your physician. A very convincing argument can be made for an attempt to convert almost every person who develops atrial fibrillation back into a sinus rhythm. There are rare exceptions, usually having to do with the size of the left atrium. We know, for example, that it is unlikely we can maintain sinus rhythm in people with a huge left atrium, especially if they have rheumatic heart disease. They need rate control and Coumadin anticoagulation.

Some physicians simply refuse to use Amiodarone for this problem. I understand their position. All it takes is one patient who misses seeing the doctor for six months or so, developing pulmonary fibrosis in the interim. The need for periodic evaluations while on Amiodarone cannot be overemphasized. Nor can the importance of education of the patient.

There are other drugs that can be used in atrial fibrillation. One approach is to use a simple beta-blocker as the sole drug. This drug blocks the beta receptors in the heart cells and reduces the impact of sudden outpouring of epinephrine. In certain patients, it alone is a very effective drug in the prevention of relapses of atrial fibrillation.

Another good drug is Propafenone or Rythmol. It is well tolerated and, while not as effective as Amiodarone, is especially helpful in those patients with lung disease who cannot take Amiodarone due to fear of causing pulmonary inflammation and can't take a beta-blocker because of wheezing. It is frequently accepted as an option by those cardiologists who will not use Amiodarone. Another good drug is Sotalol, very effective in some, and Tikosyn. Tikosyn needs to be started in the hospital but is quite effective in many patients who cannot be treated effectively with the other drugs.

Surgery for Atrial Fibrillation

Everyone wants to know if there is surgery available for atrial fibrillation. There is. It is called the Mini-Maze ablation procedure, and it is done by placing laser streaks in the left atrium. Currently, it is done at the time of open-chest surgery. We have had exceptionally good results using this technique.

A Cousin: Atrial Flutter

What are the other variations on the central theme of atrial fibrillation? The first is the relative of atrial fibrillation known as atrial flutter. In this situation, the atria develop very rapid electrical activity almost always at a fixed rate of 300 beats a minute. Additionally, it is regular as opposed to chaotic. In this instance, the ventricular rate is almost always exactly 150 beats a minute as the AV node, the "governor" or modulator of transmission of electrical impulses from the atria to the ventricles, can handle about every other electrical signal. This rhythm is almost always easily converted with low current and, as opposed to atrial fibrillation, there is an effective radiofrequency ablation technique for treating cases that are refractory to chemical suppression. Radiofrequency ablation is done with a catheter inserted through the skin in the groin with its tip within the heart. A good electrophysiologist can map the heart and the veins leading into it, discovering the pathway that is causing atrial flutter. Using the radiofrequency energy emitted from the tip of the electrode, the fiber tract is burned, eliminating it as a culprit in causing this arrhythmia. The focus of initiation of atrial flutter is frequently located in the pulmonary veins, an interesting new revelation.

Fortunately, those with atrial flutter are much less likely to form clot in the left atrial appendage and toss it to the brain. It is not too unusual, however, to have what is commonly referred to as atrial flutter–fibrillation, kind of a hybrid mixture of the two. With this, there is the ever-present possibility of clot formation.

While the ventricular response to atrial fibrillation is easy to control, it can be next to impossible to control with atrial flutter. It seems the AV node generally handles one of every two atrial flutter impulses, giving the person a heart rate of 150. It is relatively resistant to treatment with drugs. It is best to resort to radiofrequency ablation early on if this arrhythmia is recurrent.

Unique Presentations and Problems with Atrial Fibrillation

Another variation on the theme is the "non-senser" of atrial arrhythmias. While I see about 200 new patients each year with atrial fibrillation and almost all of these will sense the change in their rate and/or rhythm, I see maybe three or four people a year who don't have a clue that they have developed this arrhythmia. These are not unintelligent or non-connected people. They simply don't sense their heart action! Therefore, they don't routinely seek medical attention until they have "worn their heart out." In the days before there were drugs known to slow the ventricular rate, this condition was common. It was called "dropsy."

Tachycardia-related cardiomyopathy is how I refer to this condition. This is a situation of weakness of heart muscle contractility that has developed secondary to an undiscovered, extremely rapid heart action. Usually elderly, these people walk around with a ventricular rate of 120 to 200 beats a minute with their hearts behaving as though they were exercising constantly. Over time, with this kind of rate, the cellular energy stores are depleted and the muscle cells function poorly or in the case of some cells, not at all. Such individuals come in with congestive heart failure due to large, poorly contractile ventricles. Obviously they are quite sick and require a carefully orchestrated treatment regimen for survival and improvement.

These patients must be anticoagulated. The rate has to be controlled and, after a period of time on anticoagulants, they should be cardioverted. They should also be treated with a special type of beta-blocker, Coreg, which possesses unique properties that help the heart muscle recover. They should also be treated with an ACE-Inhibitor to unload the heart, and, just as importantly, should abstain completely from cardiotoxic compounds such as alcohol. Most, if not all, of these patients will recover substantial contractile ability with time. The hibernating muscle cells will recover. These are the most grateful patients in the world because they know they've been given a reprieve.

On the other end of the spectrum is the occasional person with atrial fibrillation who has enough scar tissue within the AV node that the ventricular rate is quite low, even with no drugs to slow conduction. It is sometimes so slow that a pacemaker is required. Some of these patients will have just enough scar tissue within the heart conduction system that the ventricular rate is perfect, 60–80 beats a minute, in response to atrial fibrillation. Lucky! Maybe not. What if you go along with a rate in that range, don't sense anything wrong and then have an embolic stroke? I think, on the whole, it is better to be in the majority that has a runaway rate, gets scared by the initial development of atrial fibrillation, and gets treatment, including anticoagulation to prevent clot formation and stroke. Like so many things in life, however, we don't get to choose.

Not uncommonly, patients have paroxysmal atrial fibrillation alternating with a slow rhythm. This is the so-called *tachy-brady variant of sick sinus syndrome*, an end result of deterioration of the cardiac conduction skeleton. This seems a strange process at first. However, in this instance, the deterioration in the cardiac conduction system has largely affected electrical impulse formation and the integrity of the atrial fiber tracts. Enough breakdowns have developed in the atrial electrical network to result in intermittent atrial fibrillation. The AV node is still intact, conducting the electrical activity offered to it at a rapid rate. However, when the person spontaneously converts back to sinus rhythm, the sinus node is faulty and fails to go along at an acceptable rate. In this circumstance, a permanent pacemaker is implanted to maintain a reliable lower-rate platform. This allows us to effectively treat the tachy, or fast, component with a drug. Every drug that we use to treat atrial fibrillation will slow conduction at the AV node. Therefore, if there is not only a fast component but also an intermittent slow rhythm, the heart rate has to be assured by artificial electrical means.

The Future

Atrial fibrillation is almost at epidemic numbers. It is a huge cardiologic problem but I feel confident that we will have much better means of dealing with it in the future.

For example, I think we will soon be treating a great deal of atrial fibrillation with circumferential radiofrequency ablation of electrical activity surrounding the pulmonary veins. Currently, this is being done in research centers for paroxysmal atrial fibrillation, the type that begins suddenly and then ends suddenly. First, the focus of the atrial fibrillation has to be found in every person. We always assumed this was in the atrium somewhere; now we learn it is frequently in close juxtaposition to the pulmonary veins, draining red, oxygen-rich blood back to the left atrium. A good operator can locate this focus and burn it with the energy of radiofrequency signals. There are some risks. However, a lot of people have such major problems with various aspects of their atrial fibrillation that they are willing to take them. I'm not sure this is going to be a treatment for the masses, as it is a labor-intensive process and there are huge numbers with this problem. Time will tell.

Another exciting and promising new treatment modality is that of exclusion of the left atrial appendage. The Mayo Clinic is running a large trial using a special umbrella-like device, inserted through a catheter introduced through the skin in the groin. The device causes the left atrial appendage—the area where this nefarious business of clot formation takes place in atrial fibrillation—to seal over smoothly, eliminating the potential for a clot to form and embolize to the brain and elsewhere.

We all look forward to an effective drug that will take the place of Coumadin. We all long for a drug that is safe, free from the need for such tight regulation of dosage, not too expensive, and is reassuringly protective from clot formation and stroke. It will likely come along.

In the meantime, we must all strive to take the best care of our bodies that we possibly can. We need to maintain ideal body weight, watch our salt intake, exercise, and stay as tranquil as we can. Will some of us still develop atrial fibrillation? Yes. In large measure, it is part of the price of living a long life. It can be treated. With education, you can live with it. Making that easier and less frightening is the purpose of this book.

REMINDERS

1. **Atrial fibrillation is a rapid, chaotic arrhythmia arising in the atrium. Rate control is important.**
2. **Anticoagulation should be used in almost all patients with atrial fibrillation to prevent clot formation and its associated complications.**
3. **Discuss with your doctor the pros and cons of trying to re-establish sinus rhythm.**
4. **You can live peacefully and happily with atrial fibrillation for many, many years!**

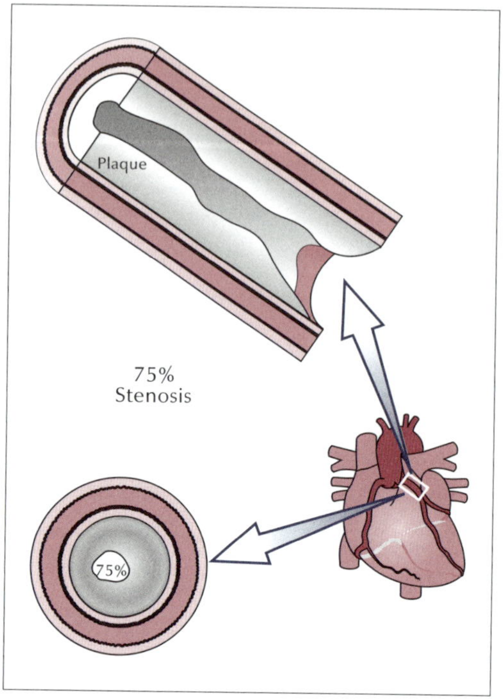

SILENT CORONARY ARTERY DISEASE AND ANGINA

Blockage of the Arteries Supplying the Heart Muscle

THERE ARE LITERALLY MILLIONS OF PEOPLE out there walking around with plaque in their coronary arteries, yet they remain asymptomatic. We commonly refer to this as *silent coronary artery disease* (silent CAD). Should these millions of people be worried? Not if we can educate them and *keep it silent*. The difference between silent CAD and a catastrophic heart attack is maintained by the fibrous cap covering the cholesterol deposit within the wall of the coronary artery supplying the heart muscle. The incidence of silent CAD is very high and has traditionally carried significant risk. The Framingham (Mass.) Heart Study, which by now has tracked heart data for over 50 years, tells us that roughly 50% of men and 60% of women who died suddenly of coronary artery disease had no previous symptoms of their disease whatsoever. You may feel more assured if you have no symptoms of your problem. You are not safer. In this context, while some with silent coronary disease simply do not have large enough plaques to cause obstruction to flow, others have inadequate warning mechanisms.

Silent CAD is in contradistinction to *symptomatic* CAD, coronary disease associated with angina (pain or discomfort due to a blocked artery). Silent CAD is totally asymptomatic; CAD with angina is usually more advanced and carries a warning signal. Angina is a broadly defined term indicating a symptom caused by oxygen starvation of the heart muscle. In its purest form, this consists of chest, jaw, or arm pain, commonly associated with shortness of breath, brought on by exertion or stress, and relieved by rest and tranquility. Any stimulus that increases the heart muscle's need for oxygen and nutrients may bring about this primitive reflex. It is due to a build-up of lactic acid in the heart tissue. The heart muscle has to keep on working in a faithful response to whatever the brain tells the body to do. If one walks rapidly, climbs stairs, has sexual intercourse, or engages in a multitude of strenuous endeavors that increase the heart rate and the force of cardiac contractility, the heart muscle, in response, demands more blood. If there is a restrictive blockage in a coronary artery (a coronary stenosis) that prevents this increased delivery of blood supply to a certain zone of heart muscle, the muscle will continue to perform valiantly, yet it will produce a larger quantity of lactic acid that is not carried away. The multiple nerve endings that invest this zone will transmit this lactic acid accumulation to the brain where it is interpreted as pain. Such discomfort is known as angina. It will keep on getting more severe if the person persists in his or her activities and the tissue accumulation of lactic acid increases. Finally, the heart muscle cells will start to falter, losing some of their contractile strength. If the individual stops all activity, the lactic acid will be washed out and the cells, now adequately supplied with oxygen and nutrients, will start to function normally again. The pain will resolve as soon as the lactic acid level falls.

Actually, we've had to re-educate ourselves somewhat. We now think of angina as more of a symptom complex in response to increased cardiac needs. In women, this symptom complex may not be pain in the chest, arms or jaw, as is the case in many men. Instead, women may experience only nausea and sweating or if discomfort occurs at all, it may be mild and located primarily in the epigastrium, the area just below the breastbone. Suffice it to say that any discomfort between the belly button and the ears that is brought on by exercise or stress, especially if associated with other symptoms such as nausea, shortness of breath, or inappropriate sweating, whether in a woman or a man, should be suspect for angina.

This particular chapter is devoted to the huge number of people who have silent CAD, plaque in their coronary arteries with no symptoms, or *mostly* silent CAD, those with occasional angina. (See Chapter 3 on CAD and heart attack.) This chapter is to make sure your silent CAD remains truly silent.

First, how will you know if you have silent CAD? It's amazing how many people just assume they have CAD because one or both parents had it. It's true that this is a strongly heritable disease. Conversely, many assume they do not have it because there is none in their family. This is not something to be taken for granted; the stakes are too high. Secondly, is it even important for you to know you have CAD if it is not causing symptoms? I'm sure you've heard the phrase, "What you don't know won't hurt you." Well, in this case it can!

Would you be okay, for example, with having a malignant tumor growing inside you and pass up a chance to know about it just because it's not hurting you at the moment? Yet every day, millions of people pass up the opportunity to know whether or not they possess silent CAD. This thinking predominates, despite the fact that CAD kills more people yearly in America than all of the tumors put together. In fact, coronary artery disease has historically been the number one killer in both men and women in America for many years. It frequently comes as a great surprise to women that heart disease, not breast cancer, is the number one cause of death in women in the United States after age 25.

The answer regarding the importance of knowing about whether one needs to know of silent coronary disease is also contained within the data from the famous Framingham study. During the last 15 years, the incidence of death from coronary artery disease has declined by about 25%.

So we're making some progress in CAD, especially regarding enhanced detection in women, reducing the incidence of primary and secondary coronary events with statin drugs (which lower cholesterol), and effective treatment of coronary blockages without open-heart surgery. However, obesity is rampant and with it comes diabetes. We know from experience that CAD is going to follow close on the heels of diabetes. Therefore, in many ways, our work has only begun. If we are in the throes of a diabetes epidemic now, we will likely see a secondary CAD epidemic follow in the next few years. In a civilized society, CAD is always going to be with us. We must learn methods of early detection that can be applied to the population-at-large. We must also continue to search for effective prevention in order to reduce the incidence of heart attacks.

If a heart attack occurs seemingly "out of the blue" in a previously asymptomatic person, what in the world happens to make this occur? The development of acute coronary occlusion and heart attack is because a cholesterol plaque within the coronary arterial wall becomes *vulnerable*. This defines a lipid-laden, bulging plaque system in which the fibrous cap, the covering over the arteriosclerotic deposit, has thinned out, setting the stage for rupture and its serious consequences. This is orchestrated by a change in the population of cells within the plaque itself, triggering release of inflammatory molecules that bring about a malicious sequence of events leading to a heart attack. When such a vulnerable plaque eventually ruptures into the central channel of the artery, platelets in the blood stream quickly aggregate at that site, leading to clot formation and, frequently, total blockage of the vessel. Heart muscle cells immediately become starved for oxygen and nutrients as they continue right on with their task of contractility to allow for uninterrupted function of the pump. This is the beginning of a heart attack.

Contrary to popular opinion, this process does not always occur with a high-grade plaque that is 75% or even 90% occluded. Roughly one-half of these acute occlusions occur at plaque systems that were only about 50% or less obstructive, partially explaining why so many people are not symptomatic preceding a heart attack. Here, the key to stability or, conversely, instability (vulnerable plaque) is a transformation of the elements that make up the plaque. This is a silent process: One day the plaque is dormant, the next it is unstable. For example, the lipid core of the plaque bulges, the fibrous cap covering the plaque thins out, the cellular makeup within the plaque changes to a preponderance of inflammatory cells, and the intense tendency for erosion of the plaque and vessel clotting is triggered by a release of cytokines, the inflammatory molecules that act as a catalyst of this devastation. While we have no good way to accurately predict just who possesses such a vulnerable plaque system within their coronary circulation, we do have excellent ways of determining who does, or does not, have silent CAD.

What is the purpose of knowing that you have silent CAD? Because we can direct treatment toward preventing its progression and, hopefully, keep it silent forever. We already know the predicted natural history of this disease. We want to modify its course. Detection of the silent process is the first step. In the past, we had no easy or effective way to non-invasively look for silent CAD. Now we do. Historically, a coronary angiogram, an invasive procedure whereby contrast material is injected through a catheter placed in the coronary artery, was thought to be the "gold standard" for determining who had CAD and who did not. We know now that this is actually a rather crude methodology because the plaque material, which accumulates within the wall of the artery, has to be protruding into the lumen, the central portion of the artery where the blood flows, to show up on angiography. In other words, you can have a very advanced case of silent coronary artery disease and still have an almost normal coronary angiogram. We obviously have needed a screening test that would alert us to the presence of "sub-clinical" disease within the coronary arteries before it becomes obstructive and certainly before it becomes unstable.

Screening Tests for Silent Coronary Artery Disease

A. Thallium Heart Scans

In this quest for a good screening test, treadmill tests utilizing radioactive tracer materials (thallium) became the first-line analysis in screening for the presence or absence of significant obstructive CAD. Now used for many years, these tests did absolutely nothing in the way of detecting silent, non-obstructive CAD. Yet silent, non-obstructive disease is exactly the sort of thing we want to detect while we still have time to treat it and prevent it from becoming a major threat to life!

When the thallium scan (named because it utilizes the radioactive tracer thallous chloride) became more prevalent, it was found to have serious limitations but was the best screening test we had. Then it got badly out of hand as thallium scans became an almost casually performed test. I'm not anti-thallium scan. I've had to order, usually reluctantly, my fair share. For a while, there was absolutely no way to non-invasively obtain needed information about whether or not the individual in question had an obstructive plaque in the coronary artery. *It has always been very important, however, to understand that this test can usually only reveal those individuals who have a 75% or greater blockage in a coronary artery.* It gave us no information whatsoever in the legions of folks who had a great amount of plaque build-up but no blockage, the epidemic of silent CAD that we need to know about and treat. Because so many people show up each day in a doctor's office with chest pain of all imaginable types, and because so many people have a multiplicity of coronary risk factors, an enormous number of these folks wound up receiving thallium scans. The use of thallium scans has increased significantly over the years with seemingly little consideration for the fact that it frequently misses the diagnosis of silent CAD. It's not enough to have a negative (normal) thallium test and to be slapped on the back and told that you don't have anything to worry about.

Let me elaborate. The thallium-201 radioactive tracer is ionically (and ironically) identical to potassium, a very important element in the blood stream. The heart muscle cells absolutely love potassium, removing it from the blood stream in one or two circulation passes through the heart. If you are put in a situation that causes increased demand on the blood supply to the heart and there has been no prior damage to the heart, the uptake should be homogenous. If a previous heart attack has occurred, there should be a "fixed" thallium defect from the old scar, simply because there is a reduced population of muscle cells in that area. Finally, if there is at least 75% blockage in one of the coronary arteries but no damage has been incurred, there should be a reversible defect, one that appears on the initial scan done using methods to provoke increased oxygen demands, but that would correct itself on the redistribution study taken sometime later. This is because there is a tight enough blockage to result in diminished blood flow to the area with increased needs of the heart muscle, but the cells are normal. They are therefore capable of bringing the radioactive tracer across the cell membrane once they have recovered from their oxygen-deprived status.

There are many problems with this concept. One is that the heart sits on the diaphragm, the bellows that bring air into the lungs. This is an area that causes attenuation of emission from radioactive decay and this may make the scan look as though there must be a tight blockage in the right coronary artery supplying the bottom surface of the heart. Additionally, if the individual is obese, the very same thing may be even more exaggerated when in actuality, the "defect" may well just represent a big belly. Another problem that can develop with thallium scans is that any woman with abundant breast tissue may well pose a "defect" in that area. It just happens to be the same area supplied by the left anterior descending coronary artery, the big artery down the front of the heart that not only supplies the front wall of the heart but also supplies the interventricular septum, the partition between the two lower chambers. One could say that if the defect on the scan doesn't also involve the septal region, it likely is breast tissue. However, we have seen any number of women with a blockage half-way down the left anterior descending coronary artery and the septum would have been spared on the thallium test.

I'm not especially down on the thallium scan. I think it has a role in the screening of high-grade blockage in a coronary artery. I just think it is a miserable test to determine whether or not silent CAD is present, and it is not very good for determining whether or not a blood vessel is blocked, unless it is very tightly blocked.

B. Coronary Calcium Scores

So what is a better screening tool for detecting silent coronary plaque material? First, let me say that not everyone needs to be screened. We know that women are relatively protected from the ravages of CAD until menopause. It makes very little sense to put a young, pre-menopausal woman through a screening test if she has no coronary risk factors whatsoever. So first, let us take a history, get some laboratory values and then if there is reason for concern, proceed with further tests.

Let's say someone has any one of a number of known coronary risk factors, such as previous or current smoking history, diabetes, hypertension, hyperlipidemia (abnormal cholesterol fractions or abnormal triglycerides), a strong family history of CAD, or evidence of metabolic syndrome (insulin resistance accompanying obesity, usually associated with abnormal lipids, such as a raised cholesterol). I think this type of person should clearly be screened for the presence of silent CAD, especially if a male or a post-menopausal female. If female and pre-menopausal, the doctor should tailor the evaluation to the severity of coronary risk factors. In other words, there are plenty of insulin-dependent diabetic women who are pre-menopausal yet have significant silent CAD. On the other hand, if a person comes in with simple hypertension and has no other significant coronary risk factors, I would not recommend screening for silent CAD. Males are a different story. They may well begin developing CAD in their teens. This was first learned about during the Korean War. Autopsy studies on a sizable number of combatants lost on the battlefield showed a substantial incidence of yellow fatty streaks in the aorta, an early marker of significant arteriosclerosis. And these were young men in their early 20s! Of course, they were under conditions of intense stress, many smoked, and their daily diet of Spam was not the best.

For many years, then, we have needed a great screening test to look for silent coronary artery disease so we could treat it accordingly and suppress it, hoping to change the natural history of the process. In order for a screening test to be effective and widely applied to a population that is totally free of symptoms, such a test has to satisfy three requirements: available and inexpensive, safe, and reliable. You can't go testing a huge population of people with something that is terribly expensive, carries significant risks, or doesn't offer reliable data.

Using these criteria, the best *screening* tool for silent CAD is, by far, the coronary calcium score. It is well known that calcium deposits develop rather soon after formation of a coronary plaque. This test is a CT scan that measures coronary calcium content within the wall of the coronary arteries. It is valid in men over 35 but, as women calcify later than men, they must be 45–50 years of age for this to be a valid test.

This score does not tell us whether or not there is a tight plaque within the coronary arteries. It just tells us, based on thousands of calcium scores, what an average score should be for each age group within each gender. This is, without a doubt, the finest screening test we have for the detection of silent CAD and it costs only $100–$200. A 50-year-old female with a calcium score of 1,200 is treated very differently from one with a zero score. We know that if you have a coronary calcium score of 100 or less (if a man; women carry calcium scores about one-half that of men up to age 60 or so, and a score of 50 in a women would be the equivalent of a score of 100 in a man), you are at very low risk of having a significant coronary blockage. Additionally, while any coronary risk factors need to be worked on, your outlook is excellent—at least for the short term. On the other hand, we know that someone with a score of greater than 400–500 has a significant risk of having a major blockage in at least one coronary artery. The catch is you have no idea what is what unless you do the screening test. The fee for this test is not much to spend on something that may well change your life and the way you view it.

Not long ago, a woman brought her husband in to see me. They were both 50. I walked in to find this well-dressed gentleman sitting on the exam table. He was chewing on a large cigar and had dribbled tobacco juice onto his white shirt. He weighed about 300 pounds. He had no coronary risk factors other than obesity, but his wife had forced him to come in because he looked like "a heart attack ready to happen." The wife was a petite, muscular woman who weighed about 120 pounds. I discussed the screening test with him and sent him off to obtain a calcium score. When they arrived at the desk to obtain the test, they were informed of two things. The insurance company would not pay for the test, although the insurance company would readily have paid for a $1,500 thallium test even though it would have been grossly inappropriate and the moral equivalent of stealing money from this man. On the flip side, when the man's wife heard that the calcium score test only costs $100 in our hospital, she exclaimed, "Honey, I think I'll get one too. My father died at age 40 of a heart attack." Despite his rather elaborate chiding, she went through with it.

The next week, they were back in my exam room. This time, the situation was reversed. The wife was on the exam table. The man was sitting in a chair with a cigar in his mouth, having drooled over on the other side of his shirt this time. His score was zero, implying no CAD whatsoever. Her score, on the other hand, was 1,230, implying extensive CAD! Her LDL-cholesterol, the bad stuff, was sky-high at 160. His was normal. Her C-reactive protein, an index of inflammation, was very high. His was normal. She had never had a single symptom, yet she had extensive coronary disease as evidenced by her high coronary calcium score.

Does it really matter whether or not she and I know that she has silent CAD? Yes! We would ordinarily have dropped her LDL-cholesterol to just below 100 with a statin drug just as a prophylactic measure. However, knowing her degree of silent CAD coupled with evidence of raging inflammation, the perfect storm for a heart attack out of the blue, made us do a couple of things differently. We dropped her LDL to about 70, because it has been shown that we have to get it this low to completely stop the arteriosclerosis process in its tracks. It is probably also the most effective therapy in treatment of the inflammatory component. Additionally, we recommended an angiogram to get a look at her coronary arteries. It turned out that she had a plaque in the left main coronary artery. It was of borderline significance by appearance—we couldn't tell whether it was 50% or closer to 75%—so we performed an intra-coronary ultrasound, bouncing sound waves off the inside of the wall of the artery, getting back a beautiful interior architectural picture of the plaque encroachment on the central canal. This showed that the plaque system was about 70% in severity of obstruction and was very complex. Since such a process is associated with a relatively high mortality, and because we have very poor methods of following this routinely and cannot predict when such a plaque will rupture and result in vessel closure, we recommended coronary bypass surgery.

This case illustrates the importance of carefully screening those people who are apt to have the disease. In her case, she had compelling coronary risk factors. She was not even my patient! She became *empowered* to look into her own care because she heard the spiel. She now knew what constituted being at coronary risk. I'm good at giving this lecture. However, only a very small fraction of the people who *should* hear about it actually hear it. The vast number of folks walking around with silent CAD is mind-boggling. One would have to become the cardiologic equivalent of Billy Graham to preach this sermon to such a huge population at risk. This is one of the reasons for this book.

To reiterate, the thallium scan very frequently does not tell you whether or not you have silent CAD. However, *silent coronary artery disease* is exactly the process we should be screening for and treating so that we can modify its course. The best screening test for this vast population is the coronary calcium score. It is the only test which shows that CAD is present—even if it is not causing any encroachment on the inside channel of the artery (the lumen)—without having some sort of an angiogram.

You can see that this topic has changed a lot in recent years. We still have physicians out there who are steadfastly ordering a thallium scan on everyone who complains of chest pain, even though it's fraught with the hazard of being wrong. Sir Winston Churchill once said, "A fanatic is one who can't change his mind and won't change the subject." In this case, the subject is here to stay. We must change our thinking about how to investigate the problem so we can detect the silent cases before they cause disaster.

C. New Technology: Multi-Slice CT Angiography

Thankfully, multi-slice CT angiography, a very meaningful tool, is also becoming readily available. This test is *relatively* non-invasive; an iodine-based contrast material is injected into a peripheral intravenous port. A total body arterial contrast study then can be analyzed.

The new CT angiogram is going to be a wonderful tool for screening. One of the things that has always bothered me about simply relying on the calcium score is that the vulnerable plaque, named by the pathologists, is one with a lipid-rich core bulging against a thinned-out fibrous cap and loaded down with inflammatory cells. These cells produce enzymes that erode the protective cap covering the plaque and also help activate the inflammatory cytokines, substances that bring about clotting and disruption of the integrity of the plaque. In this situation, our own cells are trying to give us a heart attack! Unfortunately, this prototypical plaque, the vulnerable plaque, is frequently not calcified, and we would potentially miss it by coronary calcium score testing. It is confusing, as the chance of a cardiovascular event, a heart attack, or an unstable coronary syndrome, is very low if you have a zero calcium score. However, if you're a woman, you calcify plaque later and less than men, so your doctor should recommend a CT angiogram promptly if you develop bothersome symptoms, or if a definite diagnosis needs to be established.

Multi-slice CT angiography is better than the calcium score. The only reason I still feel the calcium score is to be used as a screening tool for the majority of the population is because of the three criteria I set forth earlier: expense, safety, and reliability. Remember, we are talking about screening millions of people. For example, it is now estimated that over 30 million people have metabolic syndrome. This diagnosis is reached whenever a person has any three of the following: central obesity, elevated triglycerides, elevated LDL-cholesterol (especially of the small, dense particle variety), low HDL-cholesterol, insulin-resistance diabetes (which frequently accompanies obesity), and evidence of inflammation. When these people reach 50, they should be screened. Some will have coronary disease; some will not (most will). However, they are not having symptoms. I'm not sure we can scan them all with a multi-slice CT angiogram, nor am I sure that we should.

The cost of multi-slice CT angiography is roughly four times that of a calcium score, the radiation exposure is roughly 5 to 10 times higher, but the reliability is doubtless higher.

Using these considerations, I recommend:

1. Use the coronary calcium scoring as a screen.
2. If it is zero, go home.
3. If it is higher than about 50 (and certainly higher than 100), go ahead with the CT angiogram.

We start with an inexpensive, safe, and reliable test and move into the next stage only if the first is abnormal enough to warrant it.

Who Has a Vulnerable Plaque?

Another aspect of silent CAD bothers me a great deal. We have no way of determining which plaque system is vulnerable. In other words, we cannot tell which one is complex and, therefore, at great risk of rupture, and which is stable. We can't do this with any of our currently available techniques.

However, if we know that someone has significant silent CAD, we are going to treat that person very aggressively. For example, if we know that a 50-year-old man has diffuse, silent CAD and a large coronary calcium score, but the disease is scattered throughout the coronary arteries including the left main, it would not be wrong to pull out all the stops with regard to treatment of lipids, hypertension, and weight. We will also treat this patient with Plavix, a strong platelet-inhibitor, since we know that the first thing that happens when a plaque ruptures is platelet aggregation in the initiation of a clot. We simply have no way, at this time, of screening the general patient population with silent CAD to determine who is likely to develop a heart attack. The best tool, obviously, would be some reliable measurement of the degree of coronary inflammation, as we know this to be the trigger that initiates the complex cascade of events leading to the vessel clotting off. The high-sensivity C-reactive protein (hs-CRP) is a measure of inflammation, and we know that individuals who have a smattering of vulnerable plaques throughout their circulation frequently have gotten to that point at least partially through activation of the inflammatory mechanism. However, there are a number of other causes of an elevated hs-CRP. Because of this, we are on the hunt for a heart-specific marker of inflammation that would serve to warn us that someone with silent CAD has activated his or her *coronary* inflammatory mechanisms, making that person at risk for a heart attack.

To take this point further, we don't always know how to recognize a vulnerable plaque when we see it in the catheterization laboratory! Sometimes we can, if the partially ulcerated plaque collects some of the contrast material we inject. But we can't always be sure. I'll give you an illustration. This patient was a 35-year-old man who, as a youth, had watched his father die in a cotton field. He had "iffy" pain, and his wife chased him into my office. His tests indicated the need for an angiogram; he had two plaques that I could recognize. One was in the circumflex coronary artery leading around to the muscle on the back wall of the heart and it was about 95% blocked. The other was in the right coronary artery and appeared to be about 30% in severity. It never crossed my mind that the latter might be the culprit lesion (the vulnerable, or already ruptured, plaque). I stented the sub-totally blocked one. He came back into the hospital just four days later, on Plavix, with an acute occlusion of the right coronary artery, exactly at the spot where he had this tiny lesion. In retrospect, I'm sure that the 30% blockage in the right coronary artery represented the unstable plaque system. The much tighter circumflex blockage was a stable plaque. You guessed it: His hs-CRP was sky-high. He had activated his inflammatory molecule system in the inside layer of the artery—the endothelium—and had sticky platelets. He had eroded his right coronary plaque which clotted off, as this inflammatory wagon, once it gets rolling, is hard to stop.

Our conventional approach sometimes makes less sense than we would expect. There is little doubt that these tight lesions should be recognized and treated since we now have these drug-eluting stents that offer such durable results. However, the tight blockages are not always the culprits. It turns out that a non-obstructive lesion, sometimes 50% or less in severity, can be just as apt as the highly occlusive lesions to rupture and produce a heart attack. As a screen, we should always measure the level of inflammation, currently the hs-CRP. With the ongoing research, we should soon have a reliable heart-specific measure of inflammation.

Treatment and Intervention in Silent Coronary Disease

If someone has CAD and symptoms of angina, the methods of treatment and intervention are fairly uniform and generally accepted by the cardiac community. Nitroglycerin under the tongue, the old mainstay of treatment, used whenever the tissue oxygen supply-demand ratio is imbalanced, is a prompt way to treat an anginal attack. Remember, angina is the symptom complex of jaw, arm, chest or epigastric pressure-like discomfort, frequently associated with breathlessness, sweating, or nausea, commonly brought on by exertion or stress and relieved by rest. Since angina is due to a rigid plaque in the coronary arterial wall protruding into the lumen of the blood vessel carrying red blood to the heart muscle, flow is restricted to a certain finite quantity and the flow through this plaque cannot be increased. Normally, when the demands of the muscle increase, the supply of blood increases accordingly and a happy homeostasis is maintained. With this rigid plaque system, there is no way to dilate (enlarge) the artery and increase flow. Nitroglycerin works by dilating the veins carrying blood back to the heart, and also dilating the arteries producing the resistance against which the heart has to pump. A sharp reduction in the workload of the heart muscle follows, and the supply-demand ratio is restored. It also relaxes the coronary arteries which may or may not do any good, as the rigid plaque system producing the obstruction probably won't dilate anyway. In the clinical setting, a story of chest pain or any of its surrogates, relieved by nitroglycerin, strongly suggests that the cause of the symptoms is a blocked coronary artery.

As with almost all things in medicine, there are possible alternative explanations. Nitroglycerin will also relax smooth muscle in the wall of the esophagus. If esophageal spasm is the cause of the pain—it can mimic angina exactly—prompt relief will usually result from nitroglycerin. If, for example, a young lady comes in with chest pain and has no coronary risk factors but has taken her father's nitroglycerin and it relieved the pain, she very likely doesn't have structural (arteriosclerotic) CAD. The choices in her case are more likely esophageal spasm or coronary spasm. Remember, the wall of the coronary artery is laden with muscle and elastic fibers, and the tension in the wall of the artery, the tone, is a function of nerves that tell the muscle how much blood is needed downstream by the heart muscle. If there is inordinate tone in a segment—coronary spasm—angina will develop. It will, however, usually occur at rest and this is one of the differentiating features. Esophageal spasm usually does not occur with exertion.

Coronary spasm can be brought on by several outside influences such as cocaine, tobacco usage, or even some migraine medications. A good history is important. Since it is much more likely in women, I have discussed it extensively in Chapter 8, *Women and Heart Disease*.

In the past, we treated individuals with CAD and angina with a beta adrenergic-blocking drug, such as Inderal. These drugs are still effective, as they decrease the determinants of heart muscle oxygen demand, namely, heart rate and force of contractility. They can cause significant side effects. Because of that, we usually reserve them for those patients who have extensive CAD that can't be effectively treated with either coronary stenting or coronary artery bypass surgery—either because of age or other problems, or because of anatomy of the blockages. Sometimes we have to resort to a hybrid of treatment of coronary artery disease. For example, we either stent or bypass the vessels that are amenable, then incorporate a medical approach, decreasing oxygen demands of the heart muscle so that chest pain with exertion is kept to a minimum.

In the age of very nice results with coronary stenting in most cases, this is an early offering in the management of CAD with angina. When we become convinced that the cause of the chest pain or its equivalent is actually a blocked artery, an angiogram is performed and a stent is deployed. This almost always restores the supply-demand ratio to a happy spot and the angina goes away. This is much more preferable than just treating the symptoms of altered coronary blood supply. In the past, using bare metal stents, we were faced with a 30–40% re-stenosis rate (recurrent blockage at the site of stent deployment) due to proliferation of smooth muscle as a reaction to injury. We *always* injure the inside of the blood vessel when we deploy the stent because we are compressing a chunk of hardened debris out of the central channel of the artery into the wall and are literally recreating a wide-open channel. The reaction to that injury was case-specific and unpredictable. Now, however, with the drug-eluting stents, it is unusual to see aggressive re-stenosis at the site of stent deployment. These stents are impregnated with a cancer drug, either Taxol or Sirolimus, which is known to prevent cell replication. If cells can't replicate within the environment of the drug elution, cell proliferation cannot produce another blockage. (Some of the drug-eluting stents may clot several months after they are inserted since they don't always get covered over with a "film" of tissue like the bare metal stents do. Check with your doctor on the type of stent that is best for you.)

We deploy these stents, small stainless steel mesh devices crimped onto a balloon, at high pressure within the coronary artery. This takes a tightly blocked artery and converts it into a wide-open one, usually with a beautiful result that is predictably durable. This has clearly become the treatment of choice for high-grade plaque systems and even in obviously ruptured ones that are not obstructing flow. However, the elusive problem of which plaque will become vulnerable and rupture causing a heart attack, and which will remain stable continues to be an ongoing problem.

These patients should all be treated with aspirin and Plavix, which are strong platelet-active agents, a statin drug to regulate the cholesterol level and, frequently, an angiotensin converting enzyme-inhibitor to control blood pressure and to improve function of the inside of the blood vessel. This inside layer, the endothelium, is where the inflammatory cytokines are active, and this drug will help to settle this down and keep it happy.

Of all the medications used in the prevention of future events, a statin drug is doubtless the most important. It not only drops the LDL-cholesterol, the bad fraction, it stabilizes other plaques within the arterial circulation, whether in the carotid arteries leading to the brain, the renal arteries leading to the kidneys, or the leg vessels. It helps reduce the level of inflammation within plaque systems throughout. Remember: Plaques run in packs. If there is one vulnerable plaque, there is likely at least one more somewhere else. It is very common in someone who has had an acute coronary syndrome to find an ulcerated plaque in a carotid artery. We know now, for example, that we can reduce the incidence of stroke by using statins just as much as we can by dropping high blood pressure to normal levels, implying that plaque rupture has a lot to do with provoking a stroke. Whether we are dealing with silent coronary artery disease or silent carotid, renal, or leg-vessel arteriosclerosis, a statin drug does more than any other toward curtailing the incidence of dramatic events. We think that a great part of this action has to do with beating back the inflammatory component of this complex series of events leading to a heart attack.

Methods of further evaluation and treatment of the individual with totally silent CAD is more controversial. Over the last few years, I have fine-tuned my approach. Since all of these patients have, by definition, some degree of CAD, our first responsibility is to be sure that this is not about to lead to a calamity. Silent CAD means something entirely different in a diabetic individual, with a strong potential for having impaired pain receptors, than in a non-diabetic person. Also, individuals who have few pain receptors are not terribly uncommon. Therefore, we use the coronary calcium score in order to stratify the risk of having a tight blockage in a coronary artery.

We know that a person is at low risk of having a coronary event, such as a heart attack, if the score is less than 100. On the other hand, we know the risk of at least one coronary artery being greater than 75% blocked is substantial in those who have a score of greater than 400. This score helps greatly in determining who goes on for further testing. We treat these individuals in exactly the same fashion in trying to block further progression of CAD. In one instance, we have CAD that is severe enough that it is producing symptoms with extreme exercise. In the other category, it has not reached this level of severity. No matter what stage it is, we need to try to "freeze it in place."

If you have an unexpected coronary calcium score of 300, you should have further testing. This should be in the form of either a thallium scan, to be sure that you do not have a tight blockage that is simply not causing pain, or more likely today, a CT angiogram, which is more precise.

REMINDERS

1. Silent CAD does not have to be a killer. We need to screen asymptomatic persons who are apt to have silent disease as a result of their coronary risk factors.
2. A safe, inexpensive, and reliable test for silent CAD is the coronary calcium score. If your score is high, undergo more specific testing such as the multi-slice CT angiogram.
3. Women calcify coronary plaque less and later. If you are symptomatic or have risk factors—smoking, high LDL-cholesterol, and elevated hs-CRP—a CT angiogram should be done immediately.
4. The thallium scan should no longer be used as a screening tool for silent CAD. It's still a good test to determine if the heart muscle is starving for blood and oxygen, especially in patients who have had intervention or bypass surgery.

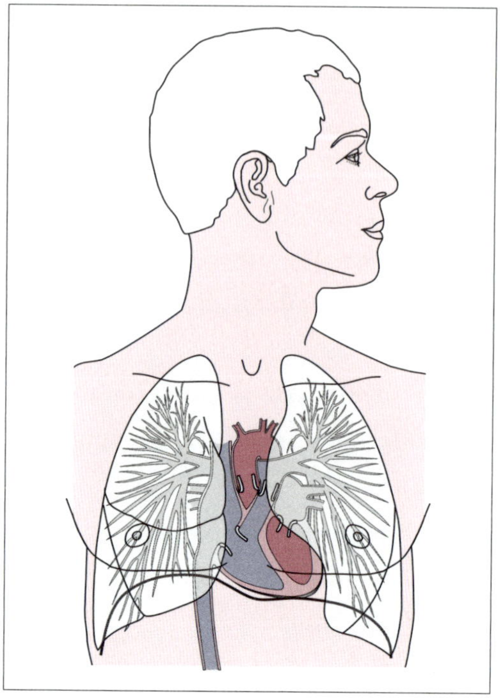

CONGESTIVE HEART FAILURE

Swelling and Fluid in the Lungs

CONGESTIVE HEART FAILURE (CHF) IS POORLY named. The term scares the bejiggers out of people. After all, when your automobile battery fails, you can't start your car and you often need the battery replaced. A failure is almost uniformly interpreted as a permanent process with no good ending.

Congestive heart failure once carried almost the same dire consequences. With the new therapeutic and electrical devices available to us, it is now a very treatable condition and can be compatible with a continued high quality of life.

CHF is already pandemic throughout the industrialized world. Currently in the U.S., there are roughly five million people with CHF! There is simply no way that physicians in this country will be able to adequately cope with the huge population of baby boomers which will ultimately develop CHF, in addition to the already large number of people who currently have it.

Two of the three causes of CHF listed above—hypertension and diabetes—can be treated and even partially prevented. The third—advanced age—obviously cannot.

Yet, of all the factors involved, advanced age is going to become ever more important in the genesis of CHF. In order to keep smiling, we must remember the humor of the great pitcher and philosopher Satchel Paige, who said, "Age is mind over matter. If you don't mind, it doesn't matter." I suspect that many of you will mind, and I know it will matter. Therefore, we'll continue our efforts to understand this age-related problem of CHF and the treatment of it.

Our paradigm for handling the ever-increasing number of people with congestive heart failure needs to change. Albert Einstein once said, "The definition of insanity is doing the same thing over and over, each time expecting a different result." With congestive heart failure, we must explore new methods, and only then can we reasonably expect a different result. One of these methods is to educate patients, empowering them to be more active participants in their cardiac care process.

Definition of Congestive Heart Failure

CHF is a process in which the left atrial or right atrial pressure is increased significantly and water is pushed out of the blood stream into the tissues. In the case of left heart failure, by far the most common, water is pushed into the lungs causing shortness of breath. In the case of pure right heart failure, water is pushed into the liver tissue causing dramatic enlargement, then into the tissues of the legs, where it is referred to as edema.

How the Heart Works: A Review

The left ventricle is the main pumping chamber of the heart. It is responsible for pumping red, oxygenated blood out the aorta to every organ in the body. Ernest Henry Starling first discovered that the heart muscle fibers contract proportionately to the amount of stretch imposed on them up to a certain point. After that threshold point, contractility diminishes as the stretch becomes excessive.

This important principle became known as the "Starling Curve." The amount of pressure and volume presented to the left ventricle is a constantly changing situation. In a youth, this filling pressure is low, between 8–10 mmHg (millimeters of mercury, the standard measurement of any bodily pressure). This doesn't change much until about age 30. Then, with advancing age, the elasticity of the left ventricle, referred to as the compliance, is reduced and the pump becomes stiffer each year. As this process marches on, the pressure necessarily exerted on the left atrium, and hence the left ventricle when the mitral valve is open, has to increase in order to stretch the muscle fibers enough for optimal contractility. In other words, the heart has to follow Starling's Curve.

Diastolic Dysfunction: The Most Common Cause of CHF (The Stiff Heart)

In an 80-year-old individual, especially if that person has had hypertension, diabetes, or a previous heart attack, the ventricle is frequently so stiff that a filling pressure of 25–30 mmHg is required to maintain optimal function of the left ventricle. The problem is that there is so little margin for increase. We usually push water across the barrier between the tiny blood vessels and the air pockets in the lungs at a pressure of 30–35 mmHg. Therefore, extra salt, which causes all of us to hold onto water, will cause this 80-year-old to push water into the air pockets, causing him to become very short of breath. This is the classic "water in the lungs" syndrome that everyone has heard about and this is also referred to as congestive heart failure. Edema refers to abnormal water accumulation. In this instance, the edema is in the lungs. If this occurs in its most severe form, called pulmonary edema, it is life-threatening.

The disturbing fact is that all of us, if we get old enough, are prime candidates for CHF based merely on the principle outlined above. That doesn't mean that our heart is necessarily failing, but it does mean that water is being pushed into the tissues because of some disturbance of normal physiology. In this case, the disturbance of normal physiology is simply a stiff heart due to aging. Now do you see why the term CHF is such a bad one? All of us will potentially have to deal with this problem if we live long enough. This is the reason we will go over principles of treatment exhaustively. I want to make the important point that CHF is dynamic and thus it is going to depend greatly on salt and water intake.

In the bulk of the population, CHF is merely going to be one of the accompaniments of advancing age. With 75 million of us turning 60 in the next few years, there are going to be a lot of people with CHF or the strong potential to develop it under the right circumstances.

There are, of course, many other causes of CHF. However, the cause I previously outlined for you, commonly referred to as diastolic dysfunction (diastole is when the ventricle is relaxed and accepts its load from the atrium), is responsible for approximately 75% of all cases. Diastolic dysfunction of the aging heart is the nemesis of the over-65 club. However, we can live with it, and we can live well!

The term CHF strikes terror in the hearts and souls of most patients. I have seen the fear in the eyes of thousands of patients over the years when they learn their diagnosis is CHF. However, just as when we were kids and heard a sound that we were sure represented the footsteps or breath of a monster outside our window, we were reassured when our parents led us outside to see that it was the branch of a willow tree brushing against the house. If you understand your disease process or simply your altered physiology, it becomes less frightening to you and you will not only cope with CHF, but you'll also learn that the term sounds scarier than living with it. You can beat it back at every turn in the road.

Hypertension and diabetes are the diseases that are most likely to increase left ventricle stiffness and cause CHF. These can cause CHF at a much earlier age than aging heart syndrome. However, if they are accompaniments of age, as they often are, they will become additive, complicating the situation and making it worse.

Hypertensive heart disease, whereby the heart muscle thickens in response to the extra burden of pumping blood against a higher pressure than is intended, is likely the next most common cause of CHF. If you lift a certain weight over and over for even ten minutes each day, the muscle mass responsible for the weight-lifting exercise will increase in size, or hypertrophy. The heart muscle frequently does the same thing. Obviously, one person will bulk up to a greater degree than another person lifting the same weight. The heart follows the same pattern. Some hearts will markedly thicken their muscle mass in response to a prevalent systolic pressure of 160 mmHg rather than a normal of 120–140 mmHg. We call this hypertensive remodeling.

A greatly hypertrophied left ventricle has been referred to as an "Arnold Schwarzenegger ventricle." Others will not hypertrophy to nearly the same degree. The thicker the heart muscle, the slower it relaxes and the higher the diastolic pressure (the pressure inside the pumping chamber when totally relaxed and filling with blood). Therefore, this person will have a high left atrial pressure and eventually, if not treated, will fill his lungs with water and become very short of breath. With any exercise, the pressure will climb even further and will result in exertional shortness of breath. Eventually, the left atrium will become larger, as it stretches in response to the higher pressure and volume it has to deal with. As this process advances, the pressure is eventually transmitted through the pulmonary vascular bed, putting the same strain on the right heart until edema develops in the tissues of the legs.

It is just now well appreciated that not only does bulk of muscle and stiffness of the ventricle play an important role in CHF, but many other mechanisms are also at play. For example, it is now well established that scar tissue is sometimes laid down between the muscle cells, the interstitium, of the pump. This is an important mechanism and can lead to fatal arrhythmias and sudden death. We are just now learning how to prevent progression of this very dangerous process. Fibrosis of the heart, this scar tissue, results in a very stiff heart, as scar tissue doesn't stretch. Since elasticity is the way the heart fills, the pressure within the left atrium goes quite high.

Diabetes causes diastolic dysfunction by an entirely different set of mechanisms, but the end result is the same. Patients with diabetes frequently have "small vessel disease." When we refer to coronary artery disease, for the most part, we are referring to the larger vessels. However, the very small vessels may also become diseased. This occurs almost exclusively in people with diabetes. These may cause tiny scarred areas of fibrosis due to blockage of one of these very small vessels. In response to these tiny little heart attacks scattered about, the left ventricle becomes stiff due to the scar tissue that is formed as a result of damage. Again, scar tissue doesn't stretch.

In fact, all of the above processes are situations with diastolic dysfunction. In other words, any process, including the mere progression of age, that tends to render the left ventricle less stretchy and distensible in its acceptance of blood, will raise the atrial pressure and potentially bring about CHF. Diastolic dysfunction can easily be considered the stiff heart syndrome. It is, by far, the most common cause of CHF.

Systolic Dysfunction as a Cause of CHF

There are also many people with heart failure who have systolic (remember, this is the contractile phase of heart action) explanations for it. These individuals all have one thing in common: They have lost muscle mass—or muscle effectiveness—by some means. The most common cause of this process is the simple heart attack. In almost all of these, a coronary artery, an artery that supplies blood to the heart muscle, has become blocked. In most instances, this process has caused the death of some of the heart muscle serviced by that artery due to oxygen starvation. Therefore, the network of interlocking heart muscle fibers has been interrupted and some degree of pump function—its squeeze—has been lost. If enough muscle is lost, the pump simply cannot move sufficient blood volume with each beat of the heart to keep the lungs clear of water.

The same situation applies to those who have experienced an invasion with a heart virus. Viruses have an affinity for certain types of cells. Just as one particular virus may produce nausea and vomiting and perhaps diarrhea, another may have an affinity for a different type of tissue, causing running nose, nasal congestion, and bronchitis. Another may cause hepatitis. Similarly, there are viruses that have an affinity for the heart cell.

They invade the heart muscle cell and cause destruction of variable numbers of cells. This is called viral myocarditis. If enough muscle cells are destroyed or stunned, a person will develop CHF. Some of these folks will have recovery of almost all of their muscle cells while others will linger on with markedly diminished contractile function and persistent CHF. This is called a post-viral cardiomyopathy. This is probably the most common cause of CHF in young people and those who have just delivered a baby, the so-called post-partum cardiomyopathy. The situation is made even more complex in such people, as they will lay down scar tissue where good, healthy muscle fibers once existed, causing diastolic dysfunction (scar doesn't stretch), as well as systolic dysfunction (loss of muscle cells). Indeed, diastolic dysfunction accompanies many situations marked by loss of systolic capacity.

Another unique cause of systolic congestive heart failure is that imposed by a leaking heart valve. This can be brought about by leakage of either the mitral or the aortic valve, leading to volume overload of the main heart pump. Eventually, muscle fibers will first stretch, then lose their intimate contractile association with other muscle cells. Finally, the over-burdened, distended left ventricle will lose its contractile function to such an extent that it cannot be reclaimed, even with valve replacement.

Other less common causes of CHF include the infiltrative diseases, such as amyloidosis and sarcoidosis, whereby these offenders replace muscle or muscle cells and are pushed away from one another so that a synchronous pumping action is altered.

Right Heart Failure

There are also instances of pure right heart failure, whereby fluid is not pushed into the lung tissue at all. The left side of things is just fine. Instead, the right heart muscle is damaged or dysfunctional with resultant accumulation of water in the tissues behind this structure. Remember, all blue blood is returned to the right atrium and is handled by the right heart pump, the right ventricle, and delivered to the lungs to pick up oxygen and leave off carbon dioxide. In reality, most right heart failure is secondary to left heart failure. In other words, the primary problem is with the left ventricle, either a systolic or a diastolic process. The build-up in pressure in the left atrium is reflected back through the lung circulation into the thin-walled right ventricle. With time, it will fail also and we recognize it as so-called right heart failure.

There are, however, plenty of causes of pure right heart failure, and it is very important to recognize these. One is pulmonary hypertension, an elevation of the blood pressure in the pulmonary artery carrying blood to the lungs. This can be in response to a connective tissue disease such as rheumatoid lung or lupus, or from so-called primary pulmonary hypertension, the cause of which is frequently unknown. Another cause of high pulmonary artery pressure that puts excessive strain on the right ventricle occurs when a massive pulmonary embolus (blood clot to the lungs) or recurrent smaller blood clots obliterate(s) much of the exchange surface of the lungs.

Still another cause is an isolated right ventricular heart attack. Pure right ventricular heart attacks are rare but do occur, and they have to be recognized and handled in a specific fashion. Right ventricular heart attacks are not rare at all when associated with left ventricular heart attacks. In fact, fully one-half of all individuals who have an inferior (bottom surface) wall heart attack, the part of the heart serviced by the right coronary artery, will have some degree of right ventricular involvement. The more right ventricular heart damage incurred, the harder the course, as the left ventricle becomes volume-starved. In other words, the damaged right ventricle can't pump adequate amounts to the left ventricle to maintain a good blood pressure.

There are other causes, but these are the most common. Any time an individual has severe edema (fluid accumulation in the abdomen and legs) but is not short of breath, these possibilities have to be considered.

Treatment of CHF

Obviously, if the accumulation of water in tissues is the main end result of CHF, the mainstay of therapy is to remove water from these same tissues. We accomplish this with diuretics or so-called water pills. Common ones are Lasix and Bumex, the "loop" diuretics that have been around for 40 years. These, in conjunction with potassium (because potassium is excreted by the kidneys when large amounts of water are lost) frequently are the only medications needed for the initial treatment of CHF. These drugs work on the elaborate tubule systems in the kidneys to allow for large quantities of water to be excreted as urine.

Historically, one of the mainstay medications used in treatment of CHF has been Digoxin. It is seldom used as a primary therapy for CHF and, at least in women, Digoxin usage in treatment of CHF increases the mortality rate. It is seldom needed unless the patient is in atrial fibrillation.

Frequently used drugs in conjunction with diuretics are beta-blockers like Inderal, Lopressor, Atenolol, and Coreg. One of the primary reasons for this is the frequent association of hypertension with CHF. Additionally, Coreg is a very fancy beta-blocker with many other properties that preserve the configuration of the ventricle; it is particularly beneficial in improving ventricular function. A large trial has shown the superiority of Coreg to other plain vanilla beta-blockers in people with CHF. Indeed, it is so effective that we refer to it as the heart failure miracle drug. There is no doubt that it is far superior to the other beta-blockers in the treatment of CHF.

Another class of drugs is the so-called ACE-Inhibitor (ACE-I) group, slang for the improbable mouthful Angiotensin Converting Enzyme-Inhibitor. These drugs block an enzyme that results in a blood pressure elevating end product. Even in people with normal blood pressures, these drugs "unload" the left ventricle by reducing its workload and dropping the filling pressure.

Additionally, the mere presence of congestive heart failure causes activation of the so-called Renin-Angiotensin-Aldosterone System (RAAS). This is a "dumb" reflex, initiated by the kidneys, that actually perpetuates the problem, causing salt and water retention along with other problems. I'm going to explain this reflex because it is so very important in the perpetuation of the endless loop of congestive heart failure.

In congestive failure, the blood feeding the tubule structure of the kidneys is inadequate. This sensitive kidney apparatus then puts out the hormone renin, which leads to the eventual production of two other compounds, both harmful. One of these, angiotensin II, is a potent vasoconstrictor—it causes small blood vessels throughout the body to get smaller—raising the blood pressure and placing even more burden on an already-struggling left ventricle. The other end compound is aldosterone, which causes the resorption of salt and water, just what the body doesn't need, as it is already water-logged. Not only that, but aldosterone in excess quantities causes the replacement of left ventricular muscle by small zones of scar tissue discussed earlier. More heart failure leads to more stimulation of this RAAS pathway. The greater the activation, the more heart failure ensues. You can see that it is not only easy but inevitable that one enters this endless loop of self-destruction—and it has to be recognized and interrupted.

Fortunately, we now have great drugs to combat this. The ACE-I drugs block one of the limbs of this dumb reflex; they block the formation of Angiotensin II. Since diabetes is frequently an accompaniment of CHF, these drugs are particularly valuable in this category as it has been shown that they preserve renal function, a problem in diabetics.

Aldosterone, the other product of this activated pathway, is blocked by an ancient drug, Aldactone. We didn't appreciate the deleterious effects of excess aldosterone production for the longest time. Now that we know its importance, the scar formation within the pump that it causes can be largely circumvented.

One of the most frustrating aspects of treatment of people with CHF lies in the fact that this is, most of all, a dynamic process. You cannot simply go see a physician, be placed on a dosage of Lasix and potassium, and think that this will forever control your CHF. If, for example, your failure is well controlled and you're leading a symptom-free existence, you can still very easily take in too much salt, hold onto water, and go right back into CHF. This is especially likely to occur if you eat out repeatedly within a small space of time. I am amazed by how salty restaurant food often is. If the chef is inadequate or if it is Chinese food, there is a possibility that a taste-enhancer called monosodium glutamate (MSG), a potent salt, is being added to the food. Salt causes you to hold onto water, and it is not unusual for someone to gain 10 or 20 pounds of water during a one-week cruise or vacation. This accumulation is an insidious process. While still taking the same dosage of diuretic you took at home, along with all of the other medications, you may suddenly develop florid CHF. And you certainly don't have to leave home to do this; it can happen right in your own house!

How to Test Yourself for Early CHF

Gravity causes water to travel to the lowest places first—it puddles. For example, the longer you are on your feet, the more water you will accumulate in the feet and ankles. Therefore, the first sign of excess fluid is finding water, or edema, in the feet usually about mid-afternoon after being up and around for several hours. It may even become a bit difficult to get your shoes back on.

Very commonly, I will ask someone with CHF if they have noticed any swelling and they will reply negatively. When I check, there is plenty of edema present.

The exam for this is embarrassingly simple. You simply pick out a point about mid-way between your knee and ankle, and press the tip of your finger against the flat surface of the large bone (the tibia) just to the inside of center. Maintain pressure for about twenty seconds. You are merely pushing any water from the tissues at the tip of your finger into the surrounding tissue. When you remove pressure, there should be no significant indentation. If there is, these tissues contain water—pre-tibial edema is present. People who live with CHF should do this daily. It takes less than thirty seconds and it will help guide your diuretic therapy. Try it on yourself. Be sure to press against the bone just a bit inside the front of your leg as the tibia lies at an angle. Soon you'll get the hang of it.

Why is this not taught to every patient with CHF? I don't have a clue! But this simple test will determine for you—on a day-to-day basis—whether your heart failure is nicely controlled or is not well controlled after all. This simple test, coupled with a daily weigh-in in your birthday suit, will give you a good day-to-day check on your volume status. If you go along blithely, you may, for example, gain four pounds of water weight over the winter holiday season without even knowing it, merely from ingesting more salt than usual. As you go into the New Year, you may gain even more. All at once, it seems you're in trouble! But it wasn't really all at once, was it? It occurred over about two weeks. However, if you had merely checked for edema and weight gain on a daily basis, you would have known it was happening and could have prevented a bad situation.

Development of Edema: What to Do About It

Since you know how to check for excess water, what do you do about it if you find that you are retaining excess water? There are basically three possible explanations: Your drugs are not effective enough; your clinical situation has changed for the worse; or, much more likely, you have somehow merely accumulated and retained salt and water. The solution is usually very simple, it can save you great emotional and physical agony, and possibly an expensive or inconvenient trip to the doctor's office or emergency room. I'll tell you what I tell my patients—but check it out with your own doctor and get approval before proceeding. My patients know to check for edema and water weight gain each day, and if they gain more than three pounds of weight over a short period of time or when they develop peripheral edema with a dent in their pre-tibial area, they take more diuretic. They usually double the diuretic for a couple of days as well as double their potassium supplement, as potassium is wasted by this enhanced elimination of water as urine. Each person who has to increase his diuretic and potassium intermittently should have sodium and potassium levels checked on one occasion to determine that this is the proper thing to do. I believe your doctors will welcome this adjunct to your care, but check with them before you do this. They will very definitely want to perform a potassium and kidney function test on you the first time you have to do this to make sure your potassium adjustments are correct and the extra diuretic is not adversely affecting your kidney function. Additionally, if you start to feel worse with this change in therapy, check with your doctor before you go any further.

What if my patients are already on fairly large amounts of diuretic drugs? There is still a good response: They use a diuretic that works on an entirely different part of the nephron in the kidney than Lasix or Bumex. Such a drug is Zaroxolyn. I routinely extend this recommendation to my patients and write on their pillboxes in large letters, BAIL-OUT MEDICINE. If they find themselves far from home, edematous and frightened, and can't think clearly, they won't have to struggle with how to manage this and head for the emergency room. They can read their label and say, "Oh yeah, the doctor told me to use this to bail out of trouble." Many use their own lingo to give them a quick read on the drug to take and when, and some put a piece of red tape on the bottle to make it even simpler. At any rate, Zaroxolyn will work quickly and effectively in many patients who are accumulating fluid despite a strong dosage of a more conventional diuretic. How long do they take it? Until there is no longer a dent when they press against the lower leg bone. I remind them that most people will require a couple of extra potassium pills during the days that they are taking Zaroxolyn. I always check my patients' electrolytes (sodium and potassium) after they have had to do this to be sure they are on track because everyone is different.

I take this emergency treatment of my patients with congestive heart failure one step farther. If this decompensation with CHF is more extreme and they wake short of breath, the quickest way to get out of trouble is to take a nitroglycerin tablet under the tongue. This promptly reduces the amount of blood returning to the heart, relieving it of its burden, and can buy the precious minutes they need to take the diuretics and allow them to start to work. Just as with nitroglycerine therapy for heart pain, they may need to take a second tablet 10–15 minutes later. This can go a long way toward preventing a pulmonary edema emergency.

What does my patient do if nothing works? He's gaining water like crazy; he's taken his bail-out medication, and he's still accumulating fluid. If he has a lot of water in the tissues in his legs and abdomen, he probably also has edema in the wall of the bowel. This can seriously impair absorption of the drug and, in this instance, he may well require a brief hospitalization for intravenous diuretics.

Treatment of CHF is a Delicate Balance

This concept of congestive heart failure being a dynamic process is very, very important. CHF is really a part of a spectrum. Imagine this: At the far right end of the spectrum is severe water overload with edema in the legs and shortness of breath due to water in the lungs. This is what we have talked about. At the far left end of the spectrum is volume contraction, dehydration. It is fairly easy to fluctuate from one extreme to the other if you're not careful. This is the very reason it is so important to take the two minutes each day to check your status. Congestive heart failure is a dynamic process!

Treatment of CHF with a diuretic always makes us search for the ideal position between these two extremes. I recently took a trip with a group of elderly folks. In fact, I was a kid in this group. One of the elderly women on that trip was very bright and accomplished and yet did something that I used to be amazed by. (I'm no longer amazed since I've seen it repeated so many times in the last 30 years.) This woman, who had chronic CHF and was on a large dosage of diuretic, developed traveler's diarrhea. She was making frequent trips to the bathroom with watery diarrhea but never stopped her diuretic. She says her doctor had forcefully told her she would need it every day for the rest of her life. After a couple of days of this, she would have made a raisin look well-hydrated. She was as dry as a stone! She came to me for advice and I stopped her diuretic, got her salty tomato juice to drink along with a fair amount of water, and advised her not to take her diuretic until she developed a slight dent in her pre-tibial area when she pressed in with her finger. She was amazed to hear you can check for water in the leg tissues. She actually helped lead to the development of this book, as she had never been told that CHF is dynamic! She certainly had no idea that she herself could monitor her current, ever-changing, situation. She was intelligent and immediately understood that water followed salt ingestion and dehydration followed protracted diarrhea, especially if she continued her diuretic. She was just faithfully following doctor's orders! Understanding the elements of checking your water volume status is key to your acknowledgement that CHF is a dynamic process, and that treatment is always a careful maneuvering on the see-saw spectrum between dehydration and CHF.

Always remember, you can check your own progress—daily. For example, not every person with CHF needs a diuretic on a daily basis. For over 30 years, I have had my CHF patients do their own pre-tibial check for excess water and they record their body weight daily to determine if they need a diuretic. At a certain point, when you have no peripheral edema and feel good and have no shortness of breath when you walk, record your weight in only your birthday suit. This is your dry weight, the weight you wish to maintain, give or take a pound or two. This, coupled with a pre-tibial check for water in the tissues and in conjunction with a taste test for salt quantities in food, will go a long way toward assuring you a safe adventure.

I have also been impressed that people are shy about requesting a low-salt meal at a restaurant. It's your money. Tell your server that your situation demands a low-salt, MSG-free meal. They will usually do their best to help you. For your own sake—remember: Congestive heart failure is a dynamic process!

Sleep Apnea and CHF

We now recognize that roughly one-half of all people with CHF also have sleep apnea. This figures out to be 2.5 million people in the United States! This is a situation marked by long periods of apnea, defined as a suspension of breathing. In the past, we thought sleep apnea was uncommon and limited to the population that was very obese. Now we think we have it figured out. There are two major groups of sleep apnea in patients with CHF: central and obstructive. The obstructive variety makes much more noise; however, it is less serious and easier to treat. If one has jowls or wattles, he or she frequently has increased adipose tissue within the oropharynx, the portion of the throat behind the soft palate that is subject to closing off with pressure, and which can fall into the back portion of the throat during deep slumber. This can obstruct the flow of air, a great deal of noise is made as a result, and the person wakes from deep sleep many times during the night. Because there is work involved in forcing air out against a collapsed airway, this variety raises the pulmonary artery pressure and brings about even more CHF.

The equally common other variety is called central sleep apnea. These individuals actually develop water in the lungs during the night. Because their blood oxygen level falls quite low, the respiratory center becomes activated and they over-breathe to get their oxygen content up. This over-breathing shuts down the respiratory center and there is a long period of apnea.

The way to learn of the presence of this common problem is to perform a sleep study, determining if there are periods during sleep when you stop breathing and if so, how many and for how long. Sometimes it's alarming when you look at the results of these tests. People with multiple prolonged episodes of apnea develop cognitive (thinking and recollection) dysfunction. They become agitated, confused, angry, and fall asleep when they are driving. It usually comes as no surprise that they develop mental disturbances since their deep slumber is so frequently punctuated by these apneic spells in which they wake constantly throughout the night. We know now that such people are also more likely to develop atrial fibrillation, a common heart rhythm disturbance, likely for the same reason.

We have learned that we can treat this problem with CPAP, Continuous Positive Airways Pressure, delivered through a machine connected to a tight-fitting mask that forces a certain volume of air into the lungs. Anytime we have an individual with CHF who develops one episode of deterioration after another, with recurrent CHF while on a good treatment program, we send the person in for a sleep study. After starting

CPAP, the patient is a different person: He or she is happier, the diuretic can usually be cut in half or discontinued, and there is much improvement from the standpoint of functional capacity, the simple measure of what can be done during the day. The obstructive form will actually turn around much more dramatically than the central variety, though they both respond. Detection and treatment are exceptionally important, as there is an increased mortality with CHF complicated by sleep apnea.

The African-American Heart Failure Trial (A-HeFT)

We cardiologists have long recognized that African-Americans were more apt than other groups to develop congestive heart failure in response to high blood pressure. This becomes doubly disconcerting when you consider that African-Americans have a disproportionate tendency to have high blood pressure. It seemed for a while that we were thwarted at every turn, as the ACE-I drugs were not as effective in African-Americans as in others. The A-HeFT trial (African-American Heart Failure Study) was performed because of these concerns, and an interesting finding emerged: This group of people with CHF, many secondary to high blood pressure, responded best to a combination of drugs, a long-acting nitrate (like nitroglycerin) plus hydralazine. These drugs both act primarily by vasodilating (enlarging) smaller arteries throughout the body, the ones we refer to as the resistance vessels. In other words, if the "tone" is higher than it should be in these millions and millions of resistance arterioles, the blood pressure is kept high. When this tone is broken, the vessels enlarge and the blood pressure falls. These individuals were also on diuretics and ACE-I drugs; however, the addition of this combination drug dramatically reduced their mortality. This is powerful data and just the sort of treatment we need to sharply reduce the detrimental influence of congestive heart failure!

Treatment of Far-Advanced CHF

There are solutions for advanced cases of CHF too. For example, we have learned that a small protein molecule called Brain-Natriuretic Peptide is present in the blood stream in markedly increased amounts in people with CHF. Understandably, we refer to this as the B-Peptide or BNP. The level of BNP is proportional to the stretch and overload of the atria. This, in turn, is roughly proportional to the degree of CHF, so we can quantify CHF by merely measuring the BNP level. For example, 300 is not bad—but 5,000 is terrible.

If there were no therapeutic solution, this finding of an elevated BNP level would be of academic interest only. However, there happens to be a great drug called Natrecor (Nesiritide) that is capable of dropping this level promptly by unloading the atria and also by promoting diuresis. It is administered by intravenous drip and it is a Godsend to those individuals who require more aggressive treatment for their CHF.

Every good cardiac program has an outpatient CHF clinic for this subset of folks with advanced CHF. My patients simply show up at their appointed time once or twice a week. They have their blood drawn to check their electrolytes and BNP level. If they have accumulated a large amount of fluid, an intravenous dosage of Lasix or Bumex will be administered. Sometimes this intensive interaction with health care providers is all that is needed for the individual with intractable heart failure to remain controlled. In the past, a large number of patients with intractable heart failure received a Natrecor infusion once or twice a week. Unfortunately, this drug is not approved for outpatient treatment of CHF. It was being given as a desperation measure for this sicker category of patients. Most cardiologists think it should be approved because it can dramatically reduce the incidence of repeated hospitalization of patients with refractory heart failure.

There was first a fear that it would shorten lives. Every single one of the patients I care for with refractory heart failure has stated emphatically that they are much more interested in quality of life, as opposed to quantity of life, at this advanced stage of CHF. Each stated, to a person, that he or she was willing to sign a waiver to that effect. There was concern that Natrecor promoted renal failure. A large clinical study failed to bear that out either. An outpatient heart failure clinic, utilizing Natrecor infusion, is expensive but, in my view, much less expensive than monthly hospitalizations for treatment of heart failure which is the case for many of these people. When Natrecor was used for outpatient management of this problem, people were able to avoid recurrent hospital stays and they had much higher-quality lives. We were only giving this drug to the sickest of the lot, those at the extreme end of heart failure, New York Heart Association functional class IV. They are a large, ever-increasing population and they deserve our finest care.

A newer form of therapy for intractable CHF is the use of a biventricular pacemaker. To qualify, one must have a blockage in the electrical circuitry within the heart. In fact, this has to be severe enough that the ventricles are contracting out of synchrony. The right and the left ventricles should contract in perfect harmony. If the conduction system is altered enough, the ventricles are like two kids in a sack race, one side making a motion, then the other. By inserting a special pacemaker that resynchronizes the ventricles, the degree of CHF is lessened considerably. I have seen dramatic improvement through the use of this device.

Sometimes a new form of therapy comes along that is inexpensive and also works. One such treatment is Aldactone, an ancient drug that has been reinvented. It prevents loss of potassium by interrupting an intricate pathway that is activated in patients with CHF. It has been around a long time, there are generic forms, and its use in low doses has been shown to improve survival in folks with CHF. Remember, we learned previously that scar tissue deposited between heart muscle fibers, myocardial fibrosis, is a dangerous phenomenon in CHF. One of the ways this happens is through the effects of aldosterone, secreted in larger amounts than needed, due to activation of a pathway as a part of CHF. In other words, aldosterone promotes fibrosis in the heart muscle—and we can block it with Aldactone for pennies a day.

Similarly, this renin-angiotensin-aldosterone pathway, activated in CHF, leads to vasoconstriction of blood vessels (makes them smaller) and increases the workload on the heart. It is a "dumb" reflex, not an uncommon entity in physiologic mechanisms gone awry. The use of ACE-Inhibitors blocks this reflex activation and dramatically improves CHF. Some people develop a chronic cough or even angioneurotic edema (shortness of breath due to swelling of the throat) with the ACE-I drugs such as Vasotec, Captopril, and Altace. Instead, these patients can use one of the Angiotensin Receptor-Blocking drugs (ARBs) such as Diovan and Avapro, which work just about as effectively to block this very bad reflex.

The Future

I have no doubt that the treatment of CHF will change markedly in the next few years. For example, we had no clue 30 years ago that Aldactone could block myocardial fibrosis, and the ACE-Inhibitors were just being discovered. It took many years before we obtained great drugs to control hypertension. Most of the drugs we use very effectively today were not even someone's dream 20 years ago.

A new form of treatment for CHF is a type of ultrafiltration that seems to be very effective and may be a good example of a new technique on the horizon for refractory heart failure. The loop diuretics that we use are now 50–60 years old and we are well aware of the kidney problems and electrolyte problems that develop with them. For this reason, we have sought different ways of treating CHF. I suspect ultrafiltration will find its true place, likely in the form of emergency treatment of decompensated DHF and, in refractory cases, perhaps in CHF clinics. It is expensive, costing about $1,000 for a single treatment. However, it is not unusual for these patients with refractory heart failure to be admitted to the hospital every 2–4 weeks with decompensation, each hospitalization costing at least $10–$20,000, so there is a certain subset of individuals for whom this will be cost-effective—and better than trying to control the fluid just with loop diuretics. It is not going to be for the majority of the five million Americans with CHF. Whatever form it takes, you can bet there will continue to be great new advances in the treatment of CHF. Until they get here, I hope this book, outlining the principles of congestive heart failure, as well as learning how I monitor and treat my patients, helps you stay out of trouble.

REMINDERS

1. Congestive heart failure is not a death sentence. You can learn to live happily and comfortably with it.
2. CHF is a dynamic and individual process. Your day-to-day requirement of diuretic may change.
3. To detect accumulated water in your legs, press your finger against the flat bone (the tibia) just to the inside of the front part of your leg, midway between the knee and the ankle. Press for 20 seconds, then run your finger down your leg. If you have a sizable dent in the tissue, you're carrying excess water.
4. If my patients develop edema in the legs or an increase in shortness of breath, they know to double their diuretic and potassium for a couple of days until it clears.
5. My patients with CHF carry a drug called Zaroxolyn, a potent diuretic that works at a different site in the kidney than more conventional diuretics. It is their "bail-out" drug. If their conventional drugs are not working and they have edema, they take a Zaroxolyn daily for a couple of days. This can prevent a hospital trip for pulmonary edema.
6. Rather than getting into a desperate situation when nothing is working, consult with your doctor and have your electrolytes checked.

7. If you have intractable CHF, ask your doctor about Natrecor treatments, ultrafiltration, or possible implantation of a biventricular pacemaker.
8. If you have difficult-to-control CHF, ask your doctor about obtaining a sleep study. Many people with CHF have sleep apnea and many people with sleep apnea have CHF. No matter which came first, CPAP will dramatically improve your quality of life if you have this problem.

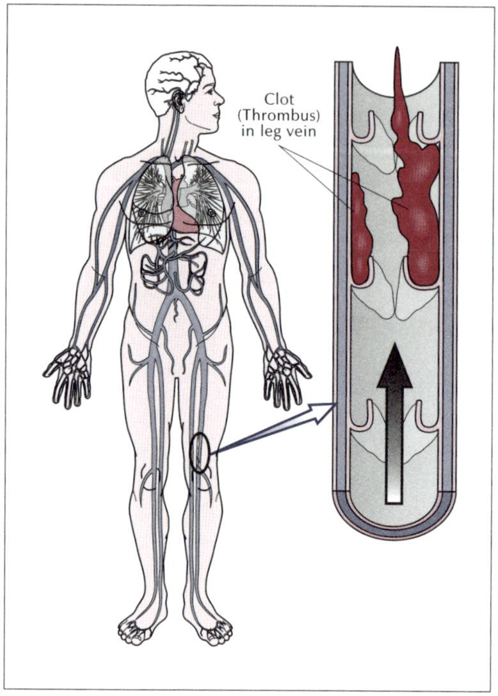

19 DEEP VENOUS THROMBOPHLEBITIS AND PULMONARY EMBOLISM

Blood Clots in the Leg Veins That Travel to the Lungs

ONE OF THE MOST DIFFICULT BLOOD VESSEL problems to diagnose early in its course is that of *deep venous thrombophlebitis* (DVT). This is basically thrombus (clot) formation in the deep veins, usually of the legs, but sometimes of the pelvic veins. The deep veins are the major conduits for blood return to the heart. Any clot that forms in these large vessels may wreak havoc in two ways:

1. By so completely obstructing the venous drainage system that fluid accumulation develops in the limb or
2. By getting loose from its attachments in the vein, traveling through the chambers of the heart, to finally lodge in the blood vessels leading to the lungs.

It is important to refine the definition of DVT and distinguish it from other terms. One term to which everyone is accustomed is *phlebitis*. Former President Richard Nixon lived with phlebitis for years. Phlebitis is *inflammation* of any vein. This is commonly a problem of the superficial veins, usually one that has deteriorated due to breakdown of the valve system, and a varicosity has formed. Superficial phlebitis is not dangerous. What we are talking about in this chapter is *deep venous thrombophlebitis*, a type of phlebitis in the deep drainage veins. Taken literally, this means a clot-forming inflammatory disorder within the veins lying deep within the tissues. This distinction is extremely important: **There is no way a clot within a superficial vein, those running just under the skin that sometimes show through it, can get loose and go to the lungs; a clot in the deep system can.**

Unique Structure and Function of Veins

Remember that the veins are very different from arteries. Arteries, which carry red or oxygenated blood to all the structures of the body, are muscular, elastic conduits. Veins, on the other hand, carry blue blood from which oxygen has been removed by the tissues. They are flimsy thin-walled structures. The larger of them possess v-shaped *valves*. (See Figures 5 and 6 on pages 30 and 31)

Arterial flow down the legs, feeding the tissue along the way, is under considerable pressure from the pulsatile force generated in the pumping chamber of the heart. This pressure is roughly the same as that obtained by a blood pressure cuff around the arm. Blood flow (blue blood) returning to the heart via the veins is a totally different process. Blood flow in veins is primarily due to a milking effect exerted by squeezing of the muscle groups surrounding the thin-walled venous structures. The pressure within the veins is quite low (approximately 5mmHg compared to the 120–140 mmHg in the arterial conduits). Therefore, when a muscle group contracts, blood is milked back toward the heart and the venous valves open, allowing unimpeded movement of blood. When a volume of blood moves along, the valves close, trapping the column of blood within that segment of vein.

Causes of DVT

If you have no discernible muscle contractility for a protracted period of time, venous return to the heart occurs solely due to persistent pressure of arterial flow, sending more and more blood to the extremity. The continuous volume of blood coming incessantly to the limb results in very slow venous return, simply through the principles of hydraulics. In other words, red blood keeps coming insistently—its force will push some blue blood back towards the heart. This is one of the ways edema develops in a limb that is immobile for a long stretch of time: Blood is being constantly pumped to the limb under pressure, but no muscle squeeze is returning this blood back to the heart. Due to this rather static situation, with increased pressure within the gravity-dependent part, water is pushed out of capillaries into the soft tissues of the limb. All of you who have developed edema on a long plane ride when you dosed off in a cramped space know exactly what I'm talking about.

For example, if you make a trans-Atlantic flight that takes twelve or so hours and you sleep for eight hours with your legs in a low-level position, blood pools in your legs and you are more prone than usual to develop deep venous clots. This tendency is aggravated by the fact that a large number of people travel in a volume-depleted or dehydrated condition. This basically concentrates the blood.

This tendency to clot is exacerbated in people who have had prior breakdown of the valves in the legs, producing venous stasis (pooling, sluggish flow) due to varicosities. People who have superficial varicosities due to degeneration of the walls of their superficial veins probably are slightly more likely to develop clot in their deep veins. Clot in the superficial veins cannot embolize (become dislodged and travel). However, clots from the deep veins can embolize and, indeed, frequently do.

Now that everyone has cancelled their long-anticipated overseas vacation, let's dig deeper into the mysteries of the leg vein. First, understand that we are all continuously forming clot and continuously breaking down clot. If these both occur at an identical rate, as they should, our clotting system is said to be in homeostasis (equal opposing forces). If one or the other process becomes dominant, trouble is in store.

What could set the stage for accentuated clotting? In day-to-day life, the most common cause is recent surgery. Folks who have surgery of any type activate their clotting mechanism. This is simply a built-in mechanism to protect against bleeding when trauma of any variety occurs. If we did not have this, any blunt trauma during the day would cause us to bleed out. The only way we can perform surgery is because of this reflex activation of the clotting process. This mechanism doesn't differentiate between stopping the bleeding from the excision of a tumor somewhere in the body and the formation of a clot in the leg. In other words, we can't selectively activate only a portion of our clotting mechanism, so any surgical procedure puts us at some risk of forming DVT. This is the reason that all post-operative patients are placed in intermittent compression devices to help "milk" the venous drainage back to the heart, simulating the compression that muscle groups routinely perform during walking.

If the clotting mechanism is activated by trauma, it stands to reason that trauma can also lead to DVT, especially if the trauma is incurred to a lower extremity. Prolonged immobilization is a particularly potent cause of DVT in these patients as well.

DVT doesn't just occur in patients with surgery or trauma, though they do constitute a large percentage. Elderly patients hospitalized with pneumonia or congestive heart failure also constitute a huge number of patients who are at risk of DVT. In the case of congestive heart failure, they may well have a lot of water in the peripheral tissues of the lower extremities. Flow may be sluggish, a known accelerant of clot formation.

Because we know that trauma, illness, and surgery all cause activation of the clotting mechanism, DVT always lurks just beneath the surface as a potential complication. In fact, we commonly place all such patients on low-dose fractionated Heparin, a drug that prevents clotting, just as soon as feasible to help prevent DVT.

What about the person who just walks in off the street with absolutely no obvious predisposition for DVT but has a swollen leg and turns out to have a lower extremity venous system chock-full of clot? This is a totally different story and always raises a red flag about the possibility of a malignancy lurking somewhere in the body. In reality, probably no more than 10% of these patients really turn out to have a problem, but we must always be attuned to that possibility if there is no other apparent reason for the DVT.

There are several tumors that are notorious for activating the clotting system. The most common are renal cell cancer, pancreatic and prostate cancer, some lung tumors, and finally, a brain tumor called *glioblastoma multiforme*. The search for a hidden malignant tumor is tailored to the clinical appearance and presentation of the patient with DVT. If someone presents with limited DVT, we don't launch an all-out effort to look for an occult malignancy. However, if a person has extensive DVT, especially if it is in both legs with no obvious cause, we look pretty hard for a hidden tumor.

There is also a group of people who have a particular predisposition toward spontaneous DVT due to accelerated clot formation. Not only that but when they have surgery, trauma, or a severe illness, they are at great risk for aggressive DVT. They have this peculiar tendency because their thrombotic (clotting)/thrombolytic (clot breakdown) system is out of whack. Remember, we are all clotting and breaking down clot every second of every day. This process needs to be in perfect balance. We have identified several syndromes consisting of enhanced clotting mechanisms. These are always out of balance in such people, but they get along with it until there is some event that triggers greater-than-normal clotting. We can measure specific markers in the bloodstream, looking for the existence of one of these disorders. The ones we know about are antiphospholipid antibody syndrome, Protein C and Protein S deficiency, antithrombin III deficiency, lupus anticoagulant, and Leiden Factor V mutation.

When I was a cardiac fellow in the 1970s, we occasionally saw patients who were excellent candidates for coronary artery bypass surgery, and they would receive a nice operation. They would then proceed to clot off one bypass graft after another, eventually dying from the process. It turns out that early graft thrombosis is a marker for possible hypercoagulation syndrome or, more correctly, a thrombophilic (clot affinity) disorder, such as those listed. These disorders pose special importance from several standpoints. Finding one of these helps explain otherwise enigmatic aggressive clotting. Additionally, family members need to be screened to see if they have the same disorder and need careful surveillance for DVT or other clotting disorders, such as a thrombotic stroke. Finally, the people who have one of these clotting disorders require substantially higher anticoagulation parameters, more aggressive treatment, than the person with a normal clotting system.

Diagnosis of DVT and PE

There is basically only one clinically feasible test used in the detection of DVT: the venous Doppler. It incorporates the principles of ultrasound, bouncing sound waves off the structures in the legs. From this, we can map the architecture of the veins, including any clot within a vein. We can follow the vein upward, assessing the extent of the clot, and whether or not it is obstructing flow. We can trace the veins draining the lower extremities all the way up to the groin and just a bit beyond; however, we cannot always investigate the large veins in the pelvis. The other location where clots hide out, especially in women who have had children, or men who have had prostate cancer, are the pelvic veins, and we can't predictably explore this system with Doppler.

A. The Spectrum of DVT: From Silent to Obvious

Since clot more commonly develops in the leg veins, I'm sure it seems that the diagnosis of DVT would be quite apparent. A physician will theoretically just examine the legs of the patient each day looking for swelling that might indicate that venous blood is prevented from readily returning to the heart. If a leg becomes swollen, a Doppler test is performed, looking for a clot within the lumen of the vein. If a clot is found to be present, the patient is given a drug to prevent further clot formation.

Alas, the surveillance end of things is not that simple. To point out just how sneaky this disease really is, if we only diagnose the obvious cases, about 75% of all DVT will be missed! It is frequently the most silent of diseases, as many of these are subtle and sub-clinical until they really cause a big problem.

Let me explain. If the entire venous drainage from the leg were obstructed from clots, it would be inexcusable to miss it, as the leg will become huge due to trapped blood and water in the tissues. The leg becomes *suffused*, engorged with blood, blue in color because there is spent unoxygenated blood trapped within it, and it is usually quite painful. These are certainly easy enough to detect. However, in many instances, the clot develops insidiously and doesn't really obstruct blood flow. A clump of clot material is merely sitting within the lumen of the vein, but blood is still able to make its way relatively unimpeded to the right heart. There is absolutely no external evidence of a clot in a leg such as this, even though a serious problem is brewing! Several things can happen to the clot: It can remain small and undetected, grow in size until it blocks return of blood from the leg, or break loose. The latter is the problem we all fear and dread.

B. Pulmonary Embolism

If that non-obstructive clot suddenly breaks loose from its moorings to the venous wall, it will travel to the right heart, into the pulmonary artery, ultimately landing somewhere in a small branch supplying lung tissue. (Figures 15a and 15b) This is called a *pulmonary embolus* (PE). Remember, an embolus is just a clot that has been formed in one place and then travels to another. In this instance, the clot formed in the leg vein and traveled through the right side of the heart to the lung circulation.

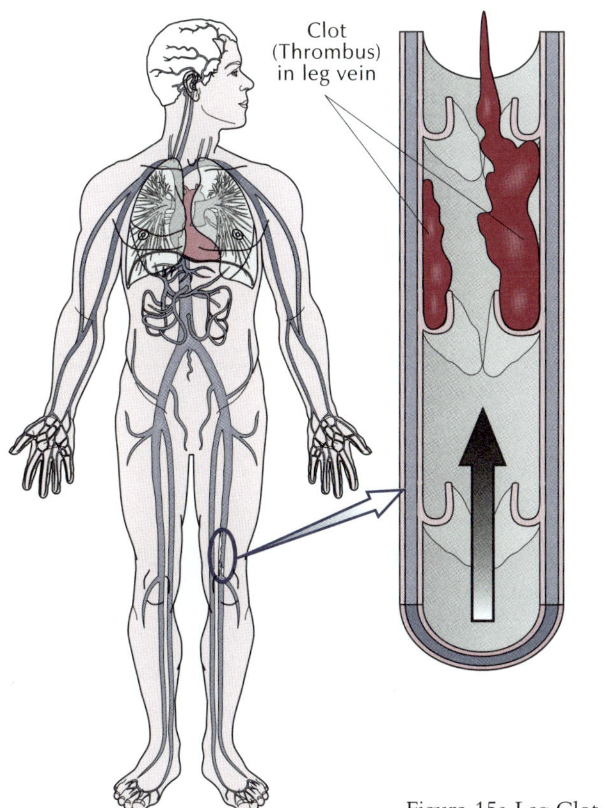

Figure 15a Leg Clot

Logically, one would think that a pulmonary embolus would always cause severe symptoms, such as intense pain or severe shortness of breath. If the clot is large or if it breaks up into many tiny pieces producing a "shower" of pulmonary emboli, it usually causes the acute onset of serious symptoms. However, in a surprisingly significant number of people, the event of pulmonary embolism is remarkably silent.

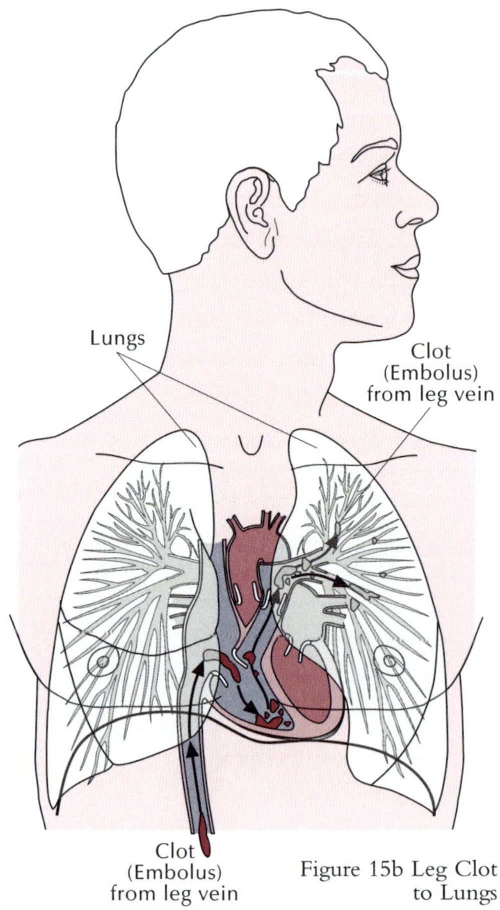

Figure 15b Leg Clot to Lungs

Keep in mind that many of the people who endure this process have undergone surgery, experienced trauma, or have an overwhelming illness of some variety. As a consequence, they are quite possibly receiving potent analgesics. Some are elderly and possibly confused. They are likely to be in some stage of already-compromised, moderately miserable existence at the time of this event. As we talk about something like this, it would seem that anything like a blood clot to the lung would immediately catch our attention. But many of the people who have these are not at their best, and something that would ordinarily cause them concern goes unrecognized as a threatening development. Therefore, these people are at the complete mercy of their doctor's observations. However, even in people who are alert, attentive, mobile, and going about their lives, the process of DVT and even PE can be very silent indeed.

The pain caused by a pulmonary embolus is located within the chest and is *pleuritic* in nature. Pleurisy means pain that is aggravated by taking a deep breath. The clot within the bloodstream meanders about, directed by turbulence. It travels as far as it can go and lodges in a branch carrying blue blood to lung tissue so oxygen can be picked up by the hemoglobin molecule within the red blood cell. The size of the branch it lodges in is dependent upon how large the clot is. Like the branches of a tree, the pulmonary arterial branches get smaller and smaller the farther out they go. If the clot is small or if a large clot breaks up into fragments as it makes its way through the heart, careening off the walls as it makes the corners, it frequently lodges in one of the distal branches causing destruction of lung tissue served by that artery. This is the cause of the pleuritic pain. It may also cause the formation of bloody sputum, as the person actually coughs up destroyed lung tissue! Such a person almost always becomes short of breath when this happens, sometimes desperately so.

If the embolus is large, it may lodge in one of the central pulmonary arteries, acutely raising pulmonary pressures. The right ventricle of the heart is thin-walled and, as such, is not prepared to handle this dramatic rise in pressure. The right heart strain from a large clot producing a high pressure, can even result in shock—a very low blood pressure. This low blood pressure may be, and usually is, due to two mechanisms:

1. The right ventricle acutely decompensates; it is unable to handle the pressure and its muscle loses much of its pump function.
2. The clot burden is blocking the flow of blood to the lungs, and therefore to the left ventricle. Since it is the main pumping chamber responsible for causing forward flow of blood to all of the organs, it can't do its job as it becomes "volume-starved."

This is a deadly duo that frequently leads to sudden vascular collapse and death. Famed author Truman Capote died in just this manner. This is truly such a medical emergency that we frequently give the patient Heparin to initiate breakdown of the clot, and then go directly to the catheterization laboratory. As we go on our way, we instruct the hospital pharmacy to mix a thrombolytic agent, a "clot-buster," as we must somehow restore blood flow to the extent that the patient has a reasonable blood pressure and can receive enough oxygen to maintain life.

In this life-threatening instance, I frequently go from a groin vein with a catheter, advance it in to the main pulmonary artery, and actually try to agitate and mechanically break up the main portion of the clot that is obstructing blood flow. This allows for better oxygenation, removes much of the pressure from the right ventricle, allowing it to recoup its function, and gets enough blood through the pulmonary circulation to the left ventricle that the blood pressure rises to a life-sustaining level. I feel sure that I have saved a few patients from death, from oxygen-starvation, and from shock using this technique.

Obviously, just as soon as the clot-buster drug arrives from the pharmacy, it is dripped right on top of the clot to disperse it as quickly as possible. These patients are always at death's door and could not possibly tolerate another embolic insult to the lungs. Therefore, I always use a filter device in the inferior vena cava. This *inferior vena cava* filter will catch a clot that escapes the leg or pelvic veins and is on its way to the pulmonary artery. In such a patient, it is important to continue acute therapy with a drug to prevent further clot formation, and break up and disperse the clot in the lung arteries. If those clots, the pulmonary emboli stuck in various branches serving the lung tissue, organize and become rigid, they will continue to restrict blood flow through these structures. This is harmful in two ways:

1. They will decrease the available lung surface for gas exchange and the person will be forever oxygen-starved.
2. The pulmonary pressure may well not return to anywhere near its normal level.

To illustrate just how silent pulmonary embolism can be: A very prominent cardiologist died of this problem. He was lecturing in Europe a number of years back and noticed that he got winded while sightseeing. He wrote it off to jet lag and age. It got progressively worse over the next week, but he had no swelling in the legs and had no pleurisy. Assuming it was nothing serious, he went on with his lecture tour. When he arrived back in the U.S., he was still aware of shortness of breath and finally had tests. Indeed, he had extensive DVT in both legs and had experienced multiple pulmonary emboli throughout the lungs. The clots had by then organized as dense rubbery casts, attaching themselves to the walls of the pulmonary arterial branches. This extensive network of organized clots decreased the surface exposure of the lung tissue so much that gas exchange (oxygen and carbon dioxide) was compromised and more importantly in his case, the pulmonary pressure was double its normal level. This placed a huge burden on the right ventricle, which was unable to compensate for this kind of pressure load. The right ventricle, thin-walled and unable to adjust quickly to pressure changes, has a maximal workload capacity. If this is exceeded, it just poops out. His right ventricle ultimately failed and this world-renowned cardiologist died. The irony of his particular disease and its outcome is that he had detected it in many others and had frequently lectured about its silent course. It was one of his major research interests, yet he failed to recognize it when it threatened *him*. Life is frequently not fair. However, the real lesson here is the silent, insidious nature of this process—what this inordinately articulate gentleman referred to on rounds one day as the *silent scream* of the patient with shortness of breath, long before this label was also appropriately used for those with severe depression.

There are two scans that can be used to detect pulmonary emboli. One is the age-old lung scan, using a radioactive tracer. This takes awhile and clots can be missed if the individual has significant lung disease, such as emphysema, that has destroyed tissue. The other is a spiral CT scan of the chest. It is quick and detects large clots easily, but may miss small clots lying within small peripheral pulmonary artery branches. We usually utilize the spiral CT scan as a screening test. As with many relatively silent diseases that impose huge punishments if missed, we must order about 20 such tests before we obtain a positive one. We need better screening tools. We usually use a lower-extremity Doppler as a routine screening tool, then check a spiral CT of the chest if the Doppler is positive for a clot. However, particularly in women, there is risk of clot within the pelvic veins and we have no reliable way to find these. Therefore, we wind up having to utilize the spiral CT scan of the chest more frequently than we would like. The cost, if you miss a pulmonary embolus, is just too great to pay for the next one may have tragic consequences.

Genetic Influence in DVT?

Why don't we all develop DVT when we travel? Beats me! I've gone to sleep with my legs in the same position for up to eight hours and didn't, to my knowledge, develop DVT. I think this has a great deal to do with muscle tone and exercise level, presence or absence of breakdown of the venous valves, state of hydration, and several other factors we don't completely understand.

I also think there may be somewhat of a genetic predisposition to it. I'm not exactly talking about one of the aggressive clot-formation disorders that we have already covered—the thrombophilic disorders. I'm talking about a relative predisposition to event-provoked DVT. For example, years ago I took care of an elderly man who walked into the clinic with chronic shortness of breath. He had, for no obvious reason, a non-occlusive clot in the deep veins in his right thigh. He also had evidence of recurrent (or a shower of) pulmonary emboli. I placed an inferior vena cava filter and put him on anticoagulant therapy. Three years later, his daughter came to see me with mild shortness of breath. She had the same thing in the same area of the same leg with multiple PE, just like her father. One situation does not make a syndrome. However, I have seen enough variations on this theme to make me suspicious that there is a genetic predisposition, even if we are unable to pick it up by blood tests.

Difficulty with Monitoring for DVT

In the hospital setting we are constantly monitoring the patient for development of DVT. Yet you can check a Doppler on a Tuesday and find it normal only to have the patient with trauma, surgery, heart attack, pneumonia, or any one of the other diseases known to predispose to DVT, develop such a process on Wednesday. In short, DVT and pulmonary embolism constitute a syndrome that has become known as one of the "silent killers" because they so often come on like a thief in the night. If I'm right and there is a genetically endowed proclivity for developing DVT, we would likely deploy an inferior vena cava filter in those within this vulnerable population who have either an illness, complicated surgery, or trauma that would expose them to a greater-than-usual risk of DVT and a potential calamity.

Birth Control Pills and DVT/PE

A word should be mentioned about birth control pills (BCP) and DVT. There is no question that BCP therapy in predisposed individuals helps bring about DVT. I just saw a 26-year-old mother of two, happily married, who was taking birth control pills and developed a large, swollen leg abruptly without apparent provocation. This usually happens in young women who also smoke, but this lady was a non-smoker. She was slender and exercised daily. I ordered the appropriate tests and she was treated aggressively with Heparin. It turned out that she had a Leiden Factor V mutation and this had predisposed her to DVT. She might have developed DVT anyway, but I strongly doubt it. In young women, the combination of cigarette smoking and birth control therapy seems to particularly predispose to DVT. Through the last 30 years, I have consistently seen one or two a year. All of these patients need a thorough laboratory survey to be sure they do not have a malignancy and to rule out a thrombophilic clotting disorder.

Treatment for DVT and Pulmonary Embolism

First, let me make it clear that DVT can occur as a very aggressive process that doesn't ever result in a pulmonary embolus if none of the clot gets dislodged from its venous anchor. The presence of DVT mandates the use of Heparin, either in a crude form or in a more sophisticated form, a fractionated derivative known as Lovenox. This is the only drug that has been shown to prevent progressive clot formation. In the young lady discussed above, I made it clear that she should be on Heparin for a full week to ten days. Her admitting physician came along, told her I was "old-fashioned," and sent her home on Coumadin after only two days of Heparin. If I was "old-fashioned," it was because I perhaps was not aggressive enough. I think, in retrospect, I should have used thrombolytic therapy, the clot-buster drug, in conjunction with a device that we can direct into the venous system to enable us to agitate the clot material, so that the device can vacuum it out. It doesn't get rid of all the clot material, but it does open the vein enough to allow good blood flow. The blood flowing through the system will then erode away the rest of the clot and the result is usually good. The admitting physician also nixed this notion. Her menses were due "any minute" and there was, of course, a chance that I could make her bleed excessively.

Normally, in patients like this with extensive DVT in the thigh vessels we do use thrombolytic therapy, not Heparin, as such patients are at high risk of being stuck with a post-phlebitic limb for the rest of their lives if the clot doesn't disperse. This is a limb that is persistently swollen, painful, and discolored following extensive DVT. It is due to chronic congestion of the limb with blue blood that has a difficult time getting back to the right heart because an old rigid clot has formed as a molded cast within the vein. It is such a crippling process that we do everything within our power to prevent it.

The young lady mentioned above, who was dismissed from the hospital during my absence, came back into the clinic a few days later with just such a huge swollen leg, the venous drainage severely limited by organized thrombus despite Coumadin therapy. I fear that she will wind up with a post-phlebitic limb. I deployed an inferior vena cava filter to prevent sudden cardiovascular collapse in the event a huge chunk got loose, as the clot had now increased in size all the way up the venous drainage system of the leg into a portion of the vena cava, the huge blood tube carrying all used blood back to the heart. The clot in the leg veins was, by now, too mature to be effectively dispersed. The lesson here is to never, never, ever give in if you are absolutely sure you are right. This will serve us in good stead in life no matter which field we are in! I actually abide by this rule; I just wasn't in a position to override the wishes of the attending physician.

This rather poorly managed case does serve one purpose: It points out the way therapy should be done, as well as what the consequences may be if we don't do it right.

To summarize acute treatment of DVT, we use Heparin or Lovenox if the process is not terribly extensive. For example, if the DVT is contained to the deep veins behind or below the knee, we feel comfortable using one of these drugs, as we feel that we can clean up the clot. In the event one gets loose, it will be small enough that it will not result in death should it lodge in a pulmonary artery branch. On the other hand, if the DVT is quite extensive, extending from the knee up into the thigh and especially into the iliac vein just above the groin, these clots are more dangerous and treatment should be tailored to match this danger. The dangers are crippling post-phlebitic limb syndrome, which we have discussed and, more urgently, the risk of a huge pulmonary embolism that might take a life. In this instance, we utilize thrombolytic therapy. If there is evidence of a pulmonary embolus when we first see the patient, or subsequently while on therapy, we quickly deploy an inferior vena cava filter. (Figure 16, page 196)

Extensive DVT: Prevention of Life-Threatening Pulmonary Embolism

About the only vascular procedure available, but performed less frequently than it really should be, is inferior vena cava filter deployment. This has been sanctioned by the powers-that-be only in cases of recurrent pulmonary embolism while the patient is being treated with an anticoagulant. *This is crazy!* If you knew, for example, that your thigh veins were chock-full of clot, would you want to wait for the "big one" before a filter was deployed? I think not. Placement of an inferior vena cava filter is very safe in most circumstances, and the modern version can be readily removed through a catheter inserted through the skin (not surgically) at some later date if desired. I have actually never seen a problem from a chronic filter, so I leave them in place unless patients are well past the threat of PE and want the filter removed because they are worried about it.

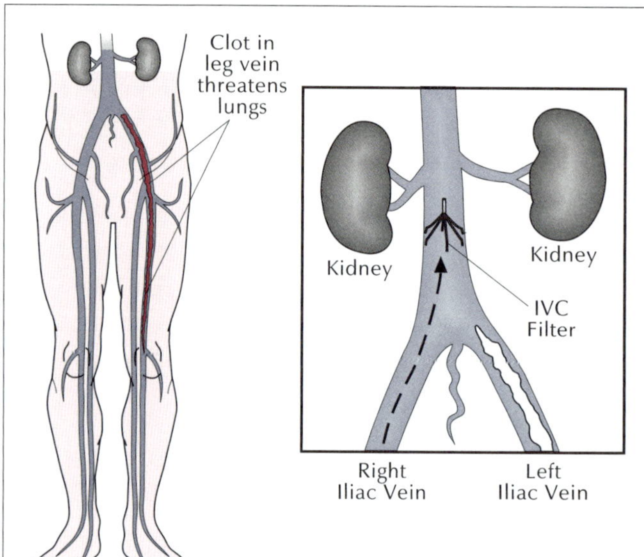

Figure 16 Catching Escaped Clot

These filters are also of great importance in the care of patients who are at high risk of developing DVT but are, for some reason, not a candidate for anticoagulation. For example, we see a lot of head and neck trauma patients who are quadriplegic. Many of them are not expected to make a full recovery and the rehabilitation process is slow and arduous. They routinely lie flaccid in bed for weeks to months. We can't perform daily Doppler tests on them, yet they pose the highest risk for DVT and PE because of trauma, absence of muscle tone, and surgery. We routinely deploy a vena cava filter in such individuals.

Chronic Treatment After DVT: With or Without Pulmonary Embolism

Following an event, whether just DVT or PE as well, the patient should remain on Coumadin anticoagulant therapy for at least three months. If the patient has one of the more threatening thrombophilic processes, they should probably never come off

Coumadin. Remember, a thrombophilic process is one of the clot-forming disorders that is present when you are making a clot much faster than you are breaking it down. Many of these are inherited disorders and such an individual will, therefore, always be susceptible to the dangers of clot formation. We adjust the dosage of Coumadin through the use of the Prothrombin Time (the Protime). In the past, every country had different standards and levels of measurement; now it is standardized worldwide and we refer to it as the INR. We routinely maintain this in the 2.0 to 2.5 range for DVT, but it should be kept around 3.5 in those individuals with an inherited or acquired increased tendency to clot. In a stable situation, we follow the Protime monthly; however, in difficult-to-control situations, we may have to measure this weekly.

For long-term patients, I feel strongly that the patient should have his or her own Protime instrument. The cost is about $600 but no one cares about you like you do, and the cost is usually partially or completely picked up by the insurance company or Medicare. Additionally, the methods medical professionals have of tracking patients on Coumadin is overwhelmed. A typical situation for people on Coumadin therapy is for them to go to the physician's office and have their blood drawn. In some instances it is sent out of that office to a laboratory. The lab then faxes or couriers over a copy of the results to the physician's office and the nurse looks at your chart to determine the range where the physician wants to maintain the INR. She then determines any dosage change and gets in touch with the patient. This can be a harrowing experience, especially if the result is sky-high and we're worried that the patient might hemorrhage; or if the result is very low, we are worried that the patient might clot. Additionally, there are six steps involved with risk of a mistake with each step.

Most cardiologists either have their own lab or send the patients to an anticoagulation clinic. Still, there are phone calls to make—with all the attendant risks inherent in a system where intricate numbers are handled repeatedly—and discussions are necessary. Alternatively, if you are on Coumadin long-term, we can provide you with an adjustment table so that you can adjust your own dosage, run the test inexpensively as frequently as necessary to provide you with peace of mind, and there is no danger of a mistake through interpretation of data or communication. Most of the terrible mishaps I see in individuals on Coumadin have to do with communication problems. I want my own machine if I ever need to go on Coumadin chronically. I know one cardiologist who has to remain on Coumadin life long. He checks his Protime every three days. He is a compulsive sort and keeps his anticoagulation right on the money.

REMINDERS

1. Don't travel long distances without moving your legs; get up frequently and walk about. This "milks" the venous blood back toward your heart and reduces the chances of developing clots in the deep veins of your legs.
2. If you can't get up frequently, flex your feet against the floor. This does much the same thing as walking, just not quite as efficiently.
3. If you develop unexplained swelling of a lower extremity, especially if on only one side, see your doctor and have a Doppler analysis to rule out DVT.
4. If you develop shortness of breath, pleurisy, or cough up bloody sputum, see your doctor so DVT with PE can be ruled out (or in).
5. If you are on Coumadin and expect to be on it for more than six months, consider purchasing your own Protime-testing machine. Ask your physician for a prescription so your insurance company or Medicare will take care of the bulk of the cost. No one will take care of you like you will!
6. If you have a first-degree relative who has had unexplained DVT or PE, consider asking for a blood test to make sure you do not have a thrombophilic (clot-forming tendency) disorder. This could save your life.

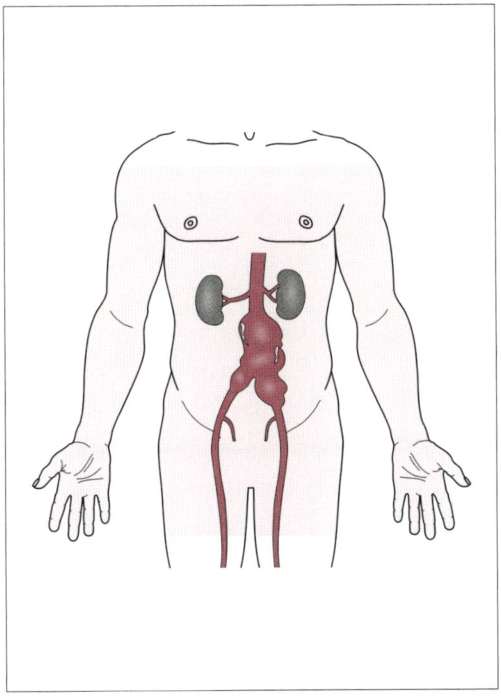

13 AORTIC ANEURYSM

Ballooning of the Wall of the Aorta

POSSIBLY ONE OF THE SCARIEST STATEMENTS a physician can make is to tell a person that he or she has an aneurysm of the aorta. Not only have most people heard the term, but almost everyone has known someone who had one and who died when it ruptured. Therefore, it is important to approach this topic with caution and reassurance.

As doctors, we need to emphasize education and awareness. So many people die of coronary artery disease in the United States that we may have failed in our public education of the less common—but significant—threat of aortic aneurysm. It has traditionally occupied the number 15 spot on the list of causes of death in the U.S. It now stands at number 11, probable testimony to a longer life span. Our public awareness campaign should be made easier by the fact that coronary artery disease, heart attack, and aortic aneurysm share many of the same risk factors. I am amazed when people come in with an overabundance of arteriosclerotic risk factors (those causing "hardening of the arteries" due to cholesterol deposits within the wall of an artery) and a family history of aneurysm formation in a close relative, but haven't considered that their family history has predisposed them to the significant likelihood of developing an aortic aneurysm.

Definition

An aneurysm means there is an out-pouching in the wall of the aorta. This can be saccular, a well-delineated process like a simple rotund party balloon, or fusiform, more of a tubular enlargement resembling a balloon that a clown might use at a party for constructing stick figures. Some are so complex that they comprise an admixture of the two but usually one form or the other prevails. Frequently, if the aneurysm is large, it will contain layered clot along the wall of the aorta. This clot seldom gets loose and embolizes to a downstream vessel in the leg.

Causes of Aortic Aneurysms

Aortic aneurysms are due to a combination of factors. They can be due to hemodynamic stress from the force of blood flowing through the aorta, creating zones of turbulence as it does, and a fault in the integrity of the wall of the aorta. Every single person is constantly bombarded by pressure against the wall of the aorta, yet only a small percentage of individuals develop aneurysms. This strongly implicates a predisposition toward developing such a ballooning of the aortic wall in those who go on to form an aortic aneurysm.

Who is at risk? Probably the biggest single risk factor is having a close family member who has had one. If your father or mother had an *abdominal aortic aneurysm* (AAA), for example, you should at some point have an abdominal aortic ultrasound to determine whether or not you have the beginnings of one. This should be done in men at about age 40 and in women at about age 50. Having a first-degree relative with an AAA is such a high risk that it cannot be ignored.

This doesn't mean you have to develop an AAA if your mother or father had one. Other risks factors are high blood pressure, an elevated cholesterol, diabetes, and cigarette or cigar smoking, most of which can be prevented or treated.

There is such a strong association of diffuse arteriosclerosis (generalized lipid deposition) in individuals with aortic aneurysm that we must assume it plays a strong role in the eventual formation of the aneurysm. I feel that the primary abnormality is one of an abnormal aortic matrix, the composition of the wall of the aorta, heavily influenced by hypertension and the other risk factors, resulting in an atherosclerotic process within the aorta itself. In such a group of predisposed individuals, aneurysm formation occurs in a substantial number.

Gender Predisposition

The women get a break with this one. Though we have seen a substantial number of women with aneurysms, they are much less likely than men to have them. This is especially true of AAAs, less so for aneurysms within other areas of the aorta. However, the one thing that should raise a red flag in women is a very high C-reactive protein, an index of inflammation. It seems likely that aneurysm formation begins as an inflammatory process. This test for a high C-reactive protein, when positive and especially when coupled with cigarette smoking and hypertension or simply with a family history of aneurysm, should be compelling enough to compel you to check for an aneurysm.

Screening

We don't emphasize screening enough. This is like anything else—if we look at a population with reasons to have an aneurysm, the number will be substantial. The reasons are the conventional risk factors of coronary artery disease, especially when coupled with a family history. The more of these risk factors you stack up, the more likely you will find an aneurysm. The number of people at screening clinics given by hospitals is abysmally low. When we screen, the number of individuals who smoke and have elevated cholesterol and hypertension is significant. One thing is certain: If you have a close relative with an aortic aneurysm, you need to be screened every 5 to10 years—5 if a man, 10 if a woman—taking into consideration the gender selection by this disease.

Abdominal Aortic Aneurysms

AAA is by far the most common site of occurrence of aortic aneurysms. In the abdominal aorta, the area just below the take-off of the renal arteries seems to be the most prone to aneurysm formation. (Figure 17, page 202) This is due to a variety of factors, but probably mostly due to the turbulence in that segment and to the fact that the aorta is not well anchored to any other structure at this point. This accessible location is certainly a lucky feature that allows us to readily repair these commonly found aneurysms.

The predominant symptom of AAA is usually that of sudden unexplained back pain. By this time, the aneurysm is either enlarging or rupturing. If you know that you have an AAA and have such a symptom, you need *immediate* evaluation. The pain may

Figure 17 Abdominal Aortic Aneurysm

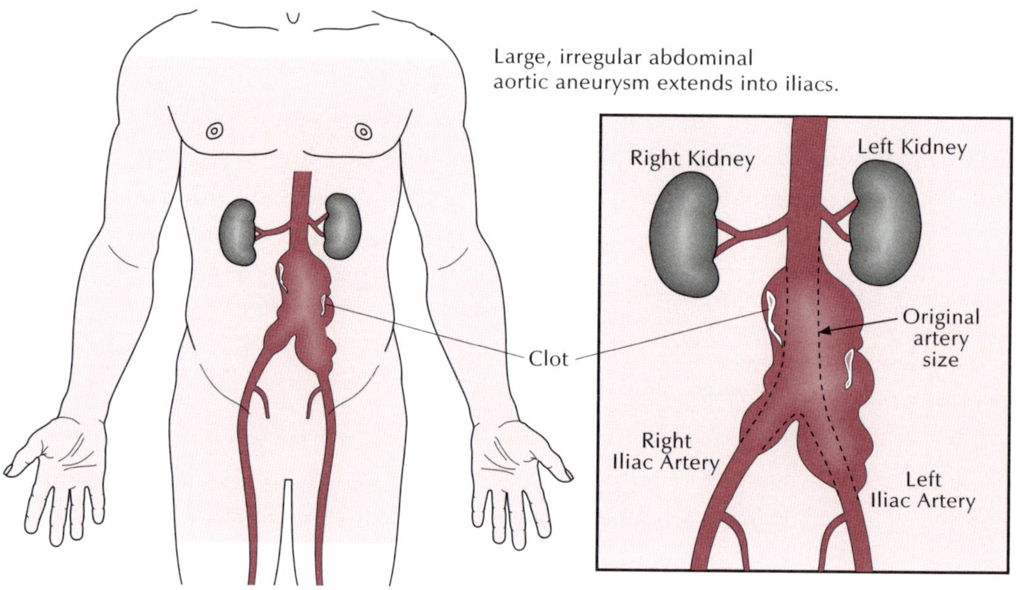

be non-vascular and, therefore, much less threatening. It may be plain old muscular pain or perhaps, a kidney stone. Fine. If you are aware that you have a small or moderate-sized AAA, you cannot afford to blame this pain on something else. You need *prompt* evaluation to be sure that the aneurysm is not enlarging.

The rupture of an AAA is usually a cataclysmic process and is associated with a very high mortality, upwards of 75% in most clinical studies. This statistic underscores the need to follow these aneurysms carefully and intervene *before* they become symptomatic. Many times there will be some degree of discomfort as the aneurysm expands. This may stop only to recur, a pattern that frequently heralds rupture. It means that the aneurysm is remodeling, thinning out its walls, and enlarging. One should not delay in obtaining a vascular evaluation if this symptom occurs.

Intervention

When we find an AAA, who gets treated with intervention? We used to wait until an aneurysm was clearly over 5.5 centimeters (cm) in transverse (cross section) diameter before we did anything. In those days, the only treatment for AAA was surgical resection. A Dacron tube graft was inserted, and the aneurysmal tissue was wrapped around the graft so that this foreign material was covered with the body's tissue as a protective maneuver. This operation was actually a good one and was effective. It's also a very big operation—at least from the patient's vantage point.

However, many of the individuals with AAAs requiring intervention are terrible surgical candidates since many smoke and have significant lung disease. Additionally, most are elderly and are in the midst of a significant number of other major disease processes. It is heartbreaking for many of these patients to be told that they are at excess risk for death if they undergo an open repair of a large AAA. Imagine getting through every day with one of these things in your abdominal aorta. Every tiny discomfort, such as gas pain, would make you worry that the end was near!

Fortunately, several years ago the Arizona Heart Institute and others began investigations into alternative ways to repair these aneurysms without surgery. Thanks to their efforts and technical refinement each year, it is now possible in a large percentage of patients to do this repair via catheters placed in exposed femoral arteries. A tube graft, called an endoluminal stent-graft, since it is comprised of material covering a stainless steel frame, can be compressed into the aorta with tentacles holding it in place once properly positioned. This still requires general anesthesia but with a good anesthesiologist, this can be very smooth. We are able to place these grafts precisely below the renal arteries and then add limbs as needed—just like putting legs on a pair of pants—into the branches of the aorta, the iliac vessels. This completely seals off the AAA, preventing its ultimate rupture. Such a patient usually leaves the hospital on the second day. (Figure 18, page 204)

We have performed this procedure with great success in exceptionally frail patients, including those who were oxygen-dependent, malnourished, and had many other medical problems. We do have to monitor these folks with yearly CT scans to rule out a leak, but this is a small price to pay for avoidance of a high-risk operation with its attendant pain and disability.

In excellent candidates, the open AAA repair through an abdominal incision is still a good option. A good vascular surgeon can perform one of these with a very low risk of death or significant complication—less than 3% in carefully selected patients. Still,

Figure 18 Stent-graft in Aortic Aneurysm

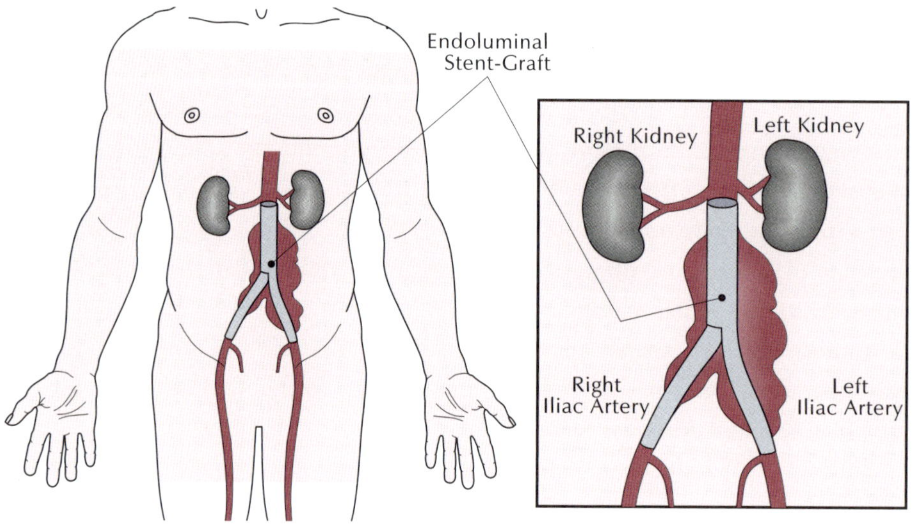

keep in mind that you will be in the hospital for almost a week and it is painful. In fact, most patients who have had both a coronary bypass operation and an open AAA repair say the coronary bypass was "a piece of cake" by comparison.

With the advent of the endoluminal stent-graft procedure, done without major surgery, we frequently offer this procedure to patients with a smaller AAA than if we were going to have to perform an open repair. We do this because many patients have a difficult time going along with their lives knowing they have a sizable AAA, and because we can also now offer a good reliable alternative to the open repair. Today, it is not uncommon across the country to see a 4.5–5 cm AAA treated with endoluminal stent-graft repair. Part of this has to do with pressure exerted by the patient. From a clinical trial, we know we can safely watch these until they are about 5–5.5 cm in transverse lumen size without any increase in mortality. However, once people learn that they have a 4.5 cm aneurysm, they almost always want it repaired, especially if we are confident we can do it with a stent-graft. I can understand, as I would likely fall into this category of pushing for it myself should I find that I have this problem.

I believe it's good medicine to treat any of these AAAs over 4.5 cm with a stent-graft. Why take a chance of rupture when we have identified this process and know that repair is inevitable at some point? Additionally, these behave exactly the way a balloon does when it is inflated—the larger it gets, the thinner the wall and the more likely rupture will occur. As kids, we all wanted to get in that last puff of air, enlarging a party balloon as much as possible, only to have it explode in our faces. This is similar, only the result is much worse. It is one thing to say, "Well, your AAA is 4.5 cm in size. We'll watch it. You go on with your life." It is quite another thing to take that advice calmly.

A certain percentage of folks are going to put off their follow-up ultrasound. It is not uncommon to see a 4.5 cm AAA move up to a 5 cm size within a six month check-up, totally without emergence of symptoms. If those people were to miss their check-up, they might be at significant risk. I believe it's fine to go ahead and repair a 4.5 cm AAA with a stent-graft if the doctor is confident he or she can offer a good outcome. If it's complex, probably all the more reason to proceed because it is at higher risk of rupture.

As with everything else, there is a wide range of aggressivity and conservatism within the physician population dealing with AAAs. If your doctor tells you that you have a 4.5 cm AAA and he or she can safely watch it until it gets to 5.5 cm, that's okay. However, be sure you report any back pain to your doctor and be sure you don't forget or delay your check-ups to monitor your situation.

Surveillance and Treatment of Negative Influences on Progression

With untrasound, a sound wave test that allows us to outline the walls of the aorta, we can pick up many baby aneurysms. We reassure patients and make sure their lipids and hypertension are treated. We particularly like to use a beta-blocker, since this drug reduces the tangential wall stress on the aorta and may well delay progression of the aneurysm. If they smoke, we try to get them to stop.

These small AAAs should be watched with a yearly abdominal aortic ultrasound. Many will remain the same, quite stable, for a long time. *It is unusual for an AAA less than 4.5 cm in transverse diameter to rupture.*

Aortic Aneurysms in the Aortic Arch and Thoracic Aorta

Aortic aneurysms can actually occur in any area of the aorta, including the ascending aorta, the area just above its take-off from the heart. (Figure 19, page 206) Usually these unique—and much less common—aneurysms are due to a congenitally abnormal aortic wall matrix, the underlying supporting framework of the aortic wall. In other words, the wall of the aorta is abnormal from birth. This abnormal zone merely balloons out from the hemodynamic stresses imposed upon it from the blood pressure over several years. These develop at variable ages of life. We have seen such aortic

Figure 19 Aneurysm in Ascending Aorta

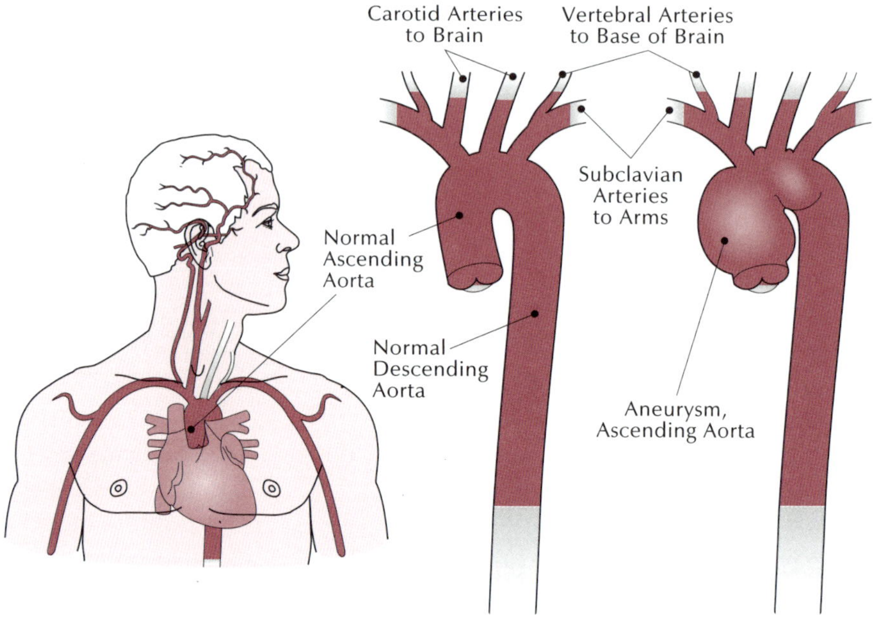

aneurysms in very young women. One type of individual who is prone to such proximal aortic aneurysms is someone with Marfan's Syndrome, marked by very abnormal connective tissue within the wall of the aorta.

There is no question that some of these proximal aortic aneurysms are due to typical arteriosclerosis. In such instances, there is almost always evidence of widespread plaque disease.

Some of these proximal and diffuse aortic aneurysms are clearly inflammatory, at least in part. For many years, I took care of an unfortunate 35-year-old lady who also had rheumatic heart disease and had previously undergone both aortic and mitral valve replacement. She had lupus and high blood pressure. The lupus had been treated for many years. She was also found to have multiple aortic aneurysms. One, which was extensive and involved the lower aorta within the chest and extended into the abdomen, was repaired. It was very complex and she barely survived. She very suddenly ruptured one of the other aneurysms (which we were watching) a few years later, and died of it. She was quite young and had no family history of aortic aneurysm. She had never smoked and had only hypertension as an atherosclerotic risk factor. I believe the lupus, which is known to incite arterial wall inflammation, probably caused the aneurysms to develop within the aorta.

I have another young woman in my practice who does not appear to have lupus or any other inflammatory process but she developed a large aortic aneurysm of the aortic arch, the area above the heart where the aorta loops over on its way down to the abdomen. It occurred right where the head vessels leading to the brain originate from the aorta. This is *not* a common site for development of aortic aneurysms. She has a family history of occurrence of aneurysm formation in unusual sites and I have no doubt that this is a heritable disorder in her case. Interestingly, she has no atherosclerotic risk factors.

We haven't performed exhaustive studies on these tissues in the past. However, in the future, offspring of these individuals will likely need genetic analysis and counseling. I think the variations in these aortic wall tissues will be especially important in this consideration and I suspect there are several, precisely unique genetic abnormalities that lead to these unusual aneurysms.

We already have genetic information on one type of aneurysm-prone individual. This is the person with a so-called spondyloarthropathy disorder, one of which is ankylosing spondylitis, a spine arthritis identified by the immunogenetic marker HLA-B27. Such individuals have aneurysms of the aortic root, including the Sinus of Valsalva in the aorta where the coronary arteries come off. They sometimes have associated aneurysms in the coronary arteries as well. This is yet another example of inflammation-incited erosion of the supporting network of the artery; this one clearly an expression of a genetic destiny. There are others.

Aortic Uncoiling: Not an Aneurysm

The wall of the aorta is made up of elastic and muscle fibers and is tightly structured. As we become older, the aorta naturally loses some of its elasticity and stretches out a bit. This is aggravated by high blood pressure. In patients with long-standing hypertension, it is not unusual to see an aorta that has lost a great deal of elasticity and now is much longer than it should be. Since there is no place for it to go vertically, it becomes tortuous, bowing out smoothly here and there and even overtly buckling where the elastic instability has become severe. *These are not aneurysms!* This is simply a formation of curves, as the aorta elongates due to loss of elastic fibers and can be compared to a man's silk stocking that has lost its elasticity and bows out in a fashion-unfriendly way.

Association of Abdominal Aortic Aneurysms with Other Arteriosclerotic Problems

As alluded to earlier, there is a strong correlation of AAAs with arteriosclerosis elsewhere in the body. This is of utmost importance, as I have seen patient after patient who had an AAA being carefully watched, hypertensive as he could be, yet no screening tests had been carried out to determine if:

A. There was another aneurysm somewhere else.

B. There might be a blockage in one of the renal arteries.

C. There is any evidence of major atherosclerotic disease in those areas where it could lead to life-changing or life-ending events, namely, the cerebral and coronary circulations.

If you have an AAA, you have a good chance of also having significant atherosclerotic disease in the carotid arteries, and also in the coronary arteries. These two systems can be evaluated non-invasively, without risk, within about an hour performing a carotid duplex ultrasound to see if there is any major blockage in one of the carotids supplying the brain and a coronary calcium score to determine if there is significant disease in the coronary circulation feeding the heart. Even better, especially in this unique situation, would be a multi-slice CT angiogram, which will yield information about all the arterial systems within the body—and it can be performed within minutes! We know that if you have an AAA, you have a statistical probability of having significant blockage of at least one of the renal arteries—the arteries supplying the kidneys—somewhere in the neighborhood of 30–40%. This is a huge likelihood, with potentially dire circumstances if left undiscovered. Also, we know that if you have an AAA, there is a significant risk of associated aneurysms elsewhere. Probably the most likely zone for this to occur is in the popliteal arteries, the large vessels behind the knees.

It is safe to say that the finding of a small AAA raises not one red flag, but several. Indeed, I know of no other disease process that serves as such a strong marker, raising this kind of clinical suspicion about other threatening entities. Even more compelling is the fact that each of these is readily treatable.

I think a lot of these features, frequently missed in the past, will come readily to clinical attention in the future. This is not because of some newfound knowledge; however, the CT angiogram is going to be employed so much more frequently in the future that most of these associated problems will declare themselves as accidental passengers.

Referral of Unusual Aortic Aneurysms

In treating aortic aneurysms involving the aortic arch—the top of the aorta where it delivers to the head vessels and makes its bend to descend within the chest cavity—we exercise extreme caution. Hard-working cardiovascular surgeons will see only a couple of these a year, and that's not enough for them to become very competent in this particular surgery. Therefore, we send these complex aortic arch aneurysms to a surgeon who does almost nothing but this type of repair. Sometimes, the aneurysms that involve the arch necessitate re-implantation of the head vessels. These are large, complex surgeries and, in my view, should only be done in institutions where they are done frequently.

Aneurysms in the descending aorta within the chest are less of a challenge; however, they still require a great deal of experience. Fortunately, the endoluminal stent-graft is currently being extended to this use and I think it will soon be an option.

REMINDERS

1. The diagnosis of AAA is not a death sentence. Don't be frightened.
2. We can efficiently and safely watch a small AAA.
3. Endoluminal stent-graft repair is a safer option for repair of an AAA in patients with lung disease, advanced age, and other disease processes.
4. Aortic aneurysms (other than those in the abdomen) should be handled by someone who routinely does that type of surgery.
5. If you have an AAA that is being watched, sudden unexplained lower back pain is the most common symptom of threatened rupture. Less commonly, abdominal pain is present. This type of pain warrants an immediate vascular examination.
6. If you have an AAA that needs to be repaired and you are told that an open repair should be done, ask why an endoluminal stent-graft repair cannot be performed. If this is not offered in that medical facility, and you are stable, ask for a second opinion where they perform both procedures.

7. If one of your parents had an AAA, get an abdominal aortic ultrasound at age 40, if male, and at age 50, if female. If the results are negative, repeat it in 5–10 years, depending on your gender.
8. If one of your close relatives had an aortic aneurysm, it is imperative that you treat any and all atherosclerotic risk factors, especially hypertension. Above all else, do not smoke!

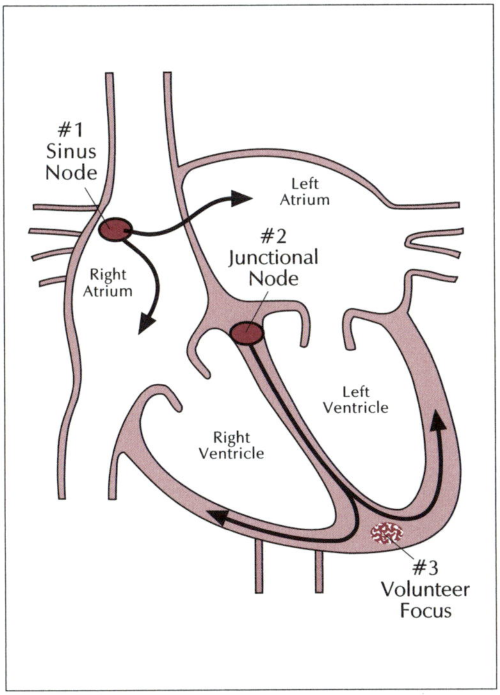

14 PALPITATIONS

The Wild and Racing Heart

IN A BUSY CARDIAC PRACTICE, THREE or so complaints emerge with incredible frequency. One is an awareness of cardiac activity, known as palpitations. Every single one of these complaints has to be taken seriously and evaluated until the problem is found or can be safely dismissed. In the majority of cases, there is no significant underlying problem and the individual just needs reassurance. Sometimes, however, there is a problem that needs further investigation and treatment. Occasionally, the underlying cause is life-threatening.

Broad Spectrum of Causes of Palpitations and Perception

Not only is there a broad spectrum of cardiac actions that can bring on an awareness of heart activity, but the *sensitivity* of awareness is a very unique property as well. Some people have tremendous awareness of their heart action and may actually sense every single *premature atrial contraction* (PAC), a benign process. We all have a certain number of these extra beats and, unfortunately, the frequency increases with age. These are simply extra beats originating from one of the upper chambers of the heart and are totally harmless, even though they can drive some people almost crazy. On the other hand, another individual, equally astute, may have long runs of *ventricular tachycardia* (VT), a potentially lethal form of arrhythmia originating from one of the bottom chambers of the heart, and may be blithely unaware of it. So, you see, the degree of awareness of heart action bears no close correlation to the severity of the underlying process, unless accompanied by other symptoms such as chest pain, shortness of breath, passing out, nausea, or sweating—all of which point to a more dangerous form of irregular heart action.

There are a variety of factors that contribute to an extraordinary sensitivity to heart action. One likely influence is the proximity of the chest bone, the sternum, to the heart. Many people who are born with a sunken sternal bone (pectus excavatum) not only have an increased number of premature beats originating from both the upper and the lower heart chambers, as they frequently have associated *mitral valve prolapse*, but they also sense them more acutely. Another contributor may be an unusually well-developed warning system, something that might easily morph into anxiety in the setting of extra beats, especially if someone close to the person has had an untoward event in such a setting. We all have unique individual levels of response to situations. Some respond to cardiac awareness with great distress; others do not.

About 90% of the time, the cause of palpitations is due to extra beats, either premature atrial contractions or premature ventricular contractions. Of these, PVCs are much more important.

In a perfect world, the heart would beat rhythmically whether sedentary or active, happy or stressed, caffeine-free or living on Starbucks Boulevard. But the world is not perfect and we know that stress, sleep-deprivation, alcohol, tobacco, and caffeine will markedly increase the frequency of both PACs and PVCs. Since these are all common in our world, frequently in some sort of combination, it is no wonder that the complaint of cardiac palpitations is a frequent one.

Not only that, but even a machine as amazing as the heart can go awry of its own accord. There is nothing in the world more elegant than the heart. Its electrical system is so beautifully formatted that no computer can compare. Within this elaborate system, however, electrical faults may exist from birth. These are abnormal electrical pathways whose patterns of conduction are inscribed in that individual's unique genome. We will explore some of these and also look at the problems that may come about by acquired pathology.

Electrical System of the Heart

The contractility of the heart depends on a collection of specialized cells high in the right atrium, the sinus node. These cells fire off a tiny electrical "spark" by intentional leakage of ions across the cell membrane. This occurs spontaneously, but nerves supplying this area can slow down or speed up the process depending on environmental influences and the way we react to them. The electrical current emitted by these specialized cells travels throughout the upper chambers—the atria—causing them to contract, squeezing their contents into the lower chambers. The electrical current then diffuses into the lower chambers—the ventricles—causing them to aggressively pump their contents into the major conduits; the right into the pulmonary artery carrying blood to the lungs, the left into the aorta. The normal course of this sequence causes a beat, then another beat, and a third, etc.

Causes of Palpitations

If there is a so-called premature beat, electrical activation in that particular location is early. This may be due to some extrinsic stimulus such as caffeine, stress, or alcohol. It may be secondary to some other problem in the heart, such as volume overload due to a leaking heart valve, stretch of the chambers due to heart muscle weakness (cardiomyopathy), increased pressure within the heart due to obstruction to emptying, or oxygen deprivation of the heart muscle due to a narrowed heart artery. It may also simply be due to the aging heart, since we each have a tendency toward more premature beats with each year of age. With any of these processes, an extra beat may originate and, indeed, may be repetitive. These may or may not be sensed by the individual.

PSVT

A substantial number of folks, most of them young, suffer from a situation known as *paroxysmal supraventricular tachycardia* (PSVT). This is a rapid, regular rhythm (tachycardia) that starts suddenly, originates within the upper chambers (supra, or above, the ventricles), and then terminates abruptly. This may develop once, never to be heard from again. On the other hand, there are many people who suffer from repeated bouts of PSVT and it can distinctly change the quality of their lives.

In PSVT, the rhythm disturbance very commonly involves a process we refer to as re-entry—it is called a re-entrant tachycardia. In this instance, differences in the silent time between electrical conduction—called the refractory time—and the ability to conduct electricity—called conductivity—allow a circular movement to be established—a "circus" electrical system. This type of process is responsible for most of the arrhythmias in the heart—both of the upper chambers, and the lower (where it can be a much more dangerous process). The ones in the atria, responsible for PSVT, frequently involve the tissue surrounding the AV Node, the bundle of electrical tissue that modulates conduction from the upper chambers to the lower. This is called an AV Nodal Reentrant Tachycardia. Most of these are not dangerous but are terrific nuisances, especially in the young, who have a naturally higher level of sympathetic drive (epinephrine output).

Some people with bouts of PSVT possess a specific bundle of electrical tissue that is frequently recognized by the electrocardiographic (ECG) recording it inscribes, such as the *Wolff-Parkinson-White Syndrome.* In such a syndrome, the aberrant electrical conduction that takes place in the re-entrant tachycardia is caused by a conduit, or tract, of conduction fibers that connect areas of the heart that should not be connected in that fashion (called an anomalous tract). Frequently, these anomalous tracts conduct at rates much greater than the usual electrical system. They "pre-excite" the ventricles and, as such, are known as part of the general group of pre-excitation syndromes. Some of these can be dangerous and can, indeed, be life-threatening. I have known three young people who have died from a rapid rhythm caused by this intrinsic electrical problem, all young doctors. *They died before we had discovered the effective ways of dealing with this that we now have.* At that time, the only conceivable way to disrupt this fiber tract was to cut it surgically. We have much better techniques today. There is no reason for anyone to die of one of these anomalous bundles.

Most of the cases of PSVT are simply great nuisances. This distinction, nuisance versus threat, obviously has to be sorted out. A very small minority of people with PSVT actually have the Wolff-Parkinson-White aberration but even if they do, it is seldom dangerous. However, we have to determine that with certainty. Many instances of PSVT are caused by a pesky conduction fiber tract, just not the more dangerous variety. While we have drugs for these situations, a procedure known as radiofrequency ablation, using an electrode inserted from the groin and taken to the site of the anomalous tract, is frequently the best therapy. This procedure employs systematic mapping of the conduction system, finding the culprit fiber tract, and emitting a small burn through the tip of the catheter. Utilizing energy harnessed in the radiofrequency current, the burn is strategically applied to the troublesome electrical conduit in the heart, putting it out of commission. This will stop the problem and is usually a life-long cure. Not only that, but it is a safe procedure. I have sent scores of people for radiofrequency ablation with no significant complication.

Once we identify a person as having one of these anomalous fiber tracts that allows the onset of a sudden arrhythmia at such a great rate that it can be life-threatening, we waste no time in getting radiofrequency ablation performed. This is almost always effective. We also refer large numbers of people who do not have a life-threatening type of problem but have simply gotten frustrated with the recurrence of the problem and want to quit taking a suppressant drug. This latter category constitutes about 95% of all the people who receive radiofrequency ablation therapy for PSVT.

If the PSVT is infrequent, one can often terminate the spell by straining down, such as you do by inflating a balloon or by initiating a bowel movement. Another good method is to fill a basin with ice water, take a deep breath, clamp your nose between your forefinger and thumb, and submerge your face in the ice water. Humans, like dolphins, possess a diving reflex. The dolphins have a better-developed reflex, as they use it and need it more than we do. But we also have a reflex. When a dolphin dives into colder depths, its heart rate plummets. Ours does too. Sometimes this reflex will snap a person right out of the PSVT arrhythmia, thereby obviating the need for drugs or a trip to the emergency room. A simple beta-adrenergic-blocker, such as Inderal, will sometimes do the trick as well. However, the chronic administration of these is not without significant side effects.

These techniques commonly work if the AV Node is involved in the re-entrant process. They are not regularly effective if there is a separate, anomalous fiber tract present.

While many patients with PSVT are treated today by radiofrequency ablation, some can be treated with drugs, such as a beta-blocker (Inderal, Atenolol). Finally, with advancing age, some degree of fibrosis (scarring) seems to occur, sharply decreasing the frequency of these devilish episodes. The great Carl Jung once said, "Nobody, as long as he moves about among the chaotic currents of life, is without trouble." If you have PSVT and choose to take drugs, you may just "out-live" these chaotic currents. Most people, however, choose to have them burned with radiofrequency current—a one-day hospital stay.

Ventricular Arrhythmias

A much more dangerous cause of palpitations is a ventricular origin of extra beats. If these PVCs are single, there is little to worry about, especially if they diminish with treadmill exercise. Repetitive forms are of more concern. We don't worry much about the occasional double. We start to worry if there are repetitive groups of three or more PVCs in a row, as this constitutes ventricular tachycardia. These deserve a thorough work-up that usually begins with a determination as to whether that person has coronary artery disease, has had a previous heart attack, or has a cardiomyopathy of some sort. Such a problem is commonly the cause of VT.

For example, consider an individual with a history of a previous heart attack who has lost enough heart muscle to greatly reduce the amount of blood pumped with each beat. This results in a reduced left ventricular ejection fraction (expressed as a percentage of the blood that the ventricle receives and subsequently pumps out with each beat). Normal would be over 55%; a severely depressed ejection fraction would be one of about 30%. We commonly refer to this as an *ischemic cardiomyopathy* because the myopathy (muscle weakness) has, in this instance, resulted from narrowed arteries with muscle death, or stunned muscle, from oxygen deprivation. A person who has severe impairment of his or her ejection fraction (especially if due to previous heart attack) and complains of palpitations requires immediate investigation. This should take place within a protective environment (a monitored bed in a hospital) because the cause is more apt to be a potentially fatal rhythm disturbance.

In each form of impairment within the left ventricle, it is certainly possible for an injured or overworked cell to fire off spontaneously. This is a PVC. It is frequently generated by a muscle cell in the transition zone of interspersed scar and viable tissue, the area skirting the epicenter of destruction from the heart attack. If the damage is severe enough, a perverted pattern of electrical activity may well be established—a rapid, very dangerous, disturbance of the heart rhythm: ventricular tachycardia of the re-entrant variety established because of differences in conductivity and refractoriness in and around the scar tissue in the heart. In well over 90% of occurrences, it will cause loss of consciousness if it persists for more than a couple of minutes. If it does persist, it frequently deteriorates into a more perverted, disorganized form of electrical activity called *ventricular fibrillation*, and this is uniformly fatal unless the person is shocked back into a normal rhythm.

If such a person with severe muscle damage has ventricular tachycardia, they are clearly at significant risk of sudden death and need to be evaluated by an electrophysiologist without delay. In this instance, an automatic implantable cardiac defibrillator (AICD) will likely be implanted without further ado. These types of palpitations are often associated with severe dizziness or black-out. This is due to the damaged heart; its ability to pump adequate amounts of blood to perfuse the brain is terribly compromised by this fast, ineffectual heart rate and rhythm.

That brings us to an important point in dealing with palpitations. If one is just aware of an occasional "skipped beat" with no other associated symptoms, the cause is usually not life-threatening. However, if the cardiac awareness is associated with other bothersome symptoms, it becomes much more important. These symptoms consist of shortness of breath, chest pain, sweating, or passing out. They suggest that cardiac performance is dramatically compromised by whatever arrhythmia is producing the palpitations and this, by definition, makes this situation much more urgent.

Trauma to the Chest Can Cause an Arrhythmia

Other arrhythmias can cause serious consequences. It is now well established that a sudden, very high velocity blow to the chest can induce ventricular tachycardia and death. This condition pertains especially to young individuals, and the prime candidate is the little league player who is struck in the chest by a fast hard ball. This is called *commotio cordis* and the only one I saw did not even leave evidence of trauma. Currently, legislation is before Congress to attempt to outlaw the use of metal baseball bats, as a hitter can produce 20–30% more velocity with a metal bat versus a wooden one. There are several documented instances of this sort of chest trauma resulting in sudden death or worse, severe brain impairment from protracted cardiac arrest. This sort of blow can also occur in our routine daily lives from a golf ball, an angry fist in the chest, or a steering wheel.

This electrical chaos resultant from a fierce blow to the chest is interesting, as we can also sometimes terminate an arrhythmia using a strong blow to the chest, the so-called "thump version" that we discussed in Chapter 6 on *Emergency Tactics*. This is seemingly a paradox. In the one instance, the transmitted energy from the blow induces the electrical storm and in the case of a pre-existent arrhythmia, the energy transmitted by the blow can convert the arrhythmia, stopping it and allowing for the emergence of a normal rhythm.

Certainly, all trauma patients who have received a blow to the chest should be monitored carefully and if they complain of palpitations right after the trauma, we take that very seriously. They usually have had some degree of cardiac contusion (bruising) and may well require drug therapy or, in serious situations, an implantable defibrillator.

Atrial Fibrillation

Another cause of palpitations is due to the occurrence of an exceptionally common arrhythmia, *atrial fibrillation*. This is so common that I devoted an entire chapter to it

(Chapter 9). If you are primarily interested in this process as a cause of palpitations, it would behoove you to read it. It is a rapid, chaotic rhythm disturbance, usually with a ventricular rate of 120–180 beats a minute.

Atrial fibrillation can develop sporadically and then disappear just as quickly, which is referred to as *paroxysmal atrial fibrillation*. We have learned that many of these originate from the pulmonary vein region, draining red blood from the lungs back into the heart. Atrial fibrillation is probably more apt to remain as a fixed process, in which case the diagnosis is obvious by simple ECG analysis. It can, however, be interspersed with another process, such as a slow sinus node beat. We call this latter process a *tachy-brady form of sick sinus syndrome*. It is a common reason for a pacemaker to be implanted, as one can hardly ever treat the tachy (fast) component without aggravating the brady (slow) component. A related arrhythmia, atrial flutter, can present in similar fashion but it is usually quite regular and not as fast. Therefore, people are more apt to walk around longer with atrial flutter than with atrial fibrillation.

Intermittent Complete Heart Block

Finally, we occasionally see a patient who has *intermittent complete heart block*. Their primary complaint is that of palpitations—usually irregular heart action. This situation is somewhat rare, as most people with a total loss of electrical conduction between the upper and lower chambers will possess a heart rate of around 25–30 and will feel awful when they try to stand. Occasionally, however, I see someone who registers a complaint like "My heart goes along fine, and then it just stops." Usually this complaint is due to one of the other more common problems we have discussed. However, just about the time I think I really have this practice of cardiology down pat, someone will utter this complaint and they have exactly what they say. In this instance, intermittent complete heart block occurs. The lowest subservient pacemaker in the heart, the ventricular focus, is running the heart for a bit. This can be detected with a Holter monitor, a 24-hour electromagnetic tape recording of the heart action.

Channelopathies

There is a group of disorders marked by some sort of disruption of the normal movement of ions—sodium, potassium, and calcium—into and out of the cells of the heart, and this normal movement is necessary for the heart to function appropriately.

Fortunately, they are rare but they drive us crazy because they express themselves as sudden death, usually in the very young to teenage category. Very frequently, the young person will complain of palpitations, commonly associated with dizziness, prior to a sudden death episode. Some can be recognized by the ECG, some cannot.

Determination of the Cause of Palpitations

The intensity of the search for an answer as to cause is more or less dictated by the symptoms. For instance, a common complaint is an occasional skipped beat, with no associated symptoms. If the ECG is normal, failing to show one of the ominous forms of anomalous electrical conduction, a Holter monitor might be a first step toward making the diagnosis. On the other end of the spectrum is someone who comes in with a frightening array of symptoms: rapid beating of the heart, associated with sweating, shortness of breath, and a sensation that they might lose consciousness. This has obviously bothered the patient a great deal and it should bother the doctor almost as much, as the associated symptoms are at least as important as the cardiac awareness. They imply that the heart beat was so rapid as to cause a fall in blood pressure, a situation seen with life-threatening processes. Such a person should be immediately placed in a protective environment, monitored, and a variety of tests should be carried out to check for possible coronary artery disease, muscle damage, or any one of several risky problems.

A Holter monitor is the tool used most often in the evaluation of a large number of the above problems. Sometimes, if the arrhythmia sounds ominous and episodes are widely separated in space, we employ a loop recorder inserted under the skin. This takes about ten minutes to implant and can be left indefinitely. Even better for a quick read, if a patient has a pacemaker and complains of palpitations, we can simply interrogate the pacemaker, download the data retrieved, and immediately learn the answer to the problem.

However, if the symptoms are scary and no primary process is found, an electrophysiologic test should be done before the patient leaves the hospital to be sure that he or she doesn't have a tendency to develop ventricular tachycardia or one of the other rapid, life-threatening arrhthmias. Only after a negative (normal) test should such a patient be released. No matter how strongly the doctor's gut instinct that the patient just got anxious, only a negative work-up is reassuring.

Treatment of Palpitations

There are almost as many treatment regimens as there are causes of palpitations. If patients have atrial fibrillation, for example, they should be treated with a drug to slow the ventricular response to this rapid rhythm. Some will convert back to sinus rhythm and some won't. The various ways of handling atrial fibrillation are discussed in depth in Chapter 9 on *Atrial Fibrillation: The Most Common Arrhythmia*, and will not be repeated here in detail. Suffice it to say that individuals who have paroxysmal atrial fibrillation, the back-and-forth arrhythmia alternating between this and sinus rhythm have recently been treated with circumferential radiofrequency ablation of the pulmonary vein with great results. This has historically been a difficult arrhythmia to treat with medications.

Occasional extra beats, such as PVCs, may well not require treatment at all. A lot depends on the presence or absence of underlying coronary or heart muscle disease and what has to be done with it. Amiodarone is a great medication for both atrial and ventricular arrhythmias; however, it carries with its usage some equally potent side effects so your doctor will have to tailor the treatment to the disease. The beta-blocking drugs, such as Inderal, Lopressor, or Atenolol, frequently are great for decreasing or obliterating PVCs, especially if found to be secondary to mitral valve prolapse.

The cardiac defibrillator, implanted beneath the skin just like a pacemaker, is reserved for life-threatening problems, such as ventricular tachycardia.

REMINDERS

1. Many episodes of palpitations are not dangerous.
2. If the palpitations are accompanied by shortness of breath, chest pain, sweating, dizziness, or passing out, they are much more important and require an immediate and thorough evaluation.
3. If frequent episodes of PSVT occur, consider drug therapy or radiofrequency ablation to stop them.
4. Ventricular tachycardia (VT) is frequently a dangerous arrhythmia and usually has a serious underlying cause which needs to be identified and treated.
5. If VT occurs in a setting of severe left ventricular dysfunction, consideration of an automatic implantable cardiac defibrillator is in order.

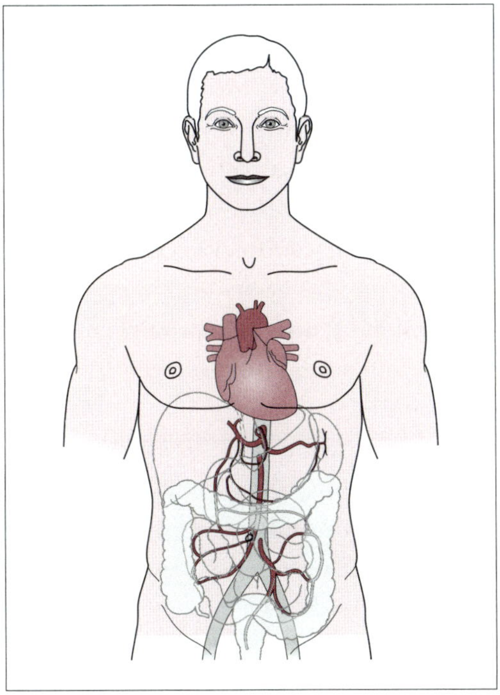

15

CHEST PAIN

Is It Dangerous, What is the Cause, and When Do I Go to the Hospital?

PROBABLY NO SYMPTOM CAUSES AS MUCH anxiety as chest pain. Perhaps it is the fear of the unknown. Everyone knows that the predominant symptom of a heart attack is chest pain. However, many other problems mimic the chest pain of a heart attack. I think that is probably why so many people wait so long to come into the emergency room with a heart attack. They simply think that their chest pain must be "heartburn" or "indigestion" or one of many other possible culprits. When they finally do make their way to the ER, some two hours after the onset of symptoms, we say things like, "Why in the world would you wait for two hours at home with a heart attack before you came to the ER?"

This chapter is all about the symptoms of a heart attack and how to differentiate it from one of the non-threatening causes of chest pain. Always remember, however, that determining whether it is a heart attack or not has be carried out expediently. And remember, too, when we are dealing with a heart attack *Time is Muscle*. As Sir Winston Churchill so eloquently put it, "One ought never to turn one's back on a threatened danger and try to run away from it. If you do that, you will double the danger. But if you meet it promptly and without flinching, you will reduce the danger by half."

In other words, the earlier one gets into an emergency room after the onset of a heart attack—due almost always to a clot blockage of the artery feeding the heart muscle—the earlier we can get the artery opened and the greater the quantity of muscle we can save. The amount of heart muscle you walk out of the hospital with following a heart attack dictates the quality of the rest of your life.

First, what are the symptoms of a coronary artery occlusion? Notice that I did not just refer to this as chest pain, for it is frequently much more than that. As we have discussed previously, the location of pain that accompanies this process is a result of where the embryonic heart is located when the nerves that supply the heart start to form. The heart starts out its journey in the neck area and, as it folds and turns, becoming its final model, it descends to its ultimate location in the chest. So, if the nerves form when the heart is still in the neck region, a person might have very little true chest pain and instead, have predominant neck or jaw pain. No matter where the pain is located, it is almost always described as a pressure-like discomfort.

Additionally, the pain typically is associated with visceral symptoms of illness, signaling that something is quite wrong. These symptoms are sweating, nausea and, occasionally, shortness of breath. The pain is typically described as a dull ache or heaviness, and it is not usually influenced by breathing.

The symptoms may come on and then dissipate, only to recur again, perhaps more strongly. This is because the artery supplying that segment of heart muscle is becoming blocked by a clot, which may then open just a bit so that the heart muscle gets adequate oxygen supply and then the clot becomes denser, more mature and firmer, repeating the cycle until it completely blocks the flow of blood.

I would like to stress the fact that this pain and its associated symptoms don't have to be terribly severe. They can be mild. This is the misleading idea in most people's mind that gets them into trouble.

If you get these symtoms, the very first thing you should do is chew a couple of aspirin because aspirin is a platelet-inhibitor. The artery becomes blocked because an arteriosclerotic plaque (a fatty deposit in the wall of the artery) has ruptured or fissured and is now in the process of completely blocking the artery. Platelet activation is the initial process involved in this phenomenon and aspirin may well prevent the maturing of this clot process by poisoning the platelets.

The next thing to do is to either take Maalox or a proton pump-inhibitor, such as Prevacid. I will explain this after discussing the major conditions that can act like a heart attack.

Reflux: The Great Mimicker

What are the other processes that might mimic a heart attack? There aren't that many. Probably the most common is *gastro-esophageal reflux*. Reflux is very common in folks over age 50. To understand the pathophysiology, you must know the normal physiology. The esophagus, the food tube that carries food from your mouth to your stomach, hates acid but loves an alkaline environment. On the other hand, hydrochloric acid is manufactured abundantly in the stomach so you can digest food. The esophagus and the stomach are partitioned off from one another by the gastro-esophageal sphincter, which is made to open to allow passage of food into the stomach and then partially close off, preventing acid from entering the esophagus. And it does, for a few years.

This sphincter is not very well developed and, with time and abuse from overeating, it becomes incompetent. When this happens, acid freely refluxes from the stomach into the esophagus, chemically burning the cells of the lower esophagus, resulting in the term "heartburn." Heartburn from this acidic erosion can be quite severe. At times, it can precipitate spasm of the smooth muscle in the wall of the esophagus, provoking an intense pain in the chest usually radiating straight into the back. It can be severe enough to cause many of the same symptoms as a heart attack, such as sweating. As an aside, chronic reflux is dangerous. It can lead to the pre-malignant condition known as Barrett's esophagus.

This pain from reflux will usually lessen when you take Maalox or a proton pump-inhibitor, such as Prevacid. Heart attack pain will not respond to these compounds and will become more unsettling with time. However, beware because as my old professor of cardiology was fond of saying, "More people have died of 'heartburn' than any other disease." What he meant by that, of course, is that many people have walked around with what they thought was heartburn, only to be having a heart attack. Put another way, there is "heartburn" and there is heart-*burn*. In the latter instance, the nerve fibers supplying the heart are carrying the message back to the brain that your muscle cells are burning, caused by the same mechanism that produces burning of the muscles of the calves of the legs with intense stair-climbing. These muscle cells produce lactic acid and, in the case of a blocked artery to the heart, blood simply doesn't flow into that area to wash away this acid. The nerves scream out to the brain that your heart muscle cells are *burning*—and they are!

Other Causes of Non-Cardiac Chest Pain

Another non-cardiac cause of chest pain often associated with sweating is that of gall bladder colic, pain caused by the lodgment of a gallstone in the common bile duct. This really hurts! It is usually not constant, but instead has a colicky component. It cramps, then lets up just a bit, then comes on hard again. It frequently causes vomiting. You may as well go on into the emergency room if you get pain like this, as you're going to need to have it diagnosed and, if caused by the gall bladder, you will likely need to have it removed.

Pleurisy is another non-cardiac cause of chest pain that also is distressing. This is chest pain, usually under the armpit, that is aggravated by deep breathing. This is almost never due to a heart attack. It is commonly due to one of several processes, such as a small blood clot to the periphery of the lung, pneumonia, viral infection of the pleural lining of the lungs, or pericarditis—an inflammation of the heart sac surrounding the heart. It usually needs prompt attention. Generally speaking, however, pain made worse by breathing is very infrequently caused by a heart attack.

There are also life-threatening processes that can simulate a heart attack but can actually be worse than a heart attack. One such is that of an aortic dissection. This is a tear in the wall of the aorta. The pain can be central, in the front of the chest, but it almost always radiates into the back, usually into the area between the scapulae, the shoulder blades. In fact, this is usually the area where the pain begins.

If one vomits and then has severe pain in the back, it can be due to an esophageal perforation or a tear in the esophagus from intense pressure exerted on the wall of the esophagus, a so-called Mallory-Weiss tear. This also needs prompt attention.

How to React

There is only one situation in which an individual with chest pain does not need to be seen promptly. That exception is when the pain resolves dramatically and completely when you take Maalox or a proton pump-inhibitor, such as Prevacid or Protonix. By this, I mean all of the symptoms should completely leave before you declare the problem resolved. **All other circumstances mandate a prompt evaluation in the emergency room.**

In other words, if the symptoms described above don't resolve to the point where you are totally pain-free and comfortable within a few minutes, you should get a ride to the emergency room. The code signifying need for emergency help is "911" all across our nation. Since the most common cause of death complicating a heart attack is a disturbance of the heart rhythm known as ventricular tachycardia, you should wait for an ambulance to take you to the ER. In the event you suffer this arrhythmia while your spouse is driving you to the ER, there would be absolutely no way he or she could provide the needed cardiac resuscitation to try to keep you alive.

I have seen many smart people stay at home, especially in the middle of the night, for two or even three hours because the pain "just didn't seem that bad." If it is keeping you awake, it probably is important enough for you to see a doctor. My father, a rancher, developed chest pain and waited for three or four hours with it. By the time he arrived at the ER, his muscle damage was complete and he succumbed to the heart attack due to rupture through the destroyed heart muscle. With a completed heart attack, the heart in that damaged area turns to mush after about three days if the heart attack is dense and involves the heart muscle through the entirety of the wall. These are just the ones that are prone to rupture through the wall of the heart, as there is precious little barrier left intact.

REMINDERS

1. Heart attack pain is unique to each individual but usually consists of several symptoms—sweating, nausea, shortness of breath, and a constant, dull, aching pain that may well radiate to the jaws, shoulders or elbows. Conversely, there may be very little pain.
2. *Time is Muscle.* The sooner you get into the ER with a heart attack, the sooner the doctor can open the artery feeding the muscle. The more muscle you have preserved in the heart attack zone when you leave the hospital, the better your quality of life.
3. The only time it is not necessary to go to the ER with chest pain is when the pain responds completely to an antacid. Otherwise, go!
4. If there is any doubt, even if the pain has responded to Maalox or a proton pump-inhibitor, go to the ER to be sure you are not closing a coronary artery. It is better to be safe than sorry.

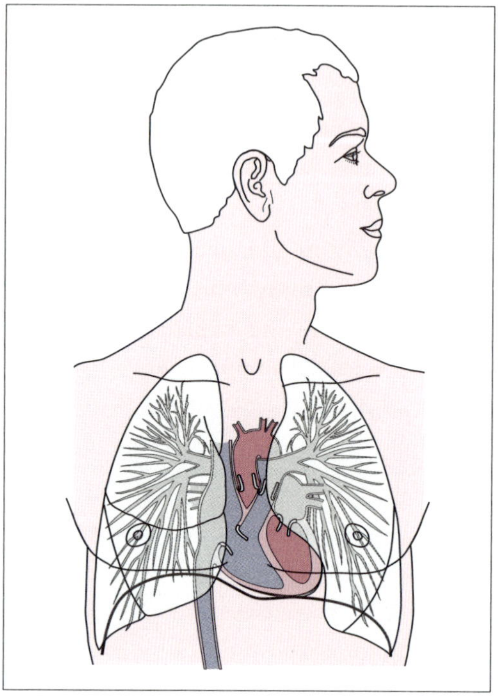

15 SHORTNESS OF BREATH

Is It a Problem and What is Causing It?

THE SYMPTOM OF SHORTNESS OF BREATH is, like most symptoms, highly variable. It can be a mere "back of the mind" awareness that we most commonly attribute to age, or it can be so sudden and severe that it is frightening in its impact. Shortness of breath is one of the most common symptoms that cause people to seek the advice of a cardiologist.

Shortness of breath is commonly referred to as *dyspnea*. It means "air hunger." Everyone experiences dyspnea at various times, usually when our exertional needs out-strip the ability of the gas exchange mechanism in the lungs to provide us with enough oxygen. In other words, everyone, no matter what age, has a rate-limiting level beyond which the body can no longer keep up with its needs of the moment. Shortness of breath ensues.

When we were children, we all ran around like crazy and it was hard for us to get totally "out of breath." The tendency to run out of breath with exercise gets more pronounced as we reach age 40, even in well-conditioned athletes. This is largely due to the fact that the heart begins to lose elasticity, the ability to stretch and take on blood volume from the lungs readily. This ability to relax and stretch is known as *compliance*. When your heart loses that ability, it is said to be *noncompliant*, or to have lost compliance.

This loss of elasticity raises the filling pressure within the heart and produces the symptom of shortness of breath at a lower level of activity. This rather complex mechanism, usually coupled with deconditioning, provides the explanation of why many people develop shortness of breath so quickly with advancing age.

It turns out that we can actually do quite a bit to prevent the progression of this problem. And, like so many other things, they are all simple measures. As Leonardo da Vinci stated, "Simplicity is the ultimate sophistication." The best way to retard loss of elasticity of the heart is to follow a healthy lifestyle. Keeping your blood pressure low will help prevent an increased wall thickness of the main pumping chamber, the left ventricle. Staying lean will reduce the metabolic requirements of the body and reduce the amount of blood the heart has to pump to satisfy those demands. Remember: There is a mile of capillaries for every pound of fat. **If you are only ten pounds overweight, that is ten miles of capillaries through which the heart has to pump blood, and this energy is totally wasted.** Exercise will not only increase the efficiency of the heart and lungs but will increase the energy producing packets within cells throughout the exercised muscle. These units are called mitochondria. They are exceptionally important. In a vigorously exercised muscle on a daily repetitive basis, these units do not reach their maximal population for about three months. It is not fair but if you stop exercising, their population will start to diminish within about three days and you lose ground rapidly after that. This is the reason that many sporadic exercise regimens are so ineffective.

A remarkable feature of the body is that the more mitochondria you have in the exercising skeletal muscle, the more efficient the muscle and the more work you can produce with your heart (the pump) and lungs (the gas exchange unit). This is one of the key reasons that exercise is so vital in patients with congestive heart failure. It has been demonstrated over and over that such patients are able to progressively increase their walking capacity if they walk daily. Much of that increased capacity is due to an enhanced mitochondrial population—a product of conditioning.

Chronic Shortness of Breath

Chronic shortness of breath in an obese, deconditioned 55-year-old person with high blood pressure is not hard to understand. The same symptom in a heavy smoker is equally obvious. Slight variations on this theme constitute roughly 50% of all patients who come to see me with shortness of breath. The other 50% are more difficult to figure out. Chronic shortness of breath has to be taken seriously because it can be the presenting symptom of something much more serious.

However, not all such people come to see a cardiologist and, if they did, there is not enough man-power in our specialty to take care of the needs of even half of them. There is an ongoing epidemic of obesity in many parts of the world including the United States, and this problem has now exceeded the 50% threshold! People frequently achieve some progress in their battle against it; however, recidivism is the norm. A gentleman I grew up with came to see me for cardiac help a couple of years ago. When I quizzed him about his weight, he chuckled and stated that he had lost over 1,500 pounds during his lifetime. On further questioning, he had lost 50 pounds at a time on many occasions, only to gain it back within the next few months. With obesity has come much more diabetes and high blood pressure, harbingers of coronary artery disease, heart attacks, and congestive heart failure. The more obese one gets, the more difficult exercise becomes. If you reach age 60 and you are markedly obese, you are more prone to the breakdown of skeletal support structures, such as joints. This compounds the issue. You get the picture. Still, there is hope!

Chronic shortness of breath can be a symptom of many serious disease processes, the most important of which is coronary artery disease. This is the most worrisome possibility since detection is so critical and might be life-saving. Many people do not possess a well-developed warning mechanism when their heart muscle becomes starved for oxygen. The first and only symptom of a narrowed coronary artery may well be shortness of breath. Therefore, it follows that one of the first tenets of evaluating this symptom is to make sure the individual doesn't have critical narrowing of a coronary vessel.

Exertional shortness of breath may be due to an equally bothersome etiology, but much less threatening to the life and safety of the individual. One such cause is *exertional asthma*. It is not that uncommon, and is marked by wheezing with exercise. One of the guys I skied with when I was in my 30s had this problem. It was the only way I could beat him down the mountain. Then he discovered what he had and started using his inhaler. That ended my triumph!

Smoking is a common cause of chronic shortness of breath. It can dramatically decrease the number of functioning alveoli, the millions of tiny air pockets that participate in oxygen and carbon dioxide exchange in the lungs. The simple truth is that some people readily develop emphysema and others don't. You have absolutely no way of knowing which category you will fit into when you start smoking except the old-fashioned way: If your mother or father developed emphysema, the progressive destruction of alveoli from cigarette smoking, you likely will do so as well.

Valvular heart disease and congenital heart disease can cause shortness of breath and are easily found with a thorough examination, coupled with an echocardiogram. Indeed, of all the tools available in the evaluation of shortness of breath, the echocardiogram is by far the most valuable. It can tell us the thickness of the left ventricular wall, contractility of the ventricle, and the structure and function of the heart valves. It will also tell us if there is a shunt (communication) between the heart chambers, and it can give us a good estimate of the pressures within the heart. If these are all normal, and noninvasive screening tests, such as a coronary calcium score or a multi-slice CT angiogram, show no evidence of occult coronary artery disease, the symptom of shortness of breath is usually not dangerous, at least in the short run. The cause still has to be found and changes have to be made to improve the quality of life of the patient.

Acute Shortness of Breath

Acute shortness of breath, a problem with breathing which comes on suddenly, is almost always important. It is one thing to run short of air at age 60, deconditioned and obese, just starting an exercise program. It is quite another to become acutely short of breath for no good reason. There are many potential causes.

Probably the most common cause of acute shortness of breath is congestive heart failure. This affects over 1% of the population of the United States, roughly 5 million people, and has traditionally been the leading cause of hospital admissions for the last several years. There is no reason to believe that the incidence will diminish in the coming years and every reason to believe that it may, indeed, increase in frequency. The simple explanation is that the population is aging. Approximately 75 million Americans will reach age 60 in the next few years. Remember: As we age, our left ventricular wall elasticity (our compliance) decreases. If a 60-year-old person picks up a pinch of skin, it will not relax as quickly as it did when that person was 20. I don't care how much cream you apply and how much you avoid the sun, the elastic properties in the skin decrease with time. This happens to your heart as well. You can accumulate a fair amount of water in the body tissues by ingesting too much salt or simply by retaining water because of a stiff heart. Finally at some point—usually when you are reclining in bed—the water redistributes from the legs, where it has pooled during the day, into the central circulation. Enough water is pushed across the membrane barrier between the capillaries and the air pockets that you awaken with acute shortness of breath. This is called *pulmonary edema*. A diuretic (medication that causes aggressive urination) will help eliminate the water quickly. However, with the initial episode, you don't usually have such a medication at hand and even if it is available, the symptom is so frightening that you can't always think clearly. A visit to the emergency room is usually the end result and can promptly result in effective treatment. The trick is to know how to prevent recurrences and, if they do develop, how to treat them.

Probably the next most common cause of acute shortness of breath is a pulmonary process such as *pneumonia* or less commonly but more threatening, a *pulmonary embolus*. An embolus is a clot that forms in a particular area, breaks loose from its moorings, and travels to another zone. In this case, a pulmonary embolus is a clot that formed elsewhere, usually the leg veins, and traveled to the lungs. Either one of these, pneumonia or pulmonary embolus, can cause pleuritic chest pain which is accentuated by breathing. Both require immediate attention.

Yet another pulmonary problem that can cause acute shortness of breath and pleurisy is that of a *spontaneous pneumothorax*, a process in which one loses the negative pressure in the pleural lining of the lung and the lung literally collapses. Fortunately, this is rare. *Traumatic pneumothorax*, which can occur with any blow to the chest wall but is most commonly an accompaniment of a rib fracture, is much more common.

Asthma, wheezing brought on frequently by constriction of the bronchi (the airways leading to the air pockets) can be triggered by environmental allergens, infection, or a variety of other causes. Along those lines, an acute allergic process such as that seen with peanut allergies or dust mites can also cause acute development of shortness of breath.

Evaluation, Treatment, and Prevention of Recurrences

The plain old chest x-ray is the first diagnostic test in evaluation of acute shortness of breath. A chest x-ray, coupled with a thorough examination, usually will promptly make the diagnosis of congestive heart failure. Pneumonia will also show up on a chest x-ray. A spontaneous pneumothorax will be immediately apparent on a film, as well. However, a blood clot, a pulmonary embolus, will not. Therefore, if a person comes in with severe shortness of breath of an acute nature, and has a clear chest by exam and x-ray, pulmonary embolus should be foremost in the mind of the examiner, and an immediate lung scan or CT scan of the chest should be done. The treatment is vastly different, and a precise diagnosis has to be reached as soon as possible.

Blood tests help. For example, if a patient has pulmonary edema, it is incumbent upon the examiner to be sure that it is not due to a silent heart attack that does not show up on the electrocardiogram. Additionally, if the doctor is not sure whether the patient has pneumonia or congestive heart failure—because they can sometimes look the same, especially if the pneumonic process is diffuse—a B-peptide elevation will help make the diagnosis of congestive heart failure. B-peptide is slang for Brain Natriuretic Peptide, a substance found in excess levels in individuals with a stretch of the right atrium and congestive heart failure.

The acute treatment of severe congestive heart failure, called pulmonary edema because the lungs are full of edema fluid, is the rapid administration of a diuretic such as Lasix or Bumex, coupled with the administration of oxygen. Occasionally such patients require intubation with a breathing tube but this is uncommon due to our modern tools of aggressive treatment. These include the use of CPAP, continuous positive airway pressure, applied by a machine that sends a certain flow of oxygen into the lungs through a tightly applied mask. An intravenous drip of nitroglycerine will acutely unload the left ventricle and will aid in the recovery of the patient in the emergency room. Another great drug that effects prompt unloading of the heart and elimination of extra water is Natrecor, currently the best drug for the job.

The treatment of a pulmonary embolus is quite different from treatment of congestive heart failure. Once this diagnosis is made, a powerful drug to anticoagulate the blood is given. This is either Heparin or a fractionated derivative called Lovenox. These drugs interrupt the progressive formation of a blood clot. If given early enough, and if the clot is freshly formed, they may also cause some dissolution of clot material.

If the blood clot is large enough to cause dramatic deterioration in the gas exchange mechanism, or enough to cause hemodynamic embarrassment (a drop in systemic blood pressure or a marked rise in pulmonary pressure), a stronger "clot-buster" drug called a thrombolytic (dissolves a clot) is given.

Once the individual is stabilized, the doctor faces the issue of more chronic treatment. For the most common of the causes, congestive heart failure, one should first and foremost throw away the salt shaker. Salt, plain old table salt, will cause you to hold onto water in an unhealthy way. Most people do not have to restrict their daily intake of water unless they have a problem with low sodium with a diuretic. The mainstay of treatment of congestive heart failure is a diuretic usually coupled with an ACE-I (Angiotensin Converting Enzyme-Inhibitor) type drug to unload the heart. For more on treatment of congestive heart failure, please see Chapter 11.

REMINDERS

1. There are many causes of chronic shortness of breath—obesity, cardiopulmonary deconditioning, a stiff heart. Serious causes of cardiac processes need to be ruled out.
2. The most common cause of acute shortness of breath is congestive heart failure. It is the most common cause of hospital admissions and will become more epidemic with the aging of the baby boomers.
3. Acute shortness of breath can also be caused by pneumonia, a blood clot to the lung, silent or painless heart attack, and asthma. Acute shortness of breath is always a medical urgency.
4. Salt causes the body to retain water in an unhealthy way. Do yourself a favor and throw out your salt shaker!

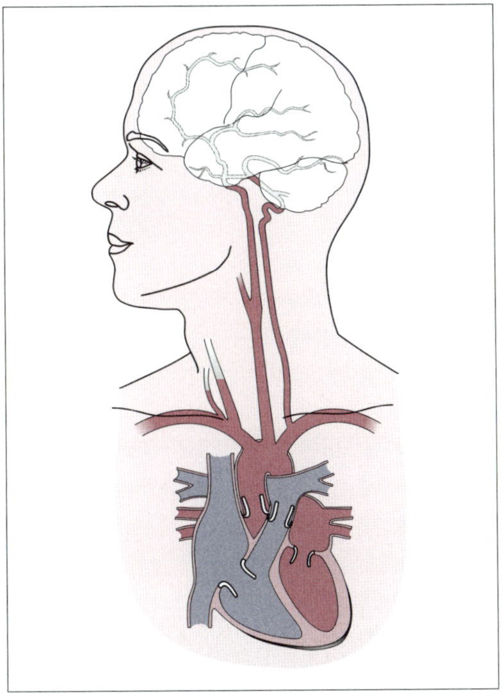

11 DIZZINESS

Please Stop the Merry-Go-Round!

THIS IS ONE OF THE THREE MOST COMMON complaints in a cardiac practice. It can be dangerous or completely innocent. It always has to be taken seriously. If we can't sort this out and find a distinct cause, which is the case in perhaps 25% of all presentations, it is almost always innocent. This group of people, followed for years, does very well. This pleasant pronouncement is possible, however, only after ruling out all of the potential dangerous causes of dizziness.

I remember an unpleasant chunk of my childhood when I would always get dizzy on the merry-go-round—we didn't call them carousels where I grew up. When I was six, I had been laid low with an ear infection, but loved the merry-go-round too much to stay off. But it made me extremely dizzy. When our particular playground bully discovered my plight, he spun it faster and faster until I ultimately got so dizzy I fell off. I have a persistent empathy for those who are afflicted by this problem.

There are many causes of dizziness. One would think that these individuals would wind up in a neurologist's office; however, they are mostly sent to us cardiologists. This is even more curious because *most* causes of dizziness are not cardiovascular in origin. I suppose we are selected to see these patients because the ones that *are* serious are frequently due to cardiac arrhythmias, intermittent heart block, or blockage in an artery, each capable of leading to reduced flow to the brain.

Actually, a very common cause of dizziness is a viral invasion of the inner ear causing vestibular dysfunction. Frequently this follows an upper respiratory tract infection and is generally accompanied by nausea. This can be diagnosed by vestibular studies performed by an ear, nose, and throat specialist.

One disease of the blood vessels that is a cause of dizziness is that of vertebrobasilar insufficiency due to arteriosclerosis. Vertebrobasilar insufficiency simply means that you don't get enough blood to the base of the brain. This area of the brain controls equilibrium and a sense of where you are with regard to other objects and people, i.e., your spatial orientation. If people with obstruction in the vertebral arteries look heavenward, they may immediately become dizzy and develop what one old Texas rancher described to me as the "blind staggers." This term sums it up as well as anything I could come up with. When he used this term, I had no difficulty realizing right away that this was not a fun-filled experience for him. I suppose his description took me briefly back to my childhood experience.

Another problem is that of subclavian stenosis with resultant subclavian/vertebral steal. This is a severe blockage in the subclavian artery, so that flow to the base of the brain is compromised with any prolonged activity of the arm on the afflicted side. This is because the vertebral artery originates from the subclavian artery supplying the arm and, if there is blockage of the subclavian artery proximal to the take-off of the vertebral artery, the arm will *steal* blood from the vertebral artery and hence from the base of the brain. This can be determined by simultaneously checking the radial pulse volume in both wrists. They should be equal.

A Doppler test is diagnostic. This is a sophisticated test performed with ultrasound, measuring the velocity and direction of blood flow. The vertebral blood flow should be of normal velocity and the direction should be toward the brain. As the subclavian blockage increases, this velocity will increase much like the velocity of water as you squeeze a garden hose. As the subclavian artery closes, the direction of flow in the vertebral artery reverses, due to the demands of the arm muscle for oxygen and nutrients. When this blood flow reversal takes place, the arm literally steals blood from the base of the brain, thus the term "subclavian-vertebral steal." The symptoms, along with the finding of differences in pulse volume between the two wrists, coupled with Doppler analysis, make the diagnosis. We love to find this situation, as we can remedy it with a stent deployed within the ostium of the subclavian artery. A good result is usually durable. An exhaustive handling of this problem, along with illustrations, can be found in Chapter 31.

A blocked carotid artery leading to the brain, called carotid artery stenosis, does not cause dizziness unless it is severe and bilateral. We are frequently asked to do a carotid Doppler to look for a carotid blockage if a patient has dizziness. This is actually how many of the subclavian stenoses are picked up.

Another cardiac cause of dizziness is associated with irregular heartbeat. This is almost always of a serious nature and requires full investigation. The dizziness is due to altered blood flow to the brain, particularly to the cerebellum, secondary to the arrhythmia. We can frequently pick this up with a 24-hour electromagnetic recording using a Holter monitor. If not, and especially if the symptoms are compelling, we can perform an electrophysiologic test and determine if the person is at high risk of having a disaster.

First, we should make sure of the primary cardiac disease process, as one is almost always present. The most likely is coronary artery blockage. Others include a heart muscle weakness, cardiomyopathy, and valvular disorders. The underlying arrhythmia causing dizziness is frequently *ventricular tachycardia* (VT) and may require an automatic implantable cardiac defibrillator (AICD) to prevent sudden cardiac death.

Other less lethal arrhythmias may also cause dizziness. These may sometimes be treated with medications, especially if the rhythm disturbance turns out to be due to a rapid heart beat in the upper cardiac chambers, such as atrial fibrillation. Occasionally, it is something that requires hybrid therapy since the primary problem itself is hybrid in causation. An example is the so-called tachy-brady variant of sick sinus syndrome, whereby the tachy (fast) limb is due to intermittent atrial fibrillation. When the atrial fibrillation stops, the heartbeat is again run by the sinus node in the top of the heart, but sometimes this area is degenerative and the beat is too slow (brady) to maintain a good perfusion pressure to the brain. Dizziness develops during these spells. In this instance, a pacemaker is installed to offer a lower rate platform, usually at 70 beats a minute. A drug can then safely be given to control the rate of atrial fibrillation. This is complex therapy for a complex problem. Usually, the outcome is quite good.

Occasionally, patients with intermittent *complete heart block* (blockage of electrical impulses from the upper to the lower chambers) will have dizziness as their only symptom. Usually they have blacked out or nearly done so, at least once. We can generally pick this up with a Holter monitor. If not, and if the index of suspicion is high enough, electrophysiologic testing will determine whether or not they have severe cardiac conduction disease and should have a pacemaker inserted.

A syndrome known as *neurocardiogenic syncope* frequently causes dizziness. In fact, after these people have had one or two blackout spells, they learn how to get down fast when this hits, and they are then just plagued by these terrific dizzy spells. Dizziness may be their only complaint when they come to a physician. These spells are due to an alteration in their hemodynamics, as the blood vessels in the legs do not appropriately constrict when they change from supine to standing and they also have a dysfunctional electrical stimulus, so the heart rate does not speed up enough in response to changes in posture. This individual frequently has dizziness and blackout, referred to as *syncope*, and the presumed clinical diagnosis can be corroborated by tilt table testing. It can frequently be at least partially treated.

Finally, almost everyone at some point in his or her life will complain of intermittent and severe dizziness. This is frequently following an illness during which you lost cardiac and blood vessel fitness, better known as conditioning. The peripheral arterioles get lazy when you have been sedentary for a long period of time, especially if you have been prone in bed. In other words, your small blood vessels should constrict (get smaller) as you rise from a prone position. You can lose this ability with bed rest and illness. It takes a while to get back appropriate function, more so in the elderly.

Additionally, many people walk around quite significantly volume (water) depleted. If you are dehydrated, you are much more likely to have dizzy spells. You always read that we need eight glasses of water a day. I think this requirement is purely arbitrary. You can very easily judge how much water you need. If your urine is yellow, you are volume contracted (dehydrated). You should drink water until your urine is clear. If you have taken in a lot of protein, you will need more water. If you are exercising, you will need more water. If you are sedentary and have a low protein diet, you will need less water. The color density of your urine will tell you how to manage your water intake.

For example, to illustrate the need for hydrating is this true story. I was looking for a smaller house to live in and the realtor showed me a particular place just as I was writing this particular chapter. When he discovered that I am a cardiologist, he told me his story: Once every three or four days in the early morning hours as he is driving his little boy to school, he will have sudden waves of dizziness. It eventually passes, but he has been forced to pull over to the side of the road on occasion. I quizzed him about his habits. He routinely has two glasses of red wine in the evening before retiring, drinks no water in the evening or during the night, nor does he have water in the morning when he rises. Instead, he drinks two to three expressos and then starts out.

By now, you too could come up with a good list of possibilities for this gentleman. I suspect he is quite dehydrated—no water and a fair amount of wine, which dehydrates you. Then he has a big hit of expresso. He very likely is developing an arrhythmia of some variety. It might be one that would not even be symptomatic were he not so volume-depleted. This is speculation but you can see how the formulation process goes. He needs a Holter monitor, a carotid duplex scan, and he needs to change his habits. Like all of us, he can learn from the teachings of Leonardo da Vinci, who lived to a very old age for his time. He counseled us to do everything in moderation and, specifically, to drink water along with wine—three glasses of water to every glass of wine.

REMINDERS

1. Severe, recurrent dizziness deserves prompt investigation.
2. Severe dizziness—without a buzzing in the ears and without vertigo—may be caused by a problem with the heart or blood vessels.
3. If you're dizzy walking around, try hydrating with water first.
4. If you drink alcohol, even wine, drink water as you go—alcohol causes significant dehydration.
5. The color of your urine will tell you how much water to drink; the lighter the better.

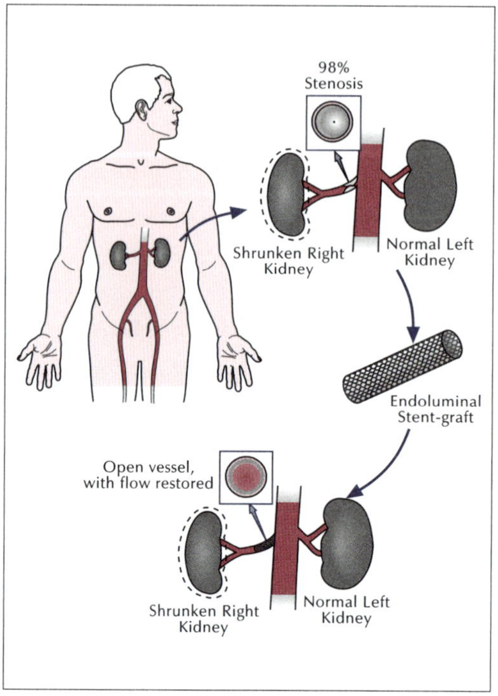

18 RENAL ARTERY STENOSIS

Blockage of the Renal Artery: The Saga of a Thirsty Kidney

A STENOSIS IS A BLOCKAGE. THE RENAL ARTERIES are the arterial conduits leading from the aorta to provide blood that is filtered by the kidneys to eliminate metabolic toxins from the blood stream. *Renal artery stenosis*, then, is a blockage in a kidney artery. It is silent and frequently missed for months, if not years. In fact, if not thought of and not looked for, it can be so silent as to completely block flow through a renal artery. As it turns out, these rather large arteries are not spared the process of cholesterol deposits within their walls (arteriosclerosis). This seems to be especially true in women.

Importance of Renal Artery Stenosis: Hypertension and Kidney Function

The reason it is so important to detect renal artery stenosis is to save kidney function and, as a plus, to help in the control of high blood pressure. As it turns out, the atheromatous plaque (the cholesterol deposit) in the wall of the renal artery doesn't really begin to cause significant reduction in overall blood flow to the kidney until it demonstrates at least a 50–60% decrease in the lumen size (the central channel) of the artery. So there is absolutely no way to know of its existence from symptoms, at an early stage. At this stage, however, it does no harm because the kidney is still receiving enough oxygen and nutrients for its needs so it is still happily performing its chore.

However, when this process becomes approximately 75% obstructive, it results in a persistently diminished supply of blood to the kidney. As this blockage becomes greater and greater, the kidney receives decreasing amounts of blood. Since its own "personal" blood flow is reduced, the kidney "thinks" its owner must be bleeding to death and that the entire body is in the same dilemma it is in. It doesn't know that its owner is a smoker or has high cholesterol or diabetes, and that these influences have led to a plaque that only reduces blood flow to the kidney. It doesn't know, or care, that the rest of the body is receiving perfectly adequate blood flow. The kidney was constructed with a built-in process to try to restore adequate blood flow to itself, the heck with the rest of the body. To be fair, since it was meant to function with a good arterial blood supply, it usually steadfastly and admirably serves for decades in its role as monitor for the water volume of the body—holding onto water when needed, eliminating it when not. When threatened by its own loss, however, it wildly releases chemicals that lead to retention of salt and water. And while the kidney may only be receiving the bare minimum of oxygen and nutrients to satisfy its own selfish needs, the final result is a marked increase in blood pressure to the rest of the body including the brain and the heart, organs that can be mightily damaged by this incessant high pressure bombarding their tissues. The process, by the way, is still silent even at this point unless you happen to get your blood pressure checked. Since end-organ damage is what we worry about most with high blood pressure—manifested as stroke or cognitive loss at the brain level, heart attack or non-elastic pump at the heart level, or destruction of functioning filtering units at the kidney level—it is imperative that we maintain good blood pressure control at all times.

The usual way we detect this problem is by finding that you are not responding appropriately to your blood pressure medications. If you have watched your salt intake, are taking increasing amounts of anti-hypertensive drugs, yet still have uncontrolled elevation of blood pressure, you may well have *renovascular hypertension* due to renal artery stenosis. This is owing to the revved-up production of renin within the structure of the kidney. Renin is constantly being produced, guiding the amount of salt each of us holds onto through the end product of this pathway, aldosterone. However, too much renin brings about too much aldosterone and, as a consequence, too much salt and water retention. Not only that, but an intermediate substance, angiotensin, brings about a vasoconstriction, a tightening of the smooth muscle in the walls of the small arteries throughout the body. This raises the systemic resistance, the resistance against which blood is pushed through the maze of arterial conduits to reach the tissues. This resistance, coupled with an increased amount of water within the conduits, brings about this difficult-to-control high blood pressure we refer to as renovascular hypertension. The pathway that is accelerated is the same one jazzed up by congestive heart failure: the *renin-angiotensin-aldosterone system* (RAAS).

A large price is sometimes paid if this obstruction goes too long undiscovered. As a consequence of reduced arterial blood supply and nutrition to the kidney, it loses some of its cell population and shrinks. This primarily involves the outer surface of the kidney, that portion referred to as the renal cortex. Even though I am diligent in watching for this problem, about twice a year I find a patient who has silently closed off a renal artery, resulting in *auto-infarction* of the kidney. This means that the artery has closed off silently, without any symptoms, and the kidney has been destroyed as a consequence. This is essentially a painless experience for the individual, but I am always dismayed when I discover that this phenomenon has occurred. The patient has lost a kidney and, even worse, it occurred on my watch! It can be a notoriously silent process.

How can such a thing happen if the doctor knows of its presence? A 50% blockage in a renal artery, non-obstructive at the time it was identified, may suffer the same fate as a similar blockage in a coronary artery. It may develop plaque rupture through erosion of the fibrous cap that covers it, platelet aggregation may occur on top of this open sore within the wall of the artery, and then a clot forms—all silently—with the end result being a totally blocked renal artery. Sometimes collaterals, tiny branches from the capsule surrounding the kidney, may develop adequately enough to save some kidney function. They always try; it is a built-in primitive mechanism. This is both good and bad. Good in that we all need as much kidney function as we can retain; bad in that there is some viable (functional) kidney tissue left to produce renin, driving up the blood pressure because the kidney is suffering for blood, but most of the kidney has already been lost. There is frequently no way for us to get through the total blockage with a wire so we can open the renal artery once again, unless the total occlusion is fresh. Just like any clot, it begins life as a soft, poorly formed collection of platelets clumped together and becomes more mature by the hour and day. With enough passage of time, it becomes almost as rigid as a stone, firmly adherent to the wall of the artery. We frequently cannot get through this sort of occlusion. These total renal artery occlusions, accompanied by capsular collaterals, can present the greatest challenges in blood pressure control due to this huge outpouring of renin. Our efforts at opening the artery are frustrated by the rock-hard blockage in the mouth of the artery.

Medical Treatment for Renovascular Hypertension

Since the major cause for this surge in blood pressure is activation of the renin-angiotensin system, we need a drug to block this pathway. We have one. It is the ACE-I, which stands for Angiotensin Converting Enzyme-Inhibitor. It blocks the conversion of Angiotensin I to Angiotensin II, the vaso-active compound that causes constriction of small arteries throughout the body. Another is the ARB, the Angiotensin Receptor-Blocker. It doesn't block the conversion of Angiotensin I to II; it blocks the effects of II at the tissue level. Both drugs serve to thwart the effects of this excessively produced material. They don't usually work too well, however, as the kidney keeps pouring out more and more renin. Additionally, we can only imagine what is happening to the poor oxygen-starved kidney. I have seen this many times. It is steadily losing tissue around its outer rim, the cortex. This has to be stopped. Just treating the high blood pressure won't cut it. We have to restore blood flow to save the kidney from destruction.

Stent Deployment in Renal Artery Stenosis

What can be done for renal artery stenosis? Plenty! We spent years using primitive biliary stents, hand-crimping them onto a balloon, trying desperately to save these kidneys. Fortunately, those days are over and we now have great stainless steel stents that we can use to open these vessels widely, restoring normal blood delivery to the kidney. (Figure 20, page 242) These are usually durable. Some will re-stenose (become blocked again with scar tissue) and, as you might expect, the smaller the artery we have to work on, the more likely scar tissue will build up in the artery within the stent to the point that it becomes occluded once again. The reason for the block, of course, is that it is impossible to wedge open this complex heap of cholesterol deposit—frequently hardened and calcified by the passage of time—without inflicting considerable damage to the inside of the renal artery. The artery reacts to this injury, another primordial

Figure 20 Renal Artery Obstruction

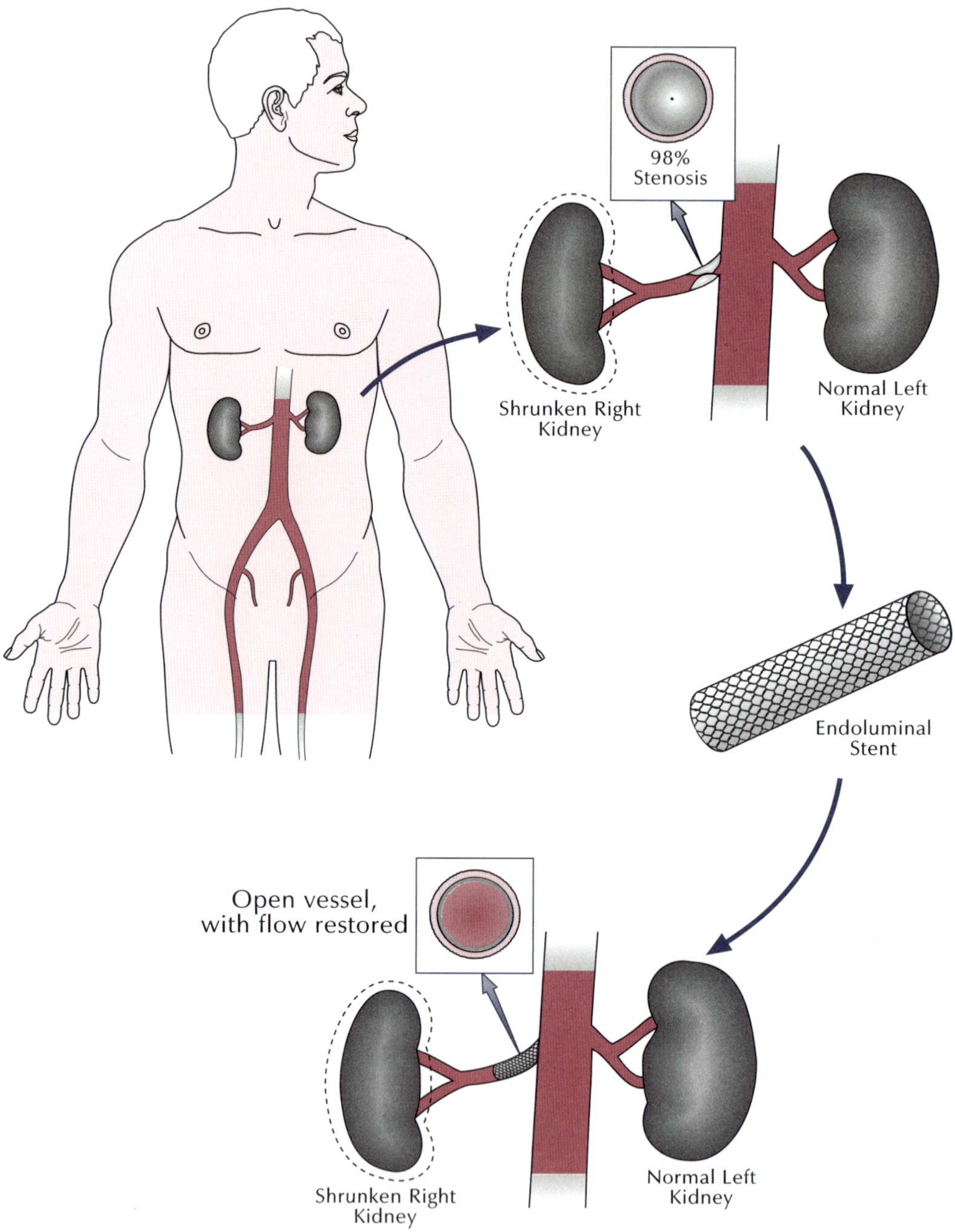

response, with proliferation of smooth muscle cells, forming a scar in the artery. If the artery is huge, it probably will not cause a problem. If it is petite, as it is in many women, it may cause a tight blockage to reappear. In the future, I believe we will likely be using drug-coated stents (similar to the ones we use in coronary arteries) in treatment of these smaller renal arteries to prevent this scar tissue blockage.

If fibrous tissue builds up within the renal stent causing it to block proper flow of blood to the kidney once again, we can use a cutting balloon, a balloon with blades within its substance. This cuts the scar tissue. If you merely use a balloon, you will frequently just stretch the scar tissue. If you cut it with a device, it is allowed to expand, this time scarring the cut zones, frequently with a durable result.

Many cases of renal artery stenosis traditionally have been discovered at the time of coronary angiography. With the advent of intravenous CT angiography, hopefully we will be detecting this disease earlier and earlier. We can readily follow the course of a non-obstructive blockage with renal Doppler, the ultrasound device that shows us velocities of blood flow within the renal arteries. The ideal situation is to watch such a blockage until it reaches approximately 75% severity and then open it with a stent. Remember, these obstructions don't begin to starve the kidney until they reach this point of severity. This is so well established that the federal government uses this percentage as its marker in the Medicare/Medicaid program. If we work on a renal artery blockage that is obviously less than 75% in severity, the burden is upon us to outline in our report just why we did this. Sometimes, for example, I will stent a 50% blockage if it appears very irregular and ulcerated because I do not want the individual to lose that kidney to a silent closure. I make this clear to the patient and in the chart record why I did it. Sometimes if the right kidney is tiny and shrunken and the left is huge but there is a 50% blockage in its equally huge renal artery, I will stent it, again for the same reasons. I do not want the individual to lose his or her only good kidney, and the artery in such a setting is usually large enough that I feel comfortable that we will achieve a good long-term result. These are special circumstances but deserve mention, as this disease can be tricky to combat.

Just as "Time is Muscle" when we are dealing with coronary arteries in preserving heart muscle, we must always keep in mind that an open artery is necessary to preserve kidney function. Some well-published physicians have historically stated that opening a renal artery does very little in correcting hypertension. Sometimes this is the case. If the renal artery is being opened just to correct hypertension, some degree of dissatisfaction and disappointment will certainly occur. I have never opened a tightly blocked renal artery with the end result being total abandonment of antihypertensive medication. It may well help in control of the blood pressure; however, the main objective in this treatment is preservation of the kidney. One thing I can guarantee: If the kidney doesn't receive enough blood flow, it will self-destruct; the end result will be a withered, poorly functional structure.

Detection and Follow-up

Anyone who has severe hypertension, especially if several high-powered drugs are being used to control it, should have a renal artery ultrasound. This is an excellent screening tool. We are now in a much better situation in terms of responding to a positive, or borderline, result from this test. In the past, if the ultrasound suggested a tight blockage in a renal artery, we could do one of two things: We could get another non-invasive test, an MRI angiogram, or we could proceed with an invasive test—a renal artery angiogram. Now we can proceed on to an excellent non-invasive test, the multi-slice CT angiogram, which will give us an outline of the renal artery showing us the encroachment of the plaque system upon the lumen of the vessel. Armed with this data, we should be able to perform an invasive angiogram only in those who have evidence of a tight blockage. Therefore, the angiogram should be performed with intent to deploy a stent.

Hazards in Renal Artery Stent Deployment

Just as any intervention poses a hazard, there are some with this one, too. The one we all worry about, embolization (downstream particles) of debris from the arteriosclerotic plaque as we open it, in reality, occurs almost every time. Fortunately, these debris particles are usually tiny and do not cause obstruction of a major segmental renal artery. Occasionally, we will see evidence of a "shower" of tiny particles with resultant obstruction of thousands of tiny branches. Fortunately, this is exceptionally unusual and sometimes will reverse with no evidence of significant lasting damage to the kidney. This is a good reason for opening only one renal artery at a time.

Another catastrophic complication is the potential for renal artery disruption with extensive bleeding into the retroperitoneum—that area behind the abdomen where the kidneys live. This is the reason to choose an interventional cardiologist who has performed many of these procedures. This is more difficult to do, in some anatomic situations, than working on a coronary artery.

Yet another hazard is losing a stent into the circulation. We still lose a few, even in this day and age when they come from the factory tightly crimped onto the balloon.

If it travels, and it frequently does, it will usually land in a leg vessel. It can frequently be removed. If not, amazingly, it usually causes no major problem.

Medical Therapy in Renal Artery Stenosis

Many people want to know about medical therapy for renal artery stenosis. There is none, except for control of the serum cholesterol and other arteriosclerotic risk factors because these blockages usually are due to cholesterol deposits, almost always right in the mouth of the renal artery. This is the point of extreme turbulence, including circular and bi-directional flow, likely the initiating cause of the ultimate plaque formation and progression since the renal artery comes off at a 90-degree angle. In cases of long-standing hypertension, the usual situation, coupled with age and its attendant loss of elastic elements not only within the arterial wall but also within the kidney suspensory elements, the take-off angle from the aorta is frequently exaggerated, resulting in even more turbulence and even more accumulation of plaque. As expected, scrupulous control of high blood pressure is terribly important as well.

Since early detection is becoming the standard, especially now with the exciting advent of the 64-slice CT angiogram, many blockages that are not tight enough to warrant stenting will be followed by renal ultrasound. Some of these will remain stable for years. Other plaque systems, no different in appearance on ultrasound, will ulcerate and become prime candidates for clot formation. Because of this, I believe these patients should be on aspirin and Plavix, platelet-active drugs that help in prevention of acute clot formation since they block the first stage in such formation, namely, platelet aggregation.

However, there is an even more important consideration. We know that this process of ulceration of a plaque doesn't just happen randomly, as we thought in the past. We know now that inflammation plays a key role in triggering this process, at least partially through the expression of what we call inflammatory cytokines, interacting with macrophage cells within a plaque system. When this happens in one plaque, it is not uncommon for it to happen to another, remote, plaque system. We can at least partially block this trigger with a drug that we use for control of the LDL-cholesterol, a statin drug. This is doubtless the most important drug in prevention of renal artery stenosis and its progression. It assumes even more importance in keeping these silent blockages really silent by preventing plaque rupture, clot formation, and total obliteration of the channel of the artery (literally starving the kidney to death).

Surgery for Renal Artery Stenosis

There is not much of a place for surgical revascularization in this disease. In the past, this was the only tool we had to correct this problem. However, this is a huge operation because the kidney is so well protected within the enclosure of the retroperiotoneum behind the abdominal cavity. It is protected from trauma and covered with a capsule and a connective tissue barrier. If the operation were durable, it would, perhaps, more frequently be worth the agony and the effort. However, there is a substantial closure rate following a very adequate surgical bypass. In this procedure, the kidney artery is either sectioned and attached to a separate portion of aorta, eliminating the diseased ostium (the opening of the renal artery where blockage almost always forms) or more likely, a segment of vein or other conduit is used to form a bypass around this blockage, going from the aorta to a segment of the renal artery that is normal. In point of fact, these are frequently not successful long term, probably because we now send only the worst salvage problems to the vascular surgeons. They know this, too, and I am sure they hate to see a referral for renal vascular grafting because they know it will be something we don't think we stand a prayer of salvaging. Even before the advent of stent deployment in opening these arteries, however, the operation was still fraught with a substantial failure rate, probably for the same reason: We only sent desperate cases. What would the success rate be if we referred the good cases for surgery? Probably a lot higher; however, we can successfully stent 99% of these within 30–45 minutes with a good durable result and a one-day hospital stay. Therefore, surgical referral for most of these would be tantamount to failure of judgment, if not patently illegal, and this is a big surgery, indeed.

Fibromuscular Hyperplasia (Dysplasia)

There are other causes of renal artery blockage. The best known is a condition called fibromuscular hyperplasia, where fibrous tissue (like scar tissue) develops in the renal artery, resulting in a "string of beads" appearance. While these can occur in many arteries throughout the body, including the carotids to the brain, most of them occur within a renal artery. Most also occur in women. Usually, only one kidney is involved. These respond to angioplasty and/or stents but not nearly as well as the arteriosclerotic variety, as they are more commonly distal in location, farther from the renal artery take-off from the aorta. The cause is unknown but, fortunately, they are rare.

REMINDERS

1. Hypertension that does not respond to aggressive treatment may be due to renal artery stenosis—blockage in the artery leading to a kidney.
2. If you have angiography for any reason and have difficult-to-control hypertension, ask your doctor if the renal arteries will be examined.
3. Renal artery blockage can almost always be effectively treated with stent deployment.
4. Stent deployment within the renal artery will frequently help, but almost never completely control, high blood pressure. Stent therapy is used primarily to save the kidney from destruction due to loss of blood supply. Any improvement in blood pressure is a plus.
5. If you have a partial blockage in a renal artery (not severe enough for a stent), make sure that you have a renal artery ultrasound at least once a year so your blockage will not progress to total occlusion and loss of the kidney.
6. Plaque rupture, with associated clot formation on top of the ruptured plaque, will take a 50% blockage in a kidney artery to complete closure of the artery. Be sure you are on a statin drug, which will block both the LDL-cholesterol and the inflammatory trigger.

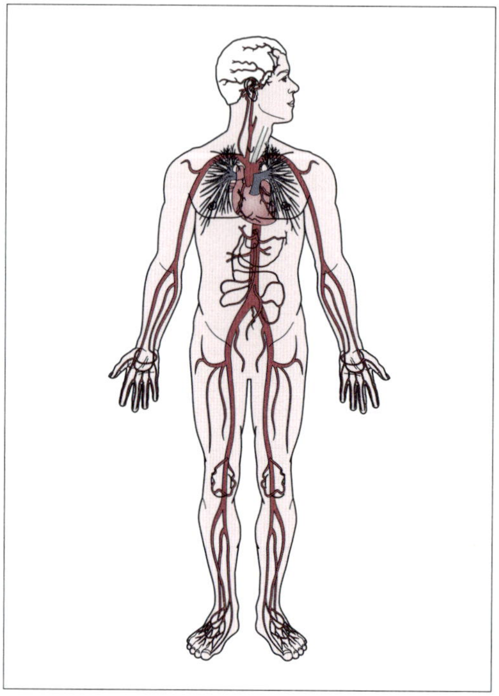

19 SYNCOPE

Blackout Spells

SYNCOPE MEANS TRANSIENT LOSS OF CONSCIOUSNESS. It can be as simple as the swoon seen when a teenager comes in contact with a rock star, or as complex as threatened sudden death from *ventricular tachycardia* (VT), a malignant rhythm disturbance arising from a focus within the left ventricular muscle after a heart attack. We always take syncope seriously. It is a common presenting symptom in any busy emergency room.

Orthostatic Syncope

A common cause of syncope has to do with standing when dehydrated. Blood is subject to the principle of gravity and it pools in the venous system. Usually, the heart rate increases markedly and the peripheral arterioles, small muscular arteries everywhere but especially in the legs, will get smaller (vasoconstrict). This combination will normally protect you from blackout. However, any number of things can alter these compensatory reflexes. One of these is defective vasoconstriction and another is a defective ability to increase the heart rate. These two, unfortunately, are common in the elderly and may frequently coexist. We call this type of blackout spell, passing out upon standing, orthostatic syncope. It is especially common in the elderly, but also happens in the below-50 crowd. A certain amount of water is necessary in the blood stream to keep the blood pressure at the level where it should be. If you are dehydrated enough, the blood becomes volume-contracted, a prelude to a blackout spell, unless your heart rate increases markedly along with constriction of the arterioles. A strong vasodilating substance is alcohol. Therefore, the culprit is sometimes alcohol, consumed at a time of volume-contraction. Instead of the arterioles constricting to keep the blood from pooling, they dilate and the glass flies into the air, as the person hits the deck. This is especially likely to happen in an elderly person, but the young are not immune to it. Da Vinci was right: "Drink water along with your wine."

It turns out that orthostatic dizziness and syncope is an incredibly common problem in the elderly, especially those who have congestive heart failure and are on a variety of pills to help eliminate water and unload the heart. If you are 25 years old and are immobilized for a couple of weeks because of an injury or surgery, you will have lost some of your compensatory reflexes when you get back on your feet and start walking, but not to the extent that you black out. If you are 75, the situation is quite different. The automatic reflexes that constrict our small arteries—raising the systemic vascular resistance in an effort to keep the blood pressure from falling when you rise from a supine to a standing position—go on vacation when you go down. They don't come roaring back, either. It takes days and days to retrain them and, if you are diabetic, this is exaggerated even more. You may require a drug to provide some tone in these peripheral arterioles falsely so that the blood pressure won't drop to disastrous levels when you stand. Pro-Amatine is such a drug. The major caveat is that in performing this task, it may inappropriately vasoconstrict a coronary artery. This doesn't usually happen, but I've seen it on one occasion. So, if you are using Pro-Amatine and get chest pain, let your doctor know without delay.

Vasovagal Syncope

A type of syncope that we are accustomed to seeing in a doctor's office or in the hospital setting, but which also occurs in everyday life, is *vasovagal syncope*. This occurs when someone, commonly a burly, muscular, macho guy, loses consciousness when he is having blood drawn for laboratory testing. He—or she, but usually he—gets sweaty, very pale, and passes out cold within a matter of 30 seconds! This person has simply brought into play both of the two mechanisms mentioned above:

1. He has slowed his heart rate inappropriately, sometimes as low as 30 beats per minute.
2. He has dilated (enlarged) the caliber of his small arteries throughout the body.

The result is a dramatic drop in blood pressure; so low, in fact, that it is inadequate to perfuse the brain, and he passes out. This is very akin to a swoon. This occurs because of an over-active vagus nerve system. This is a pair of nerves that supply the heart, lungs, and the gastrointestinal tract. It normally acts as a modulator, slowing the heart, frequently in conjunction with a visceral discharge from the stomach or colon. In this case, it is somewhat excessive. You see, there has to be some semblance of balance between the nerves that cause the heart to speed up when you are scared and slow down when you are eating, resting, or sleeping. Like all things, it can get out of whack. Anything that activates this person's vagus nerve may bring about this exaggerated reflex. Common examples are bad news, hitting your thumb with a hammer, vomiting, donating or even just seeing blood, or straining.

These individuals are simply born with these peculiar mechanisms and, while it really shouldn't, it usually embarrasses them profoundly for they are, indeed, usually men. Passing out, to a macho man, is a "girl's problem." After the first spell or two, they know to inform the medical personnel about it, and they grit their teeth and bear it. For our part, we put them flat on an exam table to draw their blood and if they get woozy, we raise their legs, dumping the pooled blood back into the central circulation and, hence, to the brain.

There used to be such a gentleman in my cardiac practice. Not only did he have the above reflex in all of its glory, but he had totally blocked off both internal carotid arteries from arteriosclerosis. All of the blood supply to his cerebral cortex, the motor center, was via collaterals, tiny branches that had developed, connecting another artery to his cerebral blood supply. This was just barely enough to get him through the day. Needless to say, we were particularly careful with him, as his brain promptly got so oxygen-starved that he would have a seizure when his blood was drawn. We carefully prepared him first by putting his head down and even gave him a small dose of Atropine (speeds the heart) to help maintain a healthy heart rate while we were taking his blood.

Strain Syncope

Obviously, if this vagus nerve system supplies not only the heart but the gastrointestinal tract, it comes as no surprise that this same group of folks may black out when they strain at stool or if they have bladder outlet obstruction, when they void. This also happens in elderly people who have degenerative changes within their conduction system.

Medications Can Play a Role

Additionally, the elderly population is frequently on medication to control congestive heart failure or high blood pressure and these drugs may play a role. In fact, they usually do. It is very tough to get the point across, for example, that if one is taking a diuretic or a blood pressure medicine, those drugs should be stopped when they might lead to volume depletion, such as during diarrhea. I can't count the times that bright but ill and usually elderly people have come into the ER having continued a diuretic until they were as dry as a raisin. And to make matters worse, there is no one to blame but the doctors. And we can't really even logically blame them because they don't have enough hours in the day to discuss every possible eventuality with every patient.

Transient Rhythm Problems Cause Syncope

Another common cause of syncope is the development of an arrhythmia. It may be transitory, such as a short burst, or even sustained atrial fibrillation. This is a benign arrhythmia in the upper chambers of the heart and is very common in the elderly. It not uncommonly alternates with a very slow rhythm, sinus bradycardia. This back and forth, fast-to-slow rhythm, kind of like an unsteady foot on the accelerator, may well land the patient on the ground, especially if that person is taking a diuretic and is therefore significantly volume-depleted. Such patients are usually treated with a pacemaker to afford them a lower rate limit platform of 60 or 70. Then the rapid limb of this process can be treated with a drug to control the rate. Unless there is a contraindication, such an individual should receive anticoagulation therapy to prevent a catastrophic stroke.

Another arrhythmia that we have to look out for very vigilantly is that of *ventricular tachycardia*. This is a potentially fatal process and, therefore, one may get only one chance at making the diagnosis and treating it. It almost never occurs in a completely normal heart. The most common underlying pathology is that of coronary artery disease and, in that instance, we must make the diagnosis and pay attention to the underlying process. Another cause of VT is cardiomyopathy (muscle loss frequently due to a virus) and yet another is a valvular disorder. Patients must never be told they have ventricular tachycardia without a full investigation into specific causation. *There is always a cause.*

There are many more possible underlying causes of blackout spells. One of particular importance occurs as a congenital problem, the *Long QT Interval Syndrome.* Another is the *Brugada Syndrome.* There are now many variations of these so-called ion channel disorders that have been categorized. They are an important group because this is a familial process. They can be readily treated, usually with an implantable defibrillator.

Ventricular tachycardia is always important. Once the cause is found, we then need to stratify, as best we can, the risk that the patient will do it again. The test for that is usually an electrophysiologic test and, if the risk is still prevalent, the patient should have an automatic implantable cardiac defibrillator (AICD) placed prior to discharge.

IHSS

One of the causes of sudden death, especially in young people, is *Idiopathic Hypertrophic Subaortic Stenosis* (IHSS). This is due to a large bulge of muscle in the left ventricular outflow tract, just below the aortic valve. With exercise, this bulge moves ever closer to the valve, producing an obstruction to the outflow of blood from the left ventricle into the aorta. These individuals are also prone to ventricular tachycardia. This can be fatal and is frequently ushered in by an antecedent blackout episode. Again, we may not get but one shot at these people. The next spell might be the last.

Pulmonary Hypertension

Pulmonary hypertension, if severe enough, can also cause syncope. This is due to a very high blood pressure within the pulmonary artery. This can be caused from a series of blood clots that have traveled to the lungs or can be due to *primary pulmonary hypertension*, an unusual disease within the small blood vessels in the lungs. This is not always an easy diagnosis. In my view, as above, every patient who has a blackout spell that is anything more than just a simple faint or swoon should have an echo with Doppler analysis to look at valves and pressures within the heart and great vessels.

Valvular Problem as Cause of Syncope

Aortic stenosis, the scarring down of the aortic valve, can cause exertional syncope. This constitutes a medical emergency, as these patients are at a high risk of dying suddenly. The aortic valve has to be very severely narrowed with only a pinhole residual opening for this to occur.

Tools to Help Make the Diagnosis of the Cause

Sometimes one can make the diagnosis of the cause of the blackout spell from a history, such as the vasovagal syncope individual outlined above. Most, however, require some investigation. The most important tools we have are the Echo-Doppler machine and the Holter monitor. With the echo, we can examine the heart valves, the thickness of the wall of the ventricle, and usually rule out a cardiac mechanical cause for the blackout spell. The Doppler will give us the velocity of the blood and will, therefore, tell us the pressures within the heart and great vessels. It will also tell us whether or not there is any blockage in the subclavian artery, an uncommon cause of syncope.

Sometimes, the Doppler test will make the diagnosis in a curious way. There is, for example, an interesting situation called carotid hypersensivity. In a male, and it seems that this is more common in males, there is usually a story of light-headedness upon shaving. If one reaches over and gently presses on the carotid bulb, a particular region of the carotid artery just above the split into internal and external branches, the heart rate will slow and the person may just try to black out right there on the spot. This makes the diagnosis of carotid hypersensitivity. Everyone's heart rate will slow when you massage the carotid bulb. These folks, however, drop their rates to the floor with even the gentlest pressure.

In one patient, I simply hadn't gotten the diagnosis upon taking a history or performing an examination. The echocardiographer did, however, when she applied the Doppler probe to his neck. She was trying to get a better picture for me to examine, turned the probe and pressed down on his neck; he blacked out right on the table with a heart rate of 20!

The Holter monitor is a common tool in the investigation of syncope in that it gives us a 24-hour—or longer if we wish—electromagnetic tape-recording of the heart rhythm. This will frequently provide the diagnosis if someone is developing a conduction or rhythm problem.

Sometimes an individual will come in with a story of blackout spells that occur infrequently, with spells widely separated by large blocks of time. In that setting, if we are concerned enough about his story, we may well implant a loop recorder under the skin so that we can examine the rhythm for a very long period of time.

We recently had such a patient. I simply could not find anything wrong after she had received a thorough investigation. She insisted that her spells were "just awful." Several 24-hour Holter recordings were normal so we implanted a loop recorder under her skin. After about a month with the loop recorder, she came in triumphant. She had experienced one of her spells. We figured it would be a benign rhythm disorder, such as paroxysmal supraventricular tachycardia (PSVT), scary but not life-threatening. When we downloaded the recorder, we were amazed to find that she had, for some reason, experienced an episode of ventricular tachycardia at a very rapid rate. This was a life-threatening arrhythmia so we implanted an AICD. We never discovered the etiology in this young lady. She had a normal heart from A to Z, as best we could tell. She adamantly denied the use of cocaine or other drugs that can affect the heart rhythm. I am nonplussed by the fact that we did not nail down the cause, but I am confident that we did what we needed to do to keep her alive. Earlier, I made a big point of saying that there is always a cause for ventricular tachycardia. There is. In her case, we just weren't smart enough to figure it out. In lieu of an explanation, we did provide her with protection. I would rather have protection and not know the cause than to have nailed down the cause but failed to provide protection. Ideally, we do both.

Arrhythmogenic Right Ventricular Dysplasia (ARVD)

This is an unusual situation whereby muscle in the right ventricle is replaced by fat tissue. The result is that the right ventricle enlarges, loses contractile power and the owner, not infrequently, has ventricular tachycardia which can be life threatening. We can usually get a hint of this problem from a rather characteristic electrocardiogram. A carefully done echocardiogram, looking for the enlarged, poorly contractile right ventricle will cinch the diagnosis. These individuals frequently experience syncope.

Seizures Can Masquerade as Syncope

Another enigmatic cause of syncope is sometimes a neurologic cause, such as a strange type of seizure. I have had a couple of patients whose cause of repeated "blackout" spells could not be found by any cardiac investigative means. During a spell, the Holter showed erratic oscillation of the baseline rhythm. It made us suspicious, and an electroencephalogram yielded the diagnosis. They were having complex seizures and needed the services of a neurologist.

Other Neurologic Causes of Syncope

Other neurologic disorders may cause syncope. These are usually the degenerative processes that, in the process of attacking the peripheral nerves, also affect the nerves that help maintain blood pressure and heart rate. One such is called the Shy-Drager syndrome. These are horribly difficult to treat.

Neurocardiogenic syncope constitutes an important group. They have ineffectual compensatory mechanisms and this can be diagnosed with tilt-table testing. It can usually be effectively treated. These people, usually young, frequently go through their day with bouts of lightheadedness and they commonly lose consciousness. An electrophysiologist should always see these patients. There are increasing numbers with this disturbing problem; I used to see perhaps three patients a year, now I see 25 a year. The condition is due to a breakdown in compensatory blood pressure regulatory function. When we assume the upright position from the supine or sitting posture, a good deal of blood immediately pools in the legs due to simple forces of gravity. In a flash, four mechanisms jump into play to prevent our blood pressure from falling:

1. An increase in heart rate
2. An increase in peripheral vascular resistance, both arterial and venous, due to constriction of the blood vessels (they get smaller)
3. An increase in force of heart muscle contractility
4. Contraction of the skeletal muscle in the legs, sometimes called the second heart, pressing venous blood back to the heart

If this elaborate loop of neurogenic signals fails at any point, the blood pressure drops and the individual becomes dizzy or may pass out. Many of these interruptions of this elaborate circuitry seem to follow a viral infection. In fact, it has now been discovered that some are caused by the formation of antibodies against some of the receptors involved in this loop, a type of autoimmune disorder.

Interruption of Electrical Circuitry in the Heart

Finally, *complete heart block* is a classic cause of syncope. This is secondary to a more or less fixed heart rate due to blockage of conduction at the AV node between the upper and lower chambers, in which case the patient comes in with an *idioventricular rhythm* at a rate of 25–35. The diagnosis is obvious from the electrocardiogram in most cases. These patients have dropped down to their lowest subservient pacemaker, a ventricular focus, as an evolutionary primitive endogenous "pacemaker." It is just enough to keep a person alive, but most are miserable until an artificial pacemaker is implanted.

This problem of complete heart block can also be intermittent and much more difficult to find. I recently saw a lady who complained bitterly and repeatedly to her doctor about blacking out. She had multiple sclerosis and was wheelchair-bound. He had done multiple Holter monitors, 24-hour electromagnetic tapes looking at the rhythm and had, in desperation from several negative tapes, told her he thought she was imagining it. She came into the emergency room with a particularly bad spell. Her electrocardiogram was normal. As I was reading her chart, the nurse cried out. The lady had a ten-second episode of complete heart block, with nothing but atrial activity on the monitor, and passed out in front of us. She subsequently did that several more times, one due to a 20-second episode. She promptly received a dual chamber pacemaker.

REMINDERS

1. Blackout spells can have many causes. They all require evaluation, ideally with an echocardiogram and a Holter monitor.
2. If you are taking a diuretic and/or blood pressure medicines, stop them if you have diarrhea.
3. If you have syncope, don't let them send you home from the ER without a plausible explanation as to exactly what caused it.
4. There is always a reason for your blackout spells. It has to be found before you can be effectively treated. If your cardiologist has performed an echocardiogram and it is okay, make sure that you are seen by a cardiac specialist who does nothing but "electrical work."

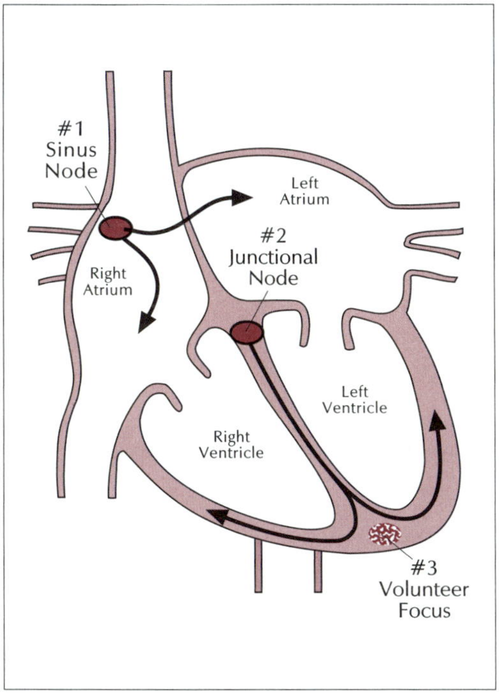

CARDIAC CONDUCTION SYSTEM DISEASE AND PACEMAKER THERAPY

You May Need to Live Better Electrically

History

The cardiac pacemaker is now in its *sixth decade* of therapeutic application. Can you even imagine the anxiety the implanting physician must have had when the first primitive pacemaker was put to use? When we look back at it, it was a truly remarkable feat. The first pacemaker had a lead implanted into the heart but was connected to an AC electrical source—the patient's mobility was limited by the length of his extension cord! But as Eugene F. Ware so famously put it, "All glory comes from daring to begin." We are now reaping the benefits of the courageous beginning established by those who came before us. Several thousand pacemakers are implanted yearly in America. Most of these are not implanted to save a life, but instead to improve the quality of life. Over the last 35 years, I have personally implanted about 2,000 pacemakers and have followed many of these people for a great many years. The percentage of folks who absolutely must have a pacemaker to live is far less than 1% of the total pacemaker population. Likewise, the number of people who develop pacemaker dependency (a lack of electrical activity if the pacemaker is turned off) is well less than 5%.

The Pathology

An impaired cardiac conduction system is the disease process that causes consideration of pacemaker therapy. This interruption of function can occur at many levels and is frequently due to pan-conduction disease—a thorough and diffuse degeneration of the conduction circuitry.

We need to know the basics of electrical current formation and delivery. The electrical impulse is generated by a collection of specialized cells high in the right atrium. These cells spontaneously leak ions across their cell membranes and this generates a tiny electrical "spark." This spark is then transmitted throughout the heart electrical system, consisting of conduits of wiring, just like you find in a house but much more elaborate. These conduits are contained within the muscular wall of the heart. This spread of electrical activity throughout first the upper chambers then the lower, in sequence, causes the muscle fibers to contract. The change in volume load causes the heart valves to open and close in response to cardiac contractility. In essence, the secondary mechanical process that pumps the blood is dependent upon the primary electrical process. If the electrical circuitry is disrupted at any place, an identifiable abnormality exists. This abnormality may or may not necessitate pacemaker intervention. This abnormality may sometimes be discovered on a simple electrocardiogram; other times, sophisticated electrophysiologic testing is required to determine the problem.

I have seen many healthy elderly people come in with cardiac electrical problems. In fact, most electrical problems requiring pacemaker therapy are a result of age-related degenerative processes within the wiring of the heart. Frequently, however, when I discuss this problem with elderly individuals, they are amazed. I probably will be too if I reach 80 and am told that I need a pacemaker.

I recently saw an 82-year-old gentleman with just this attitude. He was a high-powered contractor. When he retired, he became bored and began buying old houses with "great bones" as he put it, but apparently bad problems as a result of age. This gentleman loved to restore them to their original glory. He was aghast when I told him that the fatigue and shortness of breath that had caused him to see me was due to electrical problems in his heart (his heart rate was 35!). He actually became pretty belligerent. Nothing settled him down until I finally changed the conversation to his area of interest and asked him exactly what he did to restore the houses he worked on. He thought we were finished with the subject of his heart and gladly got into the story about how he would strip the interior, refurbish the plumbing and electrical systems completely, and then install gorgeous interiors, kitchens, and bathrooms. He puffed up with pride as he explained the process. "Soup to nuts," he boasted. "We do the whole thing. I even have a landscaping crew that puts the final polish on the project." His enthusiasm was valid and I enjoyed talking with him immensely.

I then asked him the age of the houses he refurbished. He replied that most were between 70 and 80 years old. "They only put enough lumber in them up to about 1950," he explained. I asked him if he bought any in that age group that were so good that he just left the plumbing and electrical as they were and installed new interiors. He snorted indignantly as if only a crook would do that sort of shoddy work, and informed me that the substructure was the most important part of his work. He then stopped short, his face reddened, and I thought, "Oh no, here we go again." To my immense relief, he laughed. "When do I go in for my pacemaker?" he asked, shaking his head.

A. Sick Sinus Syndrome

By far, the most common and distinct entity resulting in pacemaker implantation is that of *sick sinus syndrome* (SSS), a poorly named collection of electrical problems. The reason it is poorly named is that, taken literally, it implies a dysfunction of the sinus node, the primary pacemaker in the upper heart.

In its purest form, SSS is simply the degeneration of the specialized electrical cells comprising the sinus node, the little collection of cells in the upper right atrium that initiates the electrical spark. In this case, the sinus rate—the God-given rhythm—simply slows substantially at rest, and exercise will not increase the rate as it should. The rest of the circuitry seems just fine. Sometimes this is just the case. However, the "cockroach theory" (if you see one, there are many more where it came from) applies here too. Usually, if the sinus node is faulty, the rest of the wiring in the heart is not great either.

The first thing a doctor has to do in an elderly patient who has a very slow heart rate of 40, for example, is to make absolutely sure the patient is taking no medication that will slow the heart. The slow rate is called bradycardia—a Greek derivation for a slow heart rate, defined as less than 60 but for purposes of an inappropriate heart rate, less than 50. There are many drugs that will slow the heart rate, particularly in a heart that already has a deficient electrical system. The physician, the patient, and the patient's family all must be methodical, pursuing this avenue of detective work until all involved are sure that a pacemaker is not being offered to someone who is merely suffering from the adverse effects of a drug. Some of the well-known culprit drugs are beta-blockers, Catapres, calcium-blockers such as Diltiazem and Verapamil, the anti-arrhythmic drug Amiodarone, and many more. Sometimes it is impossible to get the individual off such a drug; however, we usually can substitute a drug that has no effect on the conduction system.

The physician also has a responsibility to the patient with a slow rate to check for a low thyroid level (hypothyroidism) or adrenal insufficiency (failure to manufacture enough cortisol in response to stress). Both of these conditions, sometimes fairly silent and hidden, can slow the heart rate, especially in an elderly person with some degree of electrical disease.

I think of myself as compulsive and vigilant but I have embarrassed myself on a couple of occasions in just this situation. One was by implanting a permanent pacemaker in an elderly patient who had adrenal insufficiency. I didn't hurt her by doing so. I could even justify it to myself by noting that she had degeneration of the sinus node and the adrenal insufficiency brought out the need for a pacemaker. The truth is, I didn't realize she had adrenal insufficiency. I just knew she had intermittent slow rates—as low as 30—and blacked out. Every time I see the particular physician who eventually made the diagnosis of adrenal insufficiency, I have to duck down the first available corridor, as he will never let me live it down! And I shouldn't. That's the reason it's called the "*practice* of medicine." We should learn from our mistakes—and some are painful. This one was just embarrassing. In point of fact, I think she really did need the pacemaker. My mistake was that I didn't make the correct diagnosis.

B. Tachy-Brady Variant of Sick Sinus Syndrome

One of the common types of SSS we see is the *tachy-brady variant.* This is pretty much what it sounds like. Namely, the heart races, developing a "tachy" arrhythmia for a while, then converts back to the sinus rhythm. The tachy element is frequently atrial fibrillation which is a fast, chaotic rhythm at a rate above 300 beats per minute in the upper chambers, the atria. This activity is conducted to the lower chambers, the ventricles, at a lower rate but is usually quite rapid nonetheless. The dysfunctional sinus node takes a while to get going again after it has been suppressed by this rapid electrical activity in the upper chambers, resulting in a long pause when the heart converts back to a sinus rhythm. Frequently, the sinus rate is quite slow for a while after conversion back to sinus rhythm, creating the "brady" component.

Such a patient may have a disturbing constellation of symptoms. These symptoms range all the way from breathlessness and chest discomfort when in atrial fibrillation with an uncontrolled rate, to getting very light-headed and nearly blacking out after converting back to sinus rhythm with the resultant long pause and initial slow rate. In some cases, such individuals will black out completely, an event we call *syncope*. There are all sorts of variations on this theme, one of which is paroxysmal atrial fibrillation, just as described above, but with a very slow ventricular response resulting in weakness and perhaps a blackout.

This rather common SSS, in one form or another, has been conventionally handled with a pacemaker because any drug treatment for the tachy limb of the syndrome is apt to make the brady limb worse. So, traditionally, a pacemaker is implanted to offer a lower rate limit platform, and then drug therapy is administered in treatment of the tachy limb of the syndrome.

Advancing age poses a problem with the beauty of this concept. In the older population, the heart has generally lost a great deal of elasticity. In other words, it has lost *compliance*—the ability to stretch to receive a load of blood. The stiff heart is said to be non-compliant, causing a high-filling pressure within the ventricle. When a right ventricular pacemaker is implanted, the electrical stimulation occurs first at the right ventricular septum (between the two lower chambers), taking septal contractility away from the left ventricle; this may cause deterioration in how the person feels and performs. With the new-paced rhythm, the septum squeezes in concert with the right ventricle rather than with the left, as was intended at birth.

This can be especially detrimental in these aging hearts and frequently brings about congestive heart failure or, if it is already present, makes it substantially worse. I have made great efforts to place the right ventricular pacing lead very high on the ventricular septum in order to simulate the electrical system that came from the factory. It has always disturbed me that someone might place a pacemaker in elderly patients who had SSS, converting them into patients whose blackout spells were replaced by severe congestive heart failure.

At the very least, the right ventricular pacemaker should be turned down to about 50 so it will perform only when the intrinsic heart rate is quite slow. With this adjustment, hopefully, the heart follows its own electrical impulse formation and conduits.

C. Complete Heart Block

A less common cause for mechanical pacemaker implantation is loss of the sinus node pacemaker and loss of the subservient junctional pacemaker. *The heart comes with its own three pacemakers built into it.* (Figure 21) The upper is the *sinus node,* the one we talked about previously as being the kingpin pacemaker. The next is the *junctional* at the level between the upper and lower chambers, the region of the AV node. It becomes dominant if the top one fails. The third and lowest is the *ventricular pacemaker,* a volunteer electrical focus within the ventricular tissue that emerges to save the day if the two more sophisticated pacemakers above it fail. Each is capable of running the heart.

Figure 21 Electrical System of the Heart

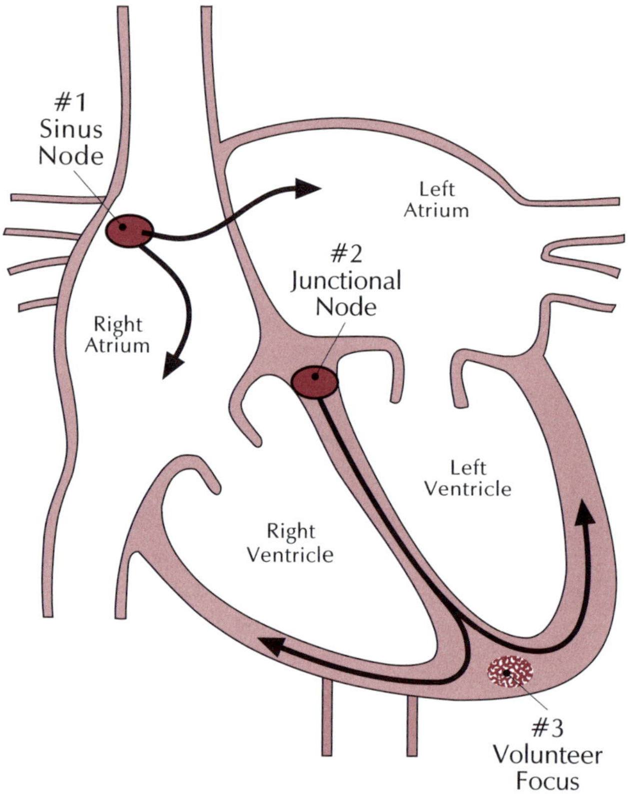

The electrical hierarchy of the heart is fashioned much like the hierarchy of government. The sinus node is quite nimble, responding to every whim and emotion of its owner with rate-adjustment. The junctional pacemaker is less adaptable, usually running along at a rather steady rate of about 40. The lowest—and least sophisticated—electrical driver in the system is the ventricular pacemaker. It rather reluctantly serves, and actually comes into play only when the intrinsically faster upper pacemakers in the heart have failed. This situation is defined as *complete (third-degree) heart block.* The ventricular rate is usually quite slow, in the 25 to 35 range. It is a self-preservation fall-back system, enough to keep a person alive and occasionally enough to prevent most symptoms if the individual remains flat. When the person tries to stand, the rate will not increase, the usual compensatory reflex, and the blood pressure will plummet. This problem should be treated with a pacemaker.

Older Hearts Need a Sophisticated Pacing System for Optimal Function

If you are in the population in which we implant most of these pacemakers, it is flat wrong for a doctor not to implant one that paces first the atrium and then the ventricle unless, of course, you are in "fixed" atrial fibrillation. This ideal pacemaker is called a *dual-chamber pacemaker*. Older persons with stiff hearts almost all need "atrial kick" or contractility. Otherwise the atrial contribution to cardiac output is lost. We know now that, as the ventricle gets sick, the atrium will increase its contribution and can contribute as much as 30% or so to the total cardiac output. The dual-chamber pacemaker more closely simulates the God-given electrical system than does a simple right ventricular pacemaker. A few years ago, the Medicare program tried to bully us into putting these only in those hearts where we could demonstrate a drop in the blood pressure when only the ventricle was paced, losing the entire contribution of the atria. (I'm sure they were merely trying to cut costs and preserve this strained system.) This drop in pressure is called a *pacemaker syndrome* and people were frequently incapacitated by it. We all rebelled as it was becoming obvious that all of these elderly, stiff hearts had lost elasticity and if we eliminated the atrial kick, we made a large percentage much worse than they were previously, at least in terms of how they felt. Furthermore, what we tested at the time of implantation was not very indicative of what might happen a year down the line. A dual-chamber system is now pretty well uniformly incorporated when installing a pacemaker in such a person.

If left ventricular function is quite severely impaired and a pacemaker is required, a triple-lead system should be implanted. One lead goes into the right atrial appendage to insure atrial activity as much as possible. Another lead goes in the conventional location in the right ventricle. A third lead goes into the coronary sinus down the great cardiac vein draining spent blood from the front portion of the heart. This latter lead, stimulating the left ventricle, is used to synchronize ventricular activity. This triple-lead system takes longer to install, but it will pay off in the long run because cardiac performance is optimized in these sick hearts.

Pacemakers to Convert Rapid Rhythms

Finally, with major advances, we have pacemaker systems that are able to recognize an algorithm generated by beats leading to the early stages of atrial fibrillation, pacing the heart out of this arrhythmia. Improvement upon this facility is going to be the next great breakthrough, I predict, and just in the nick of time, as atrial fibrillation is becoming a terribly common arrhythmia around the world. It seems to be of epidemic proportions, capable of inflicting life-changing chaos upon its unsuspecting victims in a matter of seconds. This is most commonly in the form of a clot, or thrombus, generated within the fibrillating left atrial appendage. If this thrombus dislodges and travels elsewhere, becoming an *embolus*, it can certainly cause a calamity, usually in the form of a stroke. There is no good place for an embolus to land. The best one could hope for would be for the embolus to take the bend in the aorta and travel south to the legs. However, the straight course is to go north toward the brain and lodge in one of the branches of the carotid arterial system. Hopefully, with the improvement of these pacing systems, we will be able to keep more and more people in the proper rhythm, to afford them not only the best hemodynamics possible, but the prevention of strokes and other embolic catastrophes also.

When you get your pacemaker, make sure your cardiologist checks your threshold in about three months. That is the time when all tissue swelling and scarring at the tip of the pacemaker has resolved or matured. Your system should be adjusted so you have ample protection but also so you do not use inappropriate amounts of "juice" from your pacemaker and cause battery depletion earlier than would be predicted. It is a small matter for the cardiologist to change the battery; however, it is a very large matter for you, the patient. Each time one opens the pouch, there is a chance for infection. Also, you have to receive antibiotics, which interrupts the normal bacterial flora in the gut. Finally, these batteries cost about $6,000 and the health-care dollar is already being stretched to the breaking point. Health care is currently predicted to be $1.3 trillion. In a few short years, with the baby boomer population reaching 60, it is expected to exceed $4 trillion. Soon, if we don't change the health-care paradigm in some fashion, we will break the bank.

REMINDERS

1. Fatigue, light-headedness, or shortness of breath may imply an arrhythmia, heart block, or some combination thereof.
2. Most people do not die for want of a pacemaker. However, it can vastly improve the quality of your life. Discuss the pros and cons with your doctor.
3. Ask your doctor if he or she is going to implant a pacemaker that will give you the best hemodynamics possible. It is the physician's responsibility to do so.
4. You may well wind up taking some drug combination in conjunction with pacemaker therapy to regulate your heart action.

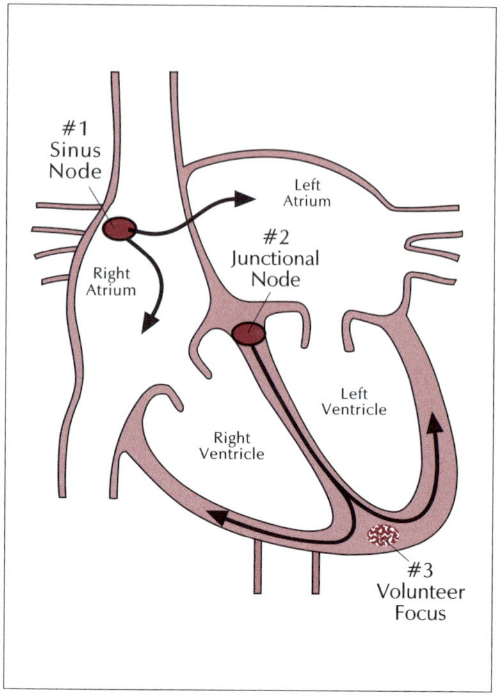

AUTOMATIC IMPLANTABLE CARDIAC DEFIBRILLATORS

A Shocking Experience That Can Save Your Life

THE AUTOMATIC IMPLANTABLE CARDIAC DEFIBRILLATOR (AICD), capable of shocking its owner out of a life-ending disturbance of heart rhythm, has turned out to be a magnificent invention. Michel Mirowski conceived of the automatic implantable cardiac defibrillator in the 1960s after his mentor died of a heart arrhythmia. The AICD has become a reality, and now there are many well-trained electrophysiologists around the world who perform the necessary testing and implantation in the at-risk population. This usually requires no more than a one-day hospital stay. As Aristotle said some 16 centuries ago, "Education is the best provision for the journey to old age." Education is the sole purpose of this book.

Who Needs an AICD?

The short answer is anyone who is at higher-than-average risk of dying from a cardiac arrhythmia. An arrhythmia is any variation from the usual regular heart beat.

Most arrhythmias are a nuisance, not life-threatening. Some are dangerous. When people are identified as having a particular tendency to develop a life-threatening electrical event, they should receive an AICD without delay. The challenge is identifying the at-risk population. Sometimes this can be exceptionally difficult. However, the cost of an oversight is frequently an unwarranted death.

The AICD is a device that is inserted in the same way as a pacemaker. It continuously reads the electrical activity of the heart on a beat-to-beat analysis. If a very rapid arrhythmia from the lower chambers develops, the AICD will fire, emitting an electrical discharge in order to restore proper sinus rhythm. The rapid rhythm we generally refer to here is *ventricular tachycardia* (VT). People generally lose consciousness fairly rapidly with this arrhythmia, but some will retain bare consciousness. If VT persists, it will frequently deteriorate into a uniformly fatal arrhythmia called *ventricular fibrillation* (VF). These are the two life-threatening arrhythmias for which an AICD is implanted, and we now have good means of predicting which individuals are at high risk for developing such arrhythmias.

In the past, it was necessary to put each individual who might need an AICD through a rigorous and rather elaborate procedure called an electrophysiology test. These were laborious. This test has become much more streamlined; however, we have found that the majority of people who require AICD implantation fit into a particular category that does not demand prior testing. Let me explain this strange development.

The *most common* patient populations at risk for VT/VF are those with coronary artery disease due to cholesterol deposits within the wall of the arteries supplying the heart muscle. When one of these arteries closes off, it produces a heart attack, usually resulting in significant muscle damage.

In general, the greater the amount of damage caused by the heart attack, the higher the risk of sudden death from VT/VF. There are certain unusual examples whereby an individual has sustained a limited amount of muscle damage and is uniquely predisposed to VT/VF. However, this potentially lethal arrhythmia has now been shown to be much more prone to develop in those who are left with a severely impaired left ventricle—the main pump of the heart.

We measure efficiency of the left ventricle by looking at the ejection fraction, the percentage of blood within the left ventricle that is pumped out into the aorta with each heartbeat. A normal figure is approximately 60%. Severe impairment is an ejection fraction of about 30%. We know from examination of large populations of individuals, that this group of people—those with a previous heart attack and a residual ejection fraction of 30% or less—has a high enough risk of dying from VT/VF to warrant an

AICD implant. Obviously, not all such individuals will ever use their AICD. I have seen several patients in this category fail to need their unit for a year or so (perhaps even grumbling good-naturedly that it wasn't really needed) only to come in after getting shocked. It had saved their lives, because they had, indeed, experienced one of these life-ending electrical storms. In other words, while we know that the greatest percentage of patients who will ultimately develop sudden cardiac death falls within this category of coronary disease with enough muscle damage to cause a dramatic decline in their muscle pumping ability, we *still* have to install a substantial number of the defibrillator devices in this population just to save a single patient. Patients who fall within the risk guidelines automatically become candidates for implantation of an AICD—and it should, at the very least, be offered to such a patient as an option. These guidelines are so well established by demographic data that Medicare/Medicaid will pay for the implantation of an AICD in folks who fall into this category.

In the individual who has had recurrent VT, we would implant the AICD but we would still treat the patient with an anti-arrhythmic drug. This is done to prevent recurrent shocks from the device.

Many of these same people are prone to develop a common arrhythmia emanating from the upper chambers of the heart, atrial fibrillation. I really dislike it when my patients get shocked with their device because of atrial fibrillation, so I usually keep them on a drug that will slow the ventricular rate if atrial fibrillation develops. While it is physically harmless for them to get shocked occasionally, it is not psychologically harmless, and I want them to receive a shock only if it is necessary to save their lives. Additionally, an occasional patient will develop atrial fibrillation and a shock will either not convert it or the patient will go right back into the atrial fibrillation, prompting another shock. Such a patient might receive multiple shocks over just a couple of hours. This is not good for the heart and even worse for the psyche. These are not happy people! Having been shocked while wide awake and working on a felled fireman while I was an intern, I can fully understand their reaction. The simple measure of providing a drug to block a rapid ventricular response to atrial fibrillation will prevent this. Too often, this is not done. I almost always choose Coreg. This is a unique beta-blocker which helps preserve, and even reclaim, ventricular performance. It doesn't have a great power as a slowing agent but it is usually enough to prevent an extremely rapid ventricular rate were the individual to develop atrial fibrillation.

An important caveat must be entered here. We are obviously most commonly implanting these devices in folks with severe left ventricular impairment. They are either in congestive heart failure or are ideal candidates for developing it. Remember, we are putting the pacemaker in the right ventricle. When the heart paces, we will be stealing septal contractility away from the left side. In other words, since the electrical impulse first activates the right ventricular septum, that segment of muscle which usually aids the left ventricle in its chore, will now work in concert with the right ventricle. This alone can precipitate heart failure in these exceptionally sick hearts. Just as we can make hemodynamic matters worse with a pacemaker, if we are not careful, we can do the same thing with an AICD. So, if the left ventricle is quite severely impaired, an additional lead should be placed in the coronary sinus and the patient should receive synchronized cardiac pacing. This adds very little risk to the procedure and can make a world of difference in terms of cardiac performance and functional ability.

There are obviously others who are at high risk for VT/VF. They are just not as obvious as this huge coronary population with severe left ventricular impairment. Since coronary artery disease is the highest percentage killer of both men and women in the United States, we have ample numbers to categorize and stratify risks statistically.

The other causes have to be sorted out as they come in. They are members of a rather diverse group. For example, the inherited sudden cardiac death syndromes, notably the Brugada and the Long QT Interval Syndromes, now the Short QT Interval Syndrome, are due to inherited disorders in the channels through which sodium, potassium, and calcium migrate. With these, there is usually a family history of others dying suddenly. Close study of the electrocardiogram will make the diagnosis. The prompt identification of these is of utmost importance, as they are usually young when they begin their innocent march toward a life-ending electrical problem. Their hearts are structurally normal; it is the electrical-signaling mechanism that is faulty, a result of a genetic endowment.

One of the problems that I worry about is *arrhythmogenic right ventricular dysplasia* (ARVD). This is a situation, usually inherited, in which right ventricular muscle is replaced by fat and scar tissue. Being obese doesn't cause it. The electrocardiogram is usually abnormal and the echocardiogram shows a large, poorly contractile right ventricle, at least in the obvious ones. I worry about missing the not-so-obvious ones. This is more common than the youth-ending sudden death syndromes just discussed. It occurs in about 1:10,000 people in America, more in some countries. Additionally, it makes up about 15–20% of all sudden deaths in the young.

Sometimes an individual comes in with no family history of sudden cardiac death, yet with an electrocardiogram strip showing ventricular tachycardia. I just had a patient with such a problem. He ran his garbage truck into a pole, managed to call 911 and when they arrived, he was in ventricular tachycardia. His electrocardiogram was entirely normal when he was in a normal rhythm. He was examined from head to toe. We did extensive electrophysiologic testing and other studies of his heart. We could find nothing abnormal; and he went home with an AICD in place. We sent off blood for laboratory testing to determine if he has one of these inherited sudden cardiac death syndromes (for his children's sake), but these require a six-month investigation. His comment was typical: "Why don't I go home and try it again; see if anything happens?" Of course, our response was that he might not be so lucky the next time around.

The saving grace in these non-coronary individuals with risk of sudden death is that commonly there is an initial history of a blackout spell (syncope) or at least bothersome palpitations with profound dizziness. This is the reason we must take every complaint very seriously. We try to segregate out the individuals who seem to be at major risk and perform electrophysiologic testing on them to determine whether or not they are at risk of sudden cardiac death. If so, they should receive an AICD posthaste.

This segregation process—who does and who doesn't require an AICD—has to be tempered by reason. It's not always so simple as to say that everyone who has rapid ventricular arrhythmias needs a defibrillator. For example, I recently saw a fellow with rapid ventricular tachycardia. But the particular pattern on the electrocardiogram made me think it might be coming from a small independent electrical source within the right ventricular outflow tract. Knowing that these respond to Verapamil, a calcium channel-blocker, when other forms will not, I gave him some and he converted. When extensively studied, he had a structurally normal heart. He had long been plagued by spells of a racing heart but had never passed out. Since starting the drug, he has not had one symptom. He doesn't need an AICD because his outlook without one is excellent.

REMINDERS

1. **Ventricular arrhythmias of life-threatening importance are most common in individuals with coronary artery disease and extensive heart muscle damage.**
2. **An Automatic Implantable Cardiac Defibrillator (AICD) should be offered to those at high risk of sudden cardiac death. They can be implanted in about an hour.**

3. Any patient with coronary artery disease and a left ventricular ejection fraction less than 30–35% should be offered an AICD. This is the group in which sudden cardiac death becomes significant.
4. Electrophysiologic testing of the heart should be performed on patients with "hard" syncope (blackout with loss of consciousness) and, if a life-threatening arrhythmia is precipitated, they should be offered an AICD.
5. Patients with very sick hearts are at high risk of developing atrial fibrillation, a benign arrhythmia that can cause the AICD to fire. Such patients should be on a drug to prevent rapid ventricular response in the event that atrial fibrillation develops.

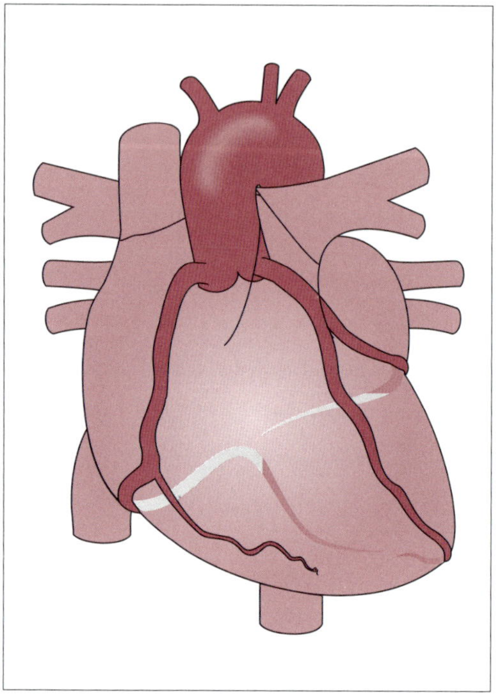

DILATED CARDIOMYOPATHY

An Enlarged Heart with Poor Function

THERE ARE SEVERAL FORMS OF CARDIOMYOPATHY, the term for heart muscle disease. Some are hereditary, some are defined by having too much muscle, but here we cover just the *dilated cardiomyopathy*. The word "dilated" means that the chambers of the heart are enlarged due to some process that has either stunned or destroyed heart muscle cells.

The heart muscle spirals around the heart and the fibers interconnect forming what we refer to as a syncytium. Contractility results from fiber shortening with a resultant decrease in the size of that chamber, accompanied by a twisting and wringing motion when the heart squeezes out blood. The left ventricle is shaped like a football with one end cut off. The apex is the very tip of the ventricle. This geometric design, and its smaller twisting, fist-like counterpart during contraction, is exceptionally important in maintaining proper function. When muscle is stunned or destroyed, this geometric shape is lost. The ventricle becomes rounded and congestive heart failure, accompanied by a fall in cardiac output (the measure of production) develops proportionately to the damage.

A significant insult to the heart muscle can actually occur without many resultant symptoms, especially if an individual is especially sedentary. Similarly, a fair amount of chamber enlargement can occur due to a malfunctioning heart valve without symptoms, especially if the process is slow and insidious. I read with sadness that the coach of the women's basketball team at West Point died at age 28 with an enlarged heart and a malfunctioning heart valve.

The condition known as *idiopathic dilated cardiomyopathy* is a form of heart muscle weakness whose true cause is unknown, but it is thought to be due to invasion of the muscle with a virus. It can become quite severe without debilitating symptoms. In fact, if the process is slow and progressive, people accommodate so reflexively that they believe this is just the way everyone else feels. Since this is sometimes so insidious in onset and progression, we often see such individuals only when they are within the framework of an advanced process.

The initial symptom of dilated cardiomyopathy is usually shortness of breath either with exertion, if early, or at rest, later in its course. The first sign of the disease is usually peripheral edema—swelling of the ankles—due to increased tissue water. Indeed, many people are waterlogged when they first seek help.

Ischemic Cardiomyopathy

There are several potential causes of dilated cardiomyopathy. The one we must rule out first is that which follows a heart attack, known as a myocardial infarction, if for no other reason than coronary artery disease is the most common disease of the heart and blood vessels. The precipitating cause could well be a silent heart attack. When confronted with this diagnosis, some people remember pain or another symptom that was simply ignored. We commonly see people who have had several such events that were relatively silent and have developed an *ischemic* (oxygen-deprived) *cardiomyopathy* as a result. In other words, one or more arteries feeding the heart muscle closed off, resulting in muscle damage. If significant heart muscle is lost, there will not be enough remaining muscle to carry on the necessary task of pumping blood effectively. As the remaining muscle struggles to carry on the load, the heart fibers stretch and the chamber enlarges as contractility becomes weaker and weaker. The left ventricle loses it ever-important geometric configuration, leading frequently to leakage of the mitral valve—and heart failure ensues. We can usually make the diagnosis of this not-uncommon situation by performing an electrocardiogram (ECG) and an echocardiogram (echo). The ECG will show a pattern of injury consistent with a recent heart attack, or more commonly, signs of an old heart attack. The echo will show segmental dysfunction of the left ventricular muscle correlating with the area(s) of previous injury.

It is particularly important to make this determination, as we have seen many patients come in with a dilated cardiomyopathy who had stunned heart muscle mixed with destroyed muscle. Many of these patients will improve markedly with restoration of good blood flow to the muscle. Obviously, we cannot reclaim destroyed muscle that has been replaced by scar tissue. However, *stunned* muscle cells that seemed destined to die off may eventually resume a contractile role, if only they are furnished with a good blood supply once again. The end result of restoring blood flow depends on the extent of destruction. The stunned cells may take a long time to recover, but it's worth the wait.

Idiopathic Dilated Cardiomyopathy

The other major form of dilated cardiomyopathy is *idiopathic* (from the Greek meaning "a disease of its own kind"). We apply this term to someone who comes in with a large, dilated heart in the setting of normal arteries and valves. Most of these situations are likely secondary to a virus entering the heart muscle, doing its damage, and then leaving. Occasionally we are able to trace back the origination of symptoms to the time of a viral process. Often, we cannot.

Every virus has tropism—an affinity for a particular type of tissue. This is the reason why, with a viral infection, you sometimes get gastrointestinal symptoms and, alternatively, sometimes have predominant upper respiratory tract symptoms. Some viruses have tropism for the heart. I personally think that, as with the common cold, everyone probably is exposed to these viruses at some point in his or her life. Those uniquely predisposed individuals stand a greater chance of the virus wreaking havoc within the heart muscle. This is sheer speculation on my part, but I have seen many individuals who had a fairly clear-cut post-viral cardiomyopathy, who lived in close proximity with other family members and office workers and yet, these people were the only ones with the problem. We must presume that the others were not as susceptible to this virus. Additionally, we know that the individual who has had one episode of invasion by this virus, called viral myocarditis, is more likely than the general population-at-large to have a subsequent episode.

There was a period of time, back in the '80s, when we did myocardial (heart muscle) biopsies via a catheter on most patients who had a dilated cardiomyopathy. There had been a report that lymphocytes, a particular type of white blood cell, would infiltrate the heart muscle in the event of viral invasion and the finding of these cells would guide therapy. This never panned out, and we have largely abandoned this procedure unless the patient is clearly deteriorating. We have also discovered that immuno-suppressant agents usually do not help, and may even hinder improvement. Certainly the old dictum "First, let us do no harm" applies here. Prednisone and other immunosuppressant agents actually can be harmful in these patients and biopsy is not without hazard. I would be very skeptical of any patients receiving either of these interventions unless they were clearly deteriorating.

What happens to these folks? With good therapy, about 50% will improve almost to the point of getting back a normal contractile pattern. About 25% will be left with some variable degree of impairment. The other 25% don't improve much. These are the ones who have suffered widespread destruction of muscle. Some of these patients may eventually require transplantation but that number is very small, especially with our new forms of therapy.

Autoimmune Cardiomyopathy

One subgroup of dilated idiopathic cardiomyopathy has drawn special interest. These are generally young people in whom we believe viral myocarditis was the initial culprit. Some of these young people will develop progressive left ventricular dysfunction, even at a time when they should be stabilizing or improving. The viral genome cannot be found, implying that the virus has cleared out of the heart muscle. However, if you look for antibodies against heart muscle, they are frequently found in this group. The supposition is that the virus destroyed heart muscle (protein) that is usually kept sequestered (out of the bloodstream), and the body's defense system built antibodies against this newly recognized protein, thinking it was an invader that could do harm. The end result of this autoimmune process is more heart muscle destruction due to antibodies that the individual has formed against his or her own heart muscle. Immunosuppressant therapy does, indeed, make sense in this group of dilated idiopathic cardiomyopathy patients. Antibodies against the heart should be proven first.

Diabetic Cardiomyopathy

Another subgroup deserves special treatment. A phenomenon called diabetic cardiomyopathy has become recognized, even in the absence of demonstrable vascular disease or a hint of previous viral invasion of the heart muscle. In the past, we felt that small vessel disease was likely to blame. It may be, in part; however, there is also evidence of a direct harmful effect from a chronically elevated glucose level causing increased cell death from oxidative stress. Oxidative stress is a result of metabolism within any cell increasing with age or under certain circumstances, such as this one. There is promising data to suggest that zinc supplementation may prevent this. We have been recommending zinc to our diabetic patients for years, as it seems to help them heal toe ulcers. Perhaps it will also help protect their hearts during those times when blood sugar gets out of control.

Cardiomyopathy of Obesity

In overweight patients, no matter the cause of the cardiomyopathy, weight loss is vital. This simply reduces the amount of work the heart has to perform to supply blood to the body. The greater the body mass, the more work the heart has to perform. There is roughly one mile of capillaries, tiny blood vessels at the end of the arterial journey, for each pound of fat. You can see that, if you are substantially overweight, you may wind up having to pump blood through several extra miles of capillaries. This requires energy on the part of the heart. The one sure way of unloading the heart is to lose weight. While "unloading" drugs are very expensive, losing weight is free.

In fact, there is no question that some forms of dilated cardiomyopathy are due entirely to obesity. I have one gentleman in my practice who weighs 400 pounds. His heart came originally equipped, based on his frame, to supply blood to a 200-pound person. His body's needs have simply placed too much demand on his heart muscle and, over time, it has lost its ability to pump effectively. The contractile elements have slipped and the chambers have become dilated. We call this the *cardiomyopathy of obesity*.

Post-Partum Cardiomyopathy

A particularly worrisome type of dilated cardiomyopathy follows childbirth and is called *post-partum cardiomyopathy*. Many believe that these individuals simply experienced a viral invasion of the heart muscle at a time of increased cardiac output. In response, fiber stretch and chamber dilatation subsequently develop.

In such situations, with a fetus growing inside the progressively more compromised mother, her heart under assault, there is simply no way to reduce demands upon heart muscle. The baby requires a certain amount of blood flow, about 30% of the demands of the mother. It is the equivalent of developing a viral invasion of the heart muscle at the same time you are forced to perform some type of exercise 24/7. By the time of delivery, many of these cases are quite severe. The emotional component always has to be addressed with compassion but with encouragement. With aggressive therapy, many of these improve substantially.

Familial Cardiomyopathy

There are a number of familial cardiomyopathies passed on from generation to generation, some in dilated form. At this time, the genome sequences in these relatively rare disorders are being analyzed. There is usually some sort of alteration in the composition of the contractile elements in the muscle. This allows for gradual stretch of muscle fibers, loss of others, disruption of the connections between muscle cells, and distortion of the syncytium resulting eventually in a grossly dilated left ventricular chamber, and loss of the important geometric form with subsequent congestive heart failure. Early recognition of this situation means early help and a slowing of the natural history of the disease process. Hopefully in the future, either stem cell treatment or genomic alteration will eliminate this disorder or appreciably change its course.

Valvular Dysfunction Cardiomyopathy

The dilated cardiomyopathy that results from an abnormal heart valve is one that we can generally improve markedly by getting prompt treatment for the primary problem: the valve. Valve repair or replacement are the indicated forms of therapy if the patient's heart situation will allow it, as much of the overwrought heart muscle will return to normal function if given the opportunity. This situation is somewhat urgent so valve surgery should not be postponed. Such forms of dilated cardiomyopathy are usually due to a leaking valve. This is either the aortic valve, the valve that is responsible for keeping the column of blood that has been pumped from the left ventricle from leaking back into that chamber, or the mitral valve between the left upper and lower chambers. Occasionally the cardiomyopathy is due to aortic stenosis, a scarred aortic valve with limited ability to open properly. This imparts a huge pressure overload on the left ventricle and more as the valve opening is reduced—and is even more urgent, as such patients need immediate replacement of the valve before complete decompensation develops.

Alcohol Cardiomyopathy

Alcohol cardiomyopathy is of particular importance because the necessary ingredient of therapy is to recognize it and comment on it. Some people are very sensitive to the effects of alcohol; others are not. As we have all recognized, some folks can drink huge amounts of alcohol and never appear drunk. Others get inebriated with a glass or two of wine. Much of this depends on one's levels of alcohol dehydrogenases, the six enzymes in the liver that are responsible for metabolism of alcohol.

Chronic alcohol consumption in excess quantities seems to activate an elaborate mechanism in the kidney called the renin-angiotensin-aldosterone system. This, interestingly enough, is usually activated when there is a blockage of a renal artery or, alternatively, seems to become activated in many people simply with congestive heart failure without renal artery blockage. In fact, this is one of the reflexes we call "dumb reflexes" because its activation clearly places the person with congestive heart failure in a vicious spiral. For some reason, it is activated in chronic alcoholism too. A number of things happen in response to this. One is particularly deleterious: Aldosterone is manufactured and sent into the blood stream in excess quantities. It can cause fibrosis (scar formation) within the heart muscle; one also tends to hold onto salt and water.

The nuances can be very important. I recently saw a woman with a severe cardiomyopathy. As with all such patients, I quizzed her about alcohol. She dismissed it by saying that she only drank a "little bit of wine." You really have to focus on this; I could easily have missed the cause of her problem, and almost did. I knew her family and was uncomfortable about grilling her. Thankfully, I persisted. When I asked her the exact amount she consumed, the result was astounding. It turned out that she drank at least two glasses of wine at lunch with friends and business associates, then had two or three glasses with dinner and, of course, had a glass of port at bedtime. I backed up and looked her over. She was quite petite. In fact, she weighed exactly 100 pounds! A burly guy might have handled such a load without trouble. However, this was a huge amount of alcohol for her. We got her to totally abstain for three months and put her on proper therapy. Her heart has now returned to a normal contractile function. This was truly an epiphany for her. She was in terrible trouble when she came in, short of breath with grotesquely swollen legs. Those signs and symptoms vanished completely. I suspect that if we did a biopsy of the heart muscle, we would discover some lost muscle cells replaced by scar tissue. However, she has preserved enough muscle to do the job—only if she continues to abstain.

I always elaborate about the causes of dilated cardiomyopathy, especially due to alcohol. You must know the cause before you can truly understand the disease and treat it. In lieu of knowing the cause, you must know all of the things it isn't.

Somebody, probably a Texas politician, once said that people always lie about sex, alcohol, and money. Well, I can tell you for sure that they frequently lie about alcohol! I had a young man in the hospital recently, and I had quizzed him extensively about alcohol consumption. He replied that he drank very little. His wife and his best friend later told me that he drank 5–6 tall scotch drinks every night and never went to bed sober. This was obviously very important information in his management. With normal heart valves and arteries, alcohol was likely the cause of his congestive heart failure. It, too, magically resolved when he stopped drinking. His wife and friend made sure he had no alcohol. The caveat is that you must completely stop alcohol; you can't just cut back.

Chemotherapy-Induced Cardiomyopathy

It has long been known that certain chemotherapeutic drugs will cause dilated cardiomyopathy. One of these is Doxorubicin. In the past, this was given by bolus injection, with all of the drug pushed through intravenously. We did heart biopsies back in the 1970s and discovered that this form of therapy literally wrecked the heart muscle cells. They looked like a bazooka had gone off! The bolus injection was then switched to continuous infusion—a slow drip infusion of the drug over several hours. This improved the situation markedly. However, we continue to have a problem, as some people who receive this drug for one of many blood and solid malignancies will develop an irreversible degenerative cardiomyopathy. Since Doxorubicin is sometimes an irreplaceable drug in the treatment of a life-threatening malignancy, we have constantly remained vigilant to protect against this. We always perform incremental studies, examining left ventricular muscle function, during the use of this drug; however, some of these still slip by. Early evidence now suggests that a cytokine, erythropoietin, produced by the kidney, may protect against this problem. We have long known that erythropoietin caused formation of red blood cells. Indeed, when the kidneys fail, this cytokine is given to prevent the overwhelming anemia that we used to see. We have also known that it played a protective role in the brain and spinal cord. We knew that erythropoietin receptors were present in the heart and might play a significant role in preventing some of the damage of heart attack. Now, it looks as though this protective effect may possibly be important in preventing the devastation of Doxorubicin cardiotoxicity as well.

Treatment of Cardiomyopathy

These patients, no matter the cause, all need to be treated aggressively with diuretics to control any extra fluid that has accumulated. If blood pressure allows, they should all be placed on an angiotensin converting enzyme-inhibitor (ACE-I) and finally, on Coreg, a very unusual and unique beta-blocking agent. Coreg has truly become known as the miracle drug in patients with congestive heart failure. This is especially true with a dilated cardiomyopathy. In conjunction with the ACE-I drugs, it helps to reclaim the geometric form so important in effective left ventricular function. These patients should be removed from all strenuous activity and alcohol—a cardiac toxin even in small amounts—for three to six months to allow for as much healing and recovery as possible. This is very important, as there are almost always muscle cells that have been injured but not destroyed, and we must preserve as many of these stunned cells as possible. The heart is the only organ that has to heal on the run, so relieving it of as much workload as possible is very beneficial. Each muscle cell is precious. The cell population at the end of your recovery period clearly will define the quality of the rest of your life.

Surgery for Dilated Cardiomyopathy

Treatment of dilated cardiomyopathy is basically identical to the treatment of congestive heart failure. However, I think one aspect of dilated cardiomyopathy requires more consideration. In the event of ischemic cardiomyopathy, there are actually two or three different surgical procedures that can improve the situation somewhat. One is the ventricular reduction operation. This is usually for an individual who has had a heart attack involving the apex of the left ventricle and has remodeled the heart, developing a large aneurysm at the apex. This impairs pump function in three ways:

1. It causes further enlargement of the left ventricular chamber, placing more burden on the remaining muscle, which then tends to deteriorate.

2. The enlargement of the left ventricle frequently causes the mitral valve ring to enlarge and spread out, creating leakage across the valve.
3. Blood swirls around in the apex, reducing the efficiency of the ventricle.

Resecting the apical aneurysm sometimes associated with bypass of the coronaries, sometimes with repair of the mitral valve, in selected cases will bring about marvelous results.

The Future

The most exciting of all therapies yet is that of potential regeneration of heart muscle using stem cells. Animal models of heart-attack-induced destruction of heart muscle treated with stem-cell deployment improve dramatically. If we can extrapolate this to humans, it may well turn into a primary therapy for cardiomyopathy. This might eventually extend to other forms including the familial, inherited form for which treatment is currently only palliative.

REMINDERS

1. Dilated cardiomyopathy has several possible causes.
2. The diagnosis is not a death sentence.
3. Make sure you are on a diuretic, an ACE-I and, most importantly, Coreg (not just any beta-blocker).
4. Salt causes you to retain water. Restrict your use of salt; salt loading can quickly get you into trouble.
5. Lose weight if you are overweight. This will unload the heart.
6. Alcohol is a cardiac toxin. Ideally, stop drinking until the condition is controlled, or have no more than one alcoholic drink per day.
7. Typically, treatment of dilated cardiomyopathy is identical to the treatment of congestive heart failure. (See Chapter 11 on *Congestive Heart Failure.)*
8. If the cardiomyopathy is due to a heart attack, surgical reconstruction may well improve your lot.
9. Stem-cell repair of heart muscle may become a primary form of therapy in life-threatening cardiomyopathy.

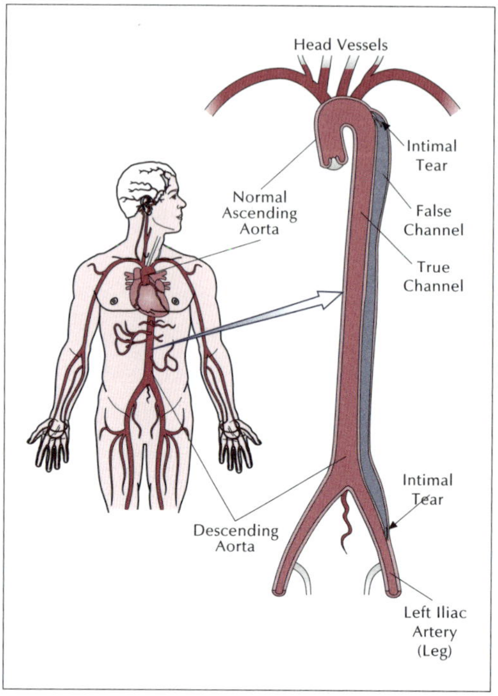

23 AORTIC DISSECTION

Separation of the Layers of the Aortic Wall

A TEAR IN THE WALL OF THE AORTA is called an aortic dissection. These are always serious. They are more apt to occur in someone who was born with a congenitally abnormal aortic wall or a person who has a degenerative process, but they can occur in just about anyone who has high blood pressure. In fact, roughly two-thirds occur in individuals who have hypertension. Fortunately, they are fairly uncommon. A flurry of attention was recently paid to this problem after the actor John Ritter died suddenly of an aortic dissection at age 54. He apparently had no idea that he possessed an underlying cardiovascular problem.

Normal and Abnormal Anatomy: How a Dissection Occurs

The composition of the wall of the aorta is three-layered, as is any artery. The middle portion, the media, is comprised of a network of elastic fibers and muscle fibers.

These are interwoven in a complex fashion, allowing muscular contraction of the wall of the aorta and elastic stretch as well. This gives the aorta the elasticity and strength it requires to handle drastic extremes of blood pressure, with its attendant stress on the aortic wall. These three layers are tightly bound, one to the other, much like decades of wallpaper on the dining room wall. In the young aorta, the elasticity of the aorta confers the ability to "yield," accepting each surge of blood with a dampening effect offered by this give in the aortic wall. With advancing age, this aortic wall elasticity is progressively lost. This results in loss of the dampening effect ("stiff pipes") causing more transmitted shear force against the aortic wall with each surge of blood.

If the integrity of the inside layer (the intima) is breeched, blood will enter the wall of the aorta. This tear creates a "flap" in the wall of the aorta. This collection of blood, called a hematoma, is subjected to the same blood pressure as that within the central channel of the aorta. Therefore, with each heartbeat, the hemodynamic stress of the blood pressure is now transmitted between the layers of the aortic wall as well as the lumen, the inside channel of the blood vessel where the blood normally flows. This "dissecting hematoma" will then continue to tear the aorta until it reaches some obstruction, such as a branch vessel. It then stops or merely reaches a point downstream where the transmitted pressure has dissipated and dampened enough to allow the dissection to halt.

Such a tear is called an *aortic dissection*. It can be compared to placing a tiny water hose underneath wallpaper and spraying it at high pressure. The water under pressure will find its course of least resistance and will dislodge the paper from the wall. In the instance of aortic dissection, the column of blood may eventually tear back into the lumen of the blood vessel, producing along its course a double-barreled structure—a true lumen and a false lumen. Many of these patients have an abnormal aortic wall matrix—some sort of fault in the underlying tissue components of the wall of the aorta. Others possess an arteriosclerotic plaque, a collection of cholesterol that has hardened within the wall of the aorta. When such a plaque ruptures due to disruption of its covering, it basically splits open like a piece of cheese that has been left uncovered in the refrigerator too long. In this instance, particularly if the wall of the aorta at that point is "brittle" due to degenerative changes within the wall, high blood pressure allows blood to enter this open lesion within the wall and separate the layers of the aorta along its course.

Such dissections may occur in any portion of the aorta. They usually occur somewhere within the up-going portion just above the heart or the downward portion after the aorta has made its loop in the chest. They rarely occur in the abdominal aorta.

The location where a dissection begins has a great deal to do with the individual's eventual outcome. There have been many efforts at categorizing dissections. The most simple and sensible for our purposes is the Stanford system, which merely divides them into two general categories.

Aortic Dissection: Stanford Type A

A dissection that originates in the ascending aorta just above the heart is by far the most dangerous. It can extend into the carotid arteries leading to the brain, causing a large stroke. It can also involve the valve support structure (the aortic annulus) causing massive leakage of the aortic valve, allowing blood already once pumped to flow copiously back into the left ventricle. It can even extend into the pericardium, the membrane covering of the heart, causing *tamponade*, strangulation of the heart pumping action due to accumulation of blood in the heart sac. Such a tear, called a Type A aortic dissection involving the ascending aorta, is the ultimate medical and surgical emergency. (Figure 22) Type A dissections carry a high mortality rate and, in the event

Figure 22 Type A Aortic Dissection Ascending Aorta

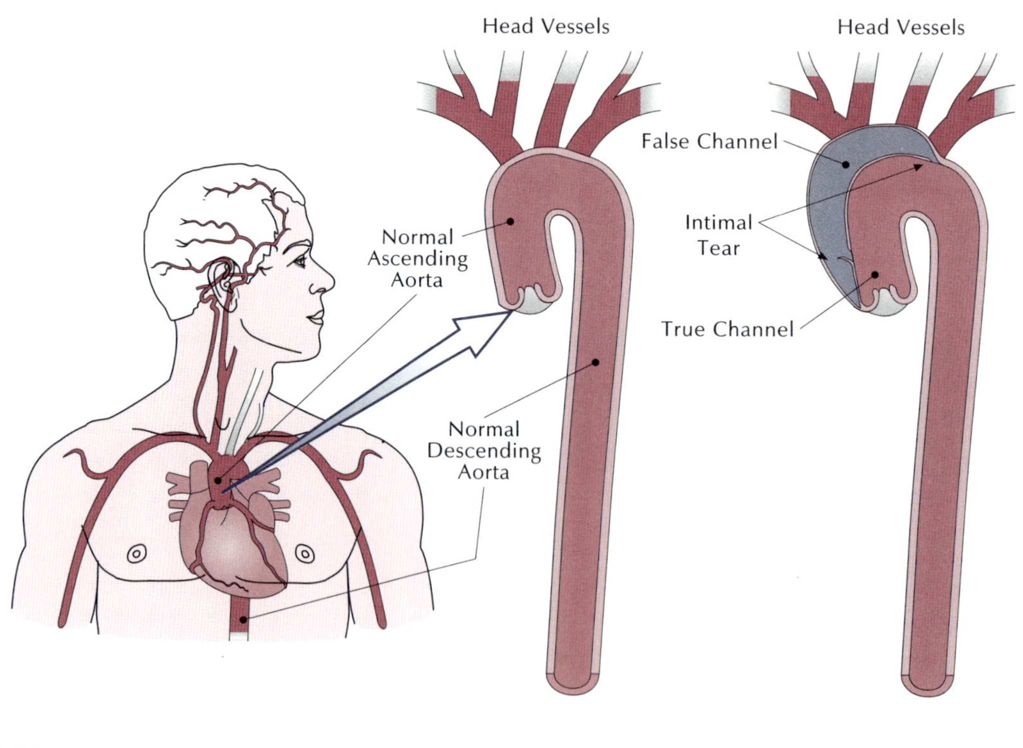

of salvage of the patient, frequently carry a high incidence of a residual problem, such as stroke—the most feared complication of this type of aortic dissection.

Aortic Dissection: Stanford Type B

Contrary to the bleak picture of the Stanford Type A aortic dissection, a dissection involving the descending aorta (the downward portion of the aorta within the chest) is called a Type B dissection and is much less ominous. (Figure 23) It begins in the aorta somewhere after it has branched off the arch vessels (the carotid arteries to the

Figure 23 Type B Aortic Dissection Descending Aorta

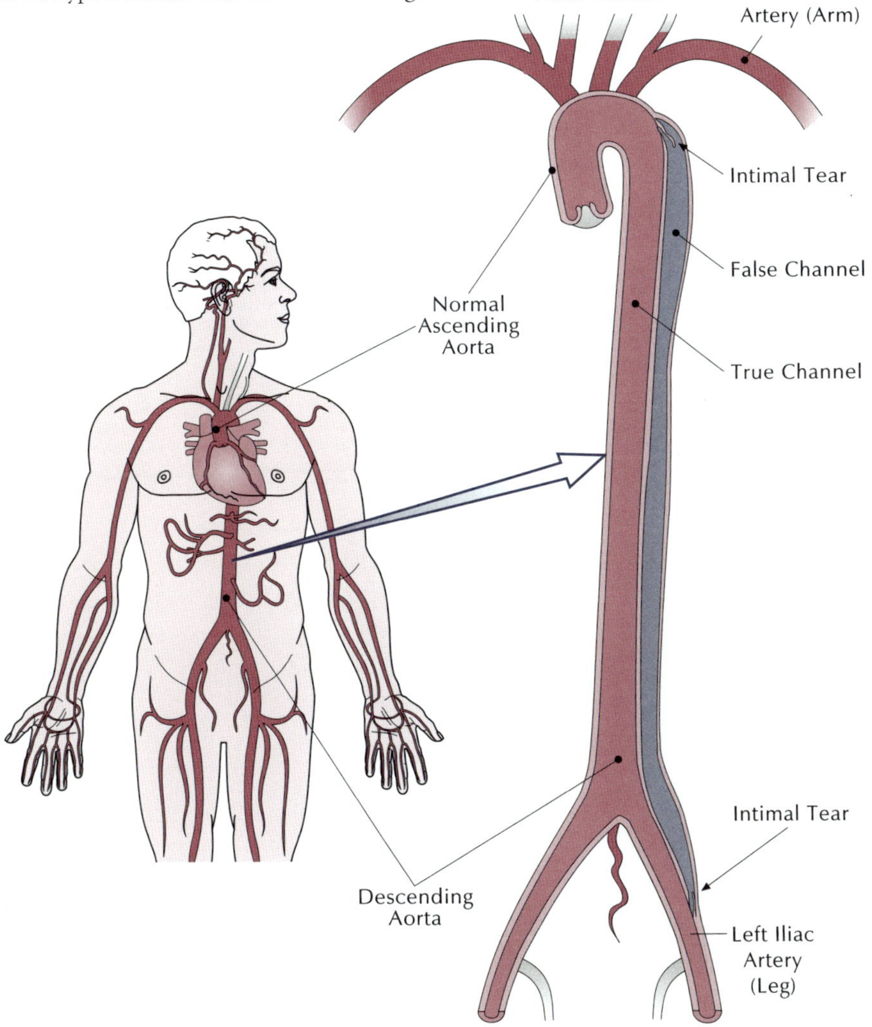

brain) and the left subclavian artery supplying the left arm. When the aorta tears in this portion, it may well continue to tear down past the diaphragm into the abdominal branches, but frequently misses the major mesenteric branches to the gut. It can also extend down into the leg vessels.

These Type B aortic dissections can typically be treated conservatively with medications. Surgery is rarely necessary. They will eventually heal and while every patient is concerned about a rupture through the wall of this damaged aorta, that would be very uncommon. I have seen some of these patients get very, very sick but in 30 years of practice, I've not seen a death from a Type B aortic dissection. There is typically, however, an established mortality rate of about 10% even in excellent medical facilities.

Type B dissection carries an excellent prognosis when properly managed. In general, surgery (which carries a mortality rate of over 25%) is reserved for those individuals who have persistent pain, threatened loss of a vital branch feeding the gut or kidney, or have a threatened rupture. Most of this high mortality—25% in a good series—is due to the fact that only the sickest and most threatened patients wind up getting referred for surgery and frequently have already compromised blood flow to a vital organ. Still, even when this 25% mortality within the surgical group is added to the total mix of patients with type B dissection (most treated medically, without surgery), the *total* mortality is only 10%, a remarkably good number when you consider the damage that such a rip in the aorta has imposed. I believe that acute stent-graft endoluminal repair, much as we treat the abdominal aortic aneurysms, will become the treatment of choice for the unstable patients within this population. As a reminder, these are material-covered stents that we can deploy via a large catheter through an exposed femoral artery. This would serve to seal off the torn segment, giving the terminal portion of the dissection a framework for healing and provide a barrier to prevent further damage.

Symptoms of Aortic Dissection

A symptom of aortic dissection is searing or ripping pain in the upper and mid back. One person told me that he was shaving and it felt as though something was being unzipped down his back. Usually, however, the pain is severe and people frequently describe it as knifelike or tearing. Whatever the adjective, descriptions of aortic dissection are almost always uttered in language that alerts us to a major problem, and it usually makes us think of aortic dissection right away. There is never any doubt in the person's mind that the pain hit suddenly and never got any better. Heart attack pain will frequently wax and wane as the artery is clotting, flow is stopped, blood pushes through the soft clot, the pain backs off, and so on. With aortic dissection, there is abrupt onset without even one second of relief until we get morphine into the patient.

Diagnosis

Usually on exam, the blood pressure is quite high in anyone with an aortic dissection. Frequently, this is the only finding unless the tear has extended into a carotid, a mesenteric vessel, or perhaps a leg vessel. While we can sometimes get an idea of the presence of aortic dissection by a plain chest x-ray, we obtain an urgent CT scan of the chest and abdomen and this almost always makes the diagnosis.

Treatment

The major thrust of treatment is to promptly and significantly drop the blood pressure so the dissection will not extend farther. In other words, blood pressure, transmitted down the dissecting column of blood within the wall of the aorta, is causing the tear to progress. We must interrupt that process. A beta adrenergic-blocker should be an integral component of the therapeutic protocol. This is the most effective drug in reducing the tangential wall stress on the aorta. The first doctor on the scene has the responsibility of dropping the systolic blood pressure so the tear will stop. However, this has to be done carefully, maintaining the pressure high enough that vital organs are adequately fed. With modern drugs and techniques, it is easier than it used to be but still fraught with hazard. Surgical consultation is required in all cases.

Unusual Forms of Aortic Wall Composition and Dissection

There are particular diseases of the aorta that cause certain individuals to be predisposed to aortic dissection. These patients should be monitored twice a year when such a disease is suspected. Such patients are primarily those with Marfan's Syndrome. These individuals—quite tall, usually with a wing span greater than their height, high arches, high palate and hyper-extensile, long, spidery fingers—have an abnormal matrix in the wall of the aorta. They are prone to aortic aneurysm formation, as well as dissection, and should be treated with beta-blocking drugs to reduce daily tangential wall stress on the aorta. They are also more likely to have relatively painless dissections. It is difficult to think that anyone could tear the aortic wall without having intense pain, but some of these patients can. The matrix, the framework within the wall of the aorta in such individuals, is so loosely joined that it allows for the accumulation of blood within the rent in the wall to move along without the intense pain that someone with a much better organized aortic wall would have. This can be compared to removal of wallpaper that is only loosely attached. Any complaint of discomfort or abnormal sensation in these patients has to be considered very important.

In Marfan's Syndrome individuals, there may be triggering events within the aortic wall that lead to aneurysm formation and the ultimate tearing of the wall, as there seems to be an imbalance between enzymes that erode tissue and the inhibitory compounds that prevent it. This is likely part of their inherited aortic wall defect, as they have an ever-diminishing population of both elastic and smooth muscle elements within the wall of the aorta. These are really the main structural elements that keep the aorta intact.

I took care of a peace officer who had gone through three previous coronary bypass operations at another hospital, the last one recently. I first met him when he moved to the city where I practice and called in the middle of the night with severe chest pain. It was located right between his shoulder blades and was described as tearing. I could hear him gasp for breath and groan when he had to breathe. When I met him in the emergency room, expecting to find him with an inflammatory reaction in the heart sac (the pericardium) from his recent bypass, I was struck by his appearance and promptly changed my diagnosis. He was well over six feet tall, had long arms with spidery fingers, his sternum went inward (pectus excavatum), and he had the highest arches I have ever seen. He was a poster child for Marfan's Syndrome. Sure enough, he had a Type A aortic dissection. The tear started right where one of the bypass grafts had been attached two weeks prior, unzipped around the aortic arch, luckily missing the head vessels, and it had re-entered the aortic lumen just above the take-off of the celiac axis supplying the stomach and liver. He did not want another operation. Yet he was only 60! We treated him conservatively, dropping his blood pressure and heart rate, allowing his aorta to heal. He developed an ICU psychosis, straining to get out of bed, hollering at the top of his lungs, which caused his blood pressure to go sky-high. Fearing that he would tear his aorta even more, he was sedated, intubated, and placed on a ventilator. He was kept in such a state for two weeks. He recovered and left the hospital on a beta-blocker. On the way out the door, he fired me, demonstrating that no good deed goes unpunished. I understand that he is still doing very well.

There are other conditions with this same predisposition for the aorta to tear due to abnormal connective tissue throughout the body including the skin, which also involves the matrix of the aorta. *Ehlers-Danlos Syndrome* is one. None of these other conditions are as susceptible to aortic dissection as the patients with Marfan's Syndrome.

There is another group of patients who have an increased tendency to tear their ascending aorta. These are the individuals with a congenital bicuspid aortic valve (a two-leaflet aortic valve rather than the normal three-leaflet valve). I have always thought it was due to an eccentric jet of blood hitting the aorta just above the valve—as the velocity of blood is increased since it is being pushed across a narrowed valve—and the jet is frequently distorted and directed toward the wall of the aorta because of the asymmetric narrowing of the valve. Or it may be due to an abnormal matrix within the aorta. I personally think this association is one of the reasons to be fairly aggressive in the replacement of these bicuspid valves.

Trauma and Aortic Dissection

Sudden deceleration, usually incurred in a motor vehicle crash, can cause the aorta to tear. This commonly occurs in the descending thoracic aorta (the down-going portion within the chest) just after it gives off the left subclavian artery supplying the arm. At this point, the aorta is firmly anchored by the ligamentum arteriosum, a fibrous band resulting from closure of a conduit carrying blood during intrauterine life. Below this, the aorta is not tethered and has much more mobility. The difference in the movement of this giant blood tube in response to sudden deceleration creates the potential for dissection.

I have seen a couple of fighter pilots who were flying unknowingly with an abnormal aortic wall matrix and developed aortic dissection. The G-forces that would ordinarily be well tolerated can disrupt the integrity of the aorta in this situation.

Surgical Repair of Aortic Dissection

Surgical repair of aortic dissection is very difficult. This is probably one of the most difficult procedures any cardiovascular surgeon will do. The Type A dissections are the ones that we usually have to operate on at some point. It is difficult to restore integrity to the aorta because the tear usually extends around the aortic arch where it branches into the vessels to the brain and upper extremities. The problem is putting the aorta back together without worsening any stroke that has resulted from the tear involving these head vessels.

Two things have become crystal clear regarding Type A aortic dissections:

1. The mortality rate is much higher if we try to treat them medically; we can improve survival dramatically by operating on these Type A aortic tears.
2. In general, the earlier the operation, the better chance they have of survival.

The problems encountered in getting these patients through surgery and discharged home in a functional state are large, but not insurmountable. It requires good coordination between the cardiac surgeon and cardiologist.

Two things have become clear regarding Type B aortic dissections, as well:

1. Most can be managed medically by dropping the blood pressure with a drug that reduces the initial thrust of the blood pressure, usually with a beta-adrenergic-blocker, such as Inderal.
2. If organ perfusion is compromised or the dissection continues, operate before the organ is dead or the aorta ruptures.

It seems that we have it stuck in our minds that Type B dissections can all be managed medically—without surgery at any point. I suppose that notion has come about because most can, indeed, be managed without surgery. However, if this dissection involves the blood supply to the gut, kidneys, or lower extremities, it should be operated on without delay.

REMINDERS

1. Aortic dissection is more common in individuals with high blood pressure.

2. Almost all also have a fault in the composition of their aorta.

3. Type A dissections, those that originate in the ascending aorta just above the heart, are typically managed with surgery.

4. Type B dissections, those that originate below the takeoff of the left arm artery, can frequently be managed medically.

5. Aortic dissection is always a medical and sometimes a surgical emergency.

6. If you have been diagnosed with Marfan's or Ehlers-Danlos Syndrome, you will require frequent monitoring and should be on a beta-blocking drug.

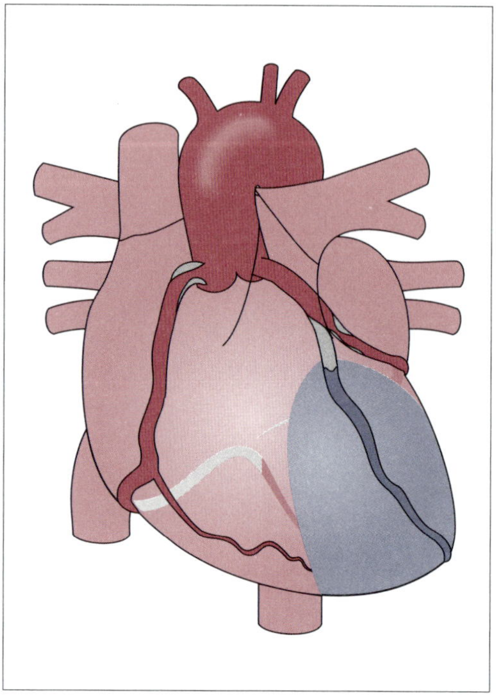

BLOOD FATS

Cholesterol and Other Lipids

WHEN MOST PEOPLE THINK OF A LIPID disorder they think of elevated cholesterol and, specifically, elevated LDL-cholesterol (LDL-C). The LDL stands for Low-Density Lipoprotein, the "bad" fraction of cholesterol. As it turns out, this is probably not the worst or even the most prevalent lipid abnormality, even though it is very significant. We have given particular emphasis to LDL-C because it is imminently treatable with today's modern medicines.

The other major fraction of cholesterol is the good one: the HDL-cholesterol (HDL-C). HDL stands for High-Density Lipoprotein. The more you have of this fraction, the better. It has several roles. The most important is serving as "garbage collector," scavenging the bad cholesterol. Another important role is as an antioxidative compound, preventing oxidation of the LDL-C. Indeed, a low HDL-C is probably a stronger risk factor for developing arteriosclerosis than is a high LDL-C. Additionally, there is no effective treatment for a low HDL-C at this time, which makes it just about as much of a menace as it was 30 years ago, whereas we have great treatment for an elevated LDL-C. The effective treatment of low HDL-C is the next great challenge in the management of lipid abnormalities for prevention of coronary artery disease and other arteriosclerotic processes.

The bulk—roughly 75%—of the cholesterol measured in the bloodstream is not ingested, but is manufactured in the body. Furthermore, one's individual handling of lipids and metabolism is as unique as one's fingerprints. I, for example, am an exercise and fitness freak, and I eat very healthy foods. When people anywhere are talking about silent coronary artery disease, they frequently comment that I will never have anything like that because I take such good care of myself. What they don't know is that I have an exceptionally low HDL-C level. The lower one's HDL-C, the greater the risk of arteriosclerosis. Ideally, you want your HDL-C above 60 milligrams per deciliter. Anything over 40 is fair. Below 40, the lower the HDL-C, the more apt you are to develop a plaque within an arterial wall; however, there are other features to consider, so don't panic.

The singular point that emerges is that, while your individual habits can significantly influence your lipid profile, your individual body metabolism, including your division of cholesterol into its good and bad components, is genetically set by your DNA just as your appearance is. That's why I can't get my HDL up with diet, exercise, and niacin. You can't fool Mother Nature.

That said; let us go on to happier thoughts. We are living in a great age! To quote Jerry Garcia, when I began this "strange and crazy trip" in the world of heart and blood vessel disease some 35 years ago, we knew only about unusual types of elevated cholesterol. Now we not only know about the good and bad fractions of the total cholesterol, but have wonderful drugs to aid us in correcting any inborn deviation from the appropriate manufacture and handling of these fractions.

It is important to understand that cholesterol has gotten a bad rap. Cholesterol is necessary:

1. It is present in large amounts in the membranes of all cells, but especially in those of the brain and spinal cord, where it is exceptionally dense.
2. It is the necessary ingredient in production of the sex hormones such as progesterone, some estrogens, and certainly in testosterone.
3. Without *some* cholesterol—and we are not totally sure what that level has to be—we could not survive.

LDL-Cholesterol

There are many people who have an elevated LDL-C. When we say it is "bad," we are referring to the fact that if it becomes oxidized (chemically changed) within the inside lining of the wall (the endothelium) of an artery, it becomes deposited there as a "fatty plaque." The amount of your LDL-C eventually oxidized into the truly bad stuff is a variable process. It is related in part to your nitric oxide content within the endothelium. Nitric oxide (NO) is called the "endothelium-derived relaxing factor," a big descriptor for a big and important job: It relaxes the wall of the artery, a good thing, as it allows more blood to flow down the artery. It is synthesized by L-Arginine, an amino acid. This amino acid is gaining greater respect from researchers every day. Your level of HDL-C also helps determine how much and at what rate your LDL-C becomes oxidized. This is important because the LDL-C doesn't really harm you unless it becomes oxidized, entering the wall of the artery. This is where the role of antioxidants comes into play: They help reduce the harmful oxidative stress, the damage to a cell by the effects of imbalances and deleterious agents within the cells. There is information on the role of antioxidants in Chapter 1 on *Preventive Maintenance*. There has been a great deal of interest in the slowing of LDL-C oxidation. It has been shown that the juice from purple grapes will slow the process.

LDL-cholesterol is always manufactured to fit a specific pattern or profile within our bodies—a genetic predisposition. The small dense particles are worst because they can more easily penetrate the wall of the artery and assume their smug position there as part of a lipid accumulation. The large fluffy particles are the least harmful for the opposite reason. It is important for you to know not only your LDL-C fraction, but also your particular particle size distribution. Ideally, we would like you to have an LDL level less than 100. Anything over 120 should be considered elevated. However, the person with an LDL fraction of 120—almost all of which are fluffy large particles—who has a low level of oxidation is less apt to develop coronary artery disease than one who has an LDL of 110, most of which is of the small particle, dense variety. This is one reason why ratios of the two fractions of LDL do not always make a lot of sense. *The particular density of your LDL is exceptionally important.*

For the great mass of people with an elevated level of LDL-C, the discovery of the HMG-CoEnzyme A-Reductase-Inhibitor (better know as statin) which blocks the formation of LDL-cholesterol, was a huge breakthrough. About 95% of people can tolerate these great drugs. This was one of the biggest drug discoveries since penicillin in terms of overall benefit to mankind. For example, the incidence of heart attacks has dropped considerably since the advent of these cholesterol-lowering drugs. I have some reservations about the widespread use of them. I'm worried that the high cholesterol population-at-large has thrown caution to the wind, eating indiscriminately and thinking that the statin will "fix" their problem. It is possible to "out-eat" the statin, plus the cholesterol is not the whole problem.

These statin drugs can be monitored carefully; we are able to set the LDL at almost the exact target level with a little fine tuning. We have all seen a sharp decline in the incidence of first heart attacks, secondary events, and strokes since they were introduced.

The most common side effect of the statins is that of muscle cramps and weakness. We can almost never pick this up simply by measuring muscle breakdown products. However, there is no doubt that it is a real phenomenon in some people. An elevation of liver enzymes is seen infrequently and is a distinctly less common problem. We usually monitor these patients and continue the drug, counsel the patient to discontinue alcohol use, and check for hepatitis or hidden liver disease of other varieties.

By far the most threatening of all of the potential side effects of the statin drugs is rhabdomyalysis. This is a dramatic injury to muscle tissue, releasing an enzyme called CPK into the blood stream in such huge quantities that it can cause acute renal failure and if severe enough, can potentially cause death. This almost always occurs in a situation in which a statin is used in conjunction with another drug, usually one used for the coexistent problem of elevated triglycerides. Therefore, whenever we use this drug combination, we observe them closely and teach the patient what to watch out for.

Initially, we doctors all worried that very low levels of LDL might lead to dementia or neuropathy, and we watched out for this. The brain tissue is made up of a great amount of exotic lipids. The nerve membranes are also about two-thirds lipid. We were worried that dropping LDL to very low levels might influence these other lipids. I am still concerned. However, the incidence of dementia seems to be strangely reduced in the population taking statin drugs. This may well have to do with the reduction of inflammation brought about by statins. This is certainly, and happily, another of its benefits. At this time, we feel that a smoldering inflammatory state (an activation of the pro-inflammatory elements within brain tissue) may be important in promoting dementia. It is also important in initiating coronary arteriosclerosis. The inflammatory combatant action of statins may be at least as important for preventing heart attacks, strokes, and dementia as for their LDL-lowering action.

We also worried about CoEnzyme Q10 levels with prolonged statin use. CoEnzyme Q10 is called the ubiquitous enzyme since it participates in almost every metabolic pathway in the body. We have seen decreased *blood* levels of this coenzyme in people taking statins. I am not aware of anyone showing decreased *tissue* levels but I figure the tissue levels will ultimately fall and, since it is not harmful, I recommend that anyone taking a statin drug also take 100 milligrams of CoEnzyme Q10 a day. It won't hurt you, and it might well prevent a problem. There have now been very infrequent poorly documented cases of neuropathy, a disorder of the nerves supplying the hands and feet, possibly associated with the statins. It must be rare if it is, indeed, "real." However, the statin drug should be promptly discontinued in any patients who think they have rapidly lost cognitive function or develops a neuropathy without some other explanation. Frequently, the patient who requires a statin for elevated cholesterol also has one of the other diseases that are well known for producing neuropathy, such as diabetes.

What is the target for LDL-C? That really depends on who you are. If you are healthy with no evidence of arteriosclerosis, it should be dropped to about 100. On the other hand, if you have established structural coronary artery disease, it should be dropped to about the 70 range, as that seems to be the level where further progression of the arteriosclerotic process is stopped in its tracks. It seems that we have worried about lower levels of LDL-cholesterol each time we have dropped the bar. We have always been reassured by the knowledge that certain populations of people throughout the world naturally carry levels of LDL of only 40 or so. A large study of almost 2,000 patients who took large amounts of statin drugs following heart attacks showed that lower is better, in terms of reducing secondary events. Out of this study, there were at least 10% who wound up with an LDL in the 40 range, and they did the best. Color me old-fashioned, but I don't think one should get his or her LDL this low and keep it there unless really threatened by a generalized arteriosclerosis process. And if you do, be sure to take some protective supplements such as Alpha Lipoic Acid and CoEnzyme Q10. *The Better Brain Book*, by Dr. David Perlmutter, is a great book on healthy brain and nerve components. He is a bit fanatical on the other side, thinking way too many people are treated with statin drugs. However, for those who have a dangerous cholesterol situation, I think we have to treat it aggressively, but also use common sense and try for both a healthy heart and a healthy brain. One works poorly without the other.

There are quite a few people who cannot get their LDL-C down to the target level even with high-dose statin therapy. The addition of Zetia, a drug which works in a completely different manner, will help achieve this target range.

HDL-Cholesterol

What about the legions of folks who were born with a low HDL-C level? There are a lot of us! Unlike an elevated LDL-C, there is no magic bullet for low HDL-C. The statins will nudge it up a bit, but not much. Eating a Mediterranean diet rich in olive oil and fish, with a small amount of red wine thrown in for good measure, will help. Good fat in walnuts and almonds are beneficial. Very dark chocolate (70% or greater since it contains very little sugar) is excellent. Grape seed extract, for those who wish to avoid alcohol, is a great source of antioxidant power. These items—walnuts, almonds, olive oil, and chocolate—all contain monounsaturated fats, good fats that increase your HDL-cholesterol. This diet, along with exercise, can usually significantly raise the HDL. I get excited when I see an HDL-C of 20 (extremely low, even lower than mine) in a smoker because discontinuation of cigarette smoking causes probably the greatest growth in the HDL level.

How important is an increase in a low HDL? The short answer is "*very*." For example, in the clinical trials, raising a very low HDL even slightly resulted in a 20–25% decrease in cardiovascular events such as heart attack.

Actually, quite a few people have a bad duo: low HDL and high LDL-cholesterol. I truly hate to use a drug that will bolster the HDL level along with a statin. This drug can also be tough on the liver in some cases. I use the statin, tell them about all of the ways to elevate the HDL through lifestyle changes, and then add another drug only if I think they are headed for a potential disaster if I do nothing further. I think you have to pull out all the stops, though, in searching for dietary means to adjust the cholesterol. Kashi makes a great breakfast cereal called Heart-to-Heart, which contains a great amount of fiber, which can help drop the LDL. It is also filled with antioxidants, grape seed extract, green tea extract, and other helpful components.

Niacin, about the only commercially available drug shown to elevate the HDL-cholesterol level, has been available for many years but until recently was so poorly tolerated that many doctors stopped prescribing it. In the old original form, it caused most people to get a sunburn reaction with tingling, burning, and itching. This has been largely eliminated using the new product, Niaspan. We use it in dosages of 500 to 2,000 milligrams daily. The administration of an aspirin one hour prior to taking it will largely eliminate any sunburn-type symptoms. We do have to check for liver dysfunction with this drug, especially when used in conjunction with the statins.

Another drug that is rapidly gaining a position for itself is fenofibrate, the most common of which is TriCor. It not only reduces the LDL, it also drops the very low-density lipoprotein (VLDL)—another proven bad actor—and it has the advantage of raising the HDL-cholesterol. Like all of the fibrates, it can (but very rarely) cause a serious muscle problem when used in conjunction with statins. However, I was very impressed with this drug because of two developments:

1. It appears to provide a beneficial influence on the insulin resistance we see in metabolic syndrome (a very common problem marked by obesity, insulin resistance, elevated LDL, elevated triglycerides, and inflammation).
2. The Fenofibrate Intervention and Event Lowering in Diabetes (FIELD) study showed it to be safe and very effective in treatment of patients with Type 2 diabetes (which is occurring in epidemic numbers, largely due to obesity).

The Italian Job!

Those of you who have seen the movie *The Italian Job* and who have a paltry HDL-C can be equally as excited by the story of this other "Italian Job."

I love Italy, especially Umbria and Tuscany in the north. There is a beautiful serene little village of about 1,000 people in Northern Italy called Limone sul Garda resting on the rocky shores of Lake Garda. It is gorgeous! It grew great lemons and olives and was relatively isolated for many years. Now it's overrun by tourists. Some of these villagers were found to have HDL-C levels that were literally on the floor! I was lamenting the fact that mine was exceedingly low at 25. Well, they commonly had levels around 10, which should have resulted in early and recurrent heart attacks. But they were remarkably free from any evidence of arteriosclerosis. Researchers in Milan found that these people carried a variant—doubtless endowed by a genetic mutation—of apolipoprotein A-1, the major protein of HDL. It has since been synthesized and has already been shown to dramatically reverse arteriosclerosis within weeks, several times the established result of the strongest statin drugs. It is called ApoA-1 Milano in tribute to the investigative persistence demonstrated by these Italian investigators. Wouldn't it be a wonderful irony if these peaceful descendents of lemon and olive farmers and fishermen—the very developers of the Mediterranean diet that has been shown to be so beneficial—also helped to combat the deadly effects of this nefarious disease by virtue of their isolation and the variant in their genome?

ApoA-1 Milano doesn't appear to cause any harm either! It is not on the market yet but I'd like my name on the list so I can use it as soon as possible. Probably an even more telling indication of its extraordinary utility is the fact that Pfizer paid $1.3

billion for it. They possess the wildly profitable drug Lipitor, and I'm sure they feel this drug might well replace it.

In the interim, Niaspan, exercise, red wine or grape seed extract, salmon, olive oil, walnuts, and dark chocolate constitute the best treatment plan we have for raising the HDL-cholesterol. If one smokes, the HDL-cholesterol can be elevated by as much as ten points just by quitting. An aerobic exercise program will drive it up farther.

Lipoprotein Lp-a—What, Another Problem?

There is one more particle that should be addressed: the lipoprotein (a). The structure of Lp-a, or little a, is very similar to an LDL particle linked to another molecule, plasminogen, which we know to be involved in the dissolution of blood clots. We have no firm idea what Lp-a does, except increase your risks of developing arterial disease if it is present in high levels. Currently, its main importance is that a high level of Lp-a makes cholesterol more "toxic" and, as such, its presence signals the need for more aggressive control of the LDL-C.

The Metabolic Syndrome

Finally, we need to address a lipid problem that wasn't even named a few years ago. It is truly the "Blood Fats from Hell Story," as its population is rapidly burgeoning and it accompanies the obesity epidemic. It is called metabolic syndrome and refers to an individual with elevated triglycerides, trunkal (abdominal) obesity, high blood pressure, low HDL-C, diabetes due to insulin resistance and, frequently, an elevation of the LDL-C (some the dreaded small dense particle size). Any three will serve to make the diagnosis of metabolic syndrome. Unfortunately, it is now estimated that it is present in at least one-fourth of all adults in the United States. It is a strong predictor of coronary artery disease and other forms of arteriosclerosis. Due to accumulating evidence that inflammation is a very important risk factor influencing vascular disease in all areas of the body, this has been added to the definition of metabolic syndrome. We check for this enhanced inflammation by measuring a high-sensitivity C-reactive protein (hs-CRP).

This disease has morphed over the few years since it was first observed. This is testimony to the incredible epidemic of obesity. Cardiologists and endocrinologists have expanded the term metabolic syndrome to the *cardiometabolic* syndrome to attempt to incorporate its multitude of end-organ damage within the confines of the disease. Its implications are huge! Epidemiologic studies have correlated this syndrome—in conjunction with its known plaque-formation, increased clotting and inflammation, protein in the urine, and more—with increased risk of developing coronary artery disease and heart attack, stroke, peripheral arterial disease, and even arrhythmias such as atrial fibrillation. I am also convinced that it sharply accelerates the rate of degeneration of the aortic valve in a process known as aortic sclerosis, which also results in death from cardiovascular cause in some cases. Non-alcoholic fatty liver disease is related. It is estimated that about 20% of the adult population in Western countries have this disease.

When you consider that millions of Americans have metabolic syndrome and the potential for these problems, you can see the future. We must corral this burgeoning problem if we are to enjoy blood vessel health. One of the ways we do this is by controlling the obesity epidemic that is ravaging our country. We are committing suicide by fork!

Metabolic syndrome can be managed with dietary alterations, blood pressure control, physical exercise, and treatment of the inflammatory component, usually with a statin. Most obesity comes from ingestion of too much simple sugar. Additionally, triglycerides derive from simple sugar. I know it dates me, but I remember the days when we drank one coke a week. We would never have considered something like the Big Gulp. Now it's commonplace to drink 30 or more ounces of sugar-saturated colas! The body has to release huge amounts of insulin to prevent our blood sugar levels from spiraling far out of control. In time, however, the cells just simply stop responding to this signal—at that point, you're insulin resistant! Additionally, all of those calories have to go somewhere; such a huge amount can't be satisfactorily processed by the body. So they go toward manufacturing fat. With this comes the rest of the syndrome. It's not fair, but women entering menopause are especially prone to developing insulin resistance due to hormonal fluctuations. A woman's health—especially her cardiovascular health—can deteriorate markedly in the early stages of menopause. This is due, in no small measure, because of the development of the lipid abnormalities that may blossom, frequently as part of metabolic syndrome.

If the individual is well motivated and consumes *no* simple sugars (like sucrose or high fructose), exercises even moderately, and sharply cuts back on starches such as potatoes, bread, and pasta, the triglycerides will plummet, insulin resistance (plenty of insulin is manufactured; it's just not able to be utilized at the tissue level) will correct, and the syndrome itself can become a thing of the past. Weight loss and stabilization have to be a large part of this treatment plan. Since inflammation is triggered, at least in part, by adipose tissue, this will partially correct as well. In the more practical clinical setting where only partial compliance (the individual tries hard and is only partially successful) is the norm, we usually treat the elevated triglycerides with a drug such as Gemfibrozil or Fenofibrate. If desperately needed, we add a statin later for the LDL-cholesterol, keeping in mind the additional risk of rhabdomyalysis with combination therapy. Remember, this is the aggressive breakdown of muscle. Most people can get along fine with this combination; just be aware of the possibility of a problem if the two drugs are combined. Obviously, if the predominant problem is a markedly elevated LDL with only a slightly elevated triglyceride level, we would start with a statin.

While almost everyone who has metabolic syndrome has an elevated triglyceride, not everyone who has an elevated triglyceride has metabolic syndrome. However, elevated triglycerides are frequently associated with excessive sugar intake and increased amounts of fat tissue, especially about the trunk. With very high triglyceride levels, pancreatitis (inflammation of the pancreas) is a risk. This usually occurs only in those individuals who have a triglyceride level greater than 1,000. We get concerned about anyone who has a level greater than 250–300 and begin to consider treatment with a drug if dietary measures will not bring down the level. It almost always will. The question is whether or not the individual is willing to make the sacrifice.

Metabolic syndrome is a scourge, silently performing its naughty task, waiting to deposit its victims in the hospital with a heart attack in a few years unless it is detected and treated. I know that no one out there wants to hear they have to pick up the reins of responsibility on this one. However, in the words of Winston Churchill, "An appeaser is one who feeds a crocodile, hoping it will eat him last." I am not an appeaser. This may be the knowledge that saves your life.

Exercise and Mediterranean Diet for Metabolic Syndrome

I don't think we have yet created enough emphasis on exercise in the management of lipid abnormalities. It seems to me that with the advent of drugs to treat both cholesterol and triglycerides, we are not stressing exercise as much or maybe I have become cynical. Anyway, it is now clear that consistent moderate-intensity exercise can play a major role in improving the lipid status in individuals with metabolic syndrome. When coupled with a dietary switch from the typical Western diet—loaded down with simple carbohydrates—to a Mediterranean diet—rich in fruits, vegetables, beans, nuts, seeds, fish, and olive oil—the results are really quite striking. We realize that with metabolic syndrome, we must do everything right to reduce the risks of cardiovascular events, such as heart attack and stroke. This means diet change, discontinuation of smoking, weight loss, and exercise. Unfortunately, medications still have to be used in most cases, but in lower doses and with fewer confusing and potentially dangerous combinations.

I want to reemphasize what a terrifying situation we are in due to 25% of our adult population having metabolic syndrome. It *dramatically* increases your likelihood of having a cardiovascular event. We're all reading these glowing predictions that the baby boomers are going to live better, work longer, be stronger, and will demand better health care. Much of our health care concepts need to come from within—a conviction that we must change our diet and our exercise habits. I'm dismayed that so many baby boomers are taking this lackadaisical attitude about eating, obesity, and inactivity. If you go to the macabre website "Baby Boomer Death Counter Clock," you will find a real-time countdown on us. It is troublesome, listing the percentage of baby boomers who are dead (6.5%); total boomers left alive (71 million); seconds before the next boomer dies (58.2); and the number of boomers who died during the last 24 hours (1,485). We must do our best to thwart this death clock! Perhaps I get hysterical about this because I am one of the baby boomers.

I am not one of the high-protein diet proponents. I think we need a balanced diet. However, most people in modern society ingest way too much carbohydrate and much of it seems to be in the form of simple sugars. I personally believe that high-fructose corn syrup is responsible for much of this huge epidemic of obesity we are seeing. Hopefully, as we divert more corn toward the production of automobile fuel, we will have less of this in our foods. Right now, it is virtually impossible to avoid it in America. Who said there was no advantage to having an oil shortage?

One of the most worrisome health concerns to devolve from this obesity epidemic is middle-aged incidence of diabetes. This is such a strong risk factor that a middle-aged diabetic woman, normally protected from the ravages of cardiovascular events until menopause, assumes the same risk as a man the same age. Obesity is not always a prerequisite for Type 2 diabetes, but it is a strong contributor.

Trans-Fatty Acids

I would be remiss not to address one of the features of lipid abnormality that can also be treated by altering your diet. That is the ingestion of trans-fatty acids. These are the worst of the bad, one of the true poisons of our time. When the low-fat diet craze was in vogue about 20 years ago, the food manufacturers labeled everything "low fat," and we flocked to it. That is precisely the time when the obesity epidemic began; all of that low fat was really high sugar, and frequently high trans-fat in content.

The market for low fat was huge, and our size quickly followed. In order to make the food taste good once the fat was removed, they had to add sugar, and a lot of it. It tasted even better if they added partially hydrogenated vegetable oil. We all looked at the label, saw "vegetable," knew that our mothers thought vegetables were good for us, and bought it by the ton. Then we grew by the ton. The Atkins Diet, while fraught with problems, did alert us to this problem. We owe the late Dr. Atkins a great vote of thanks for that, as he stuck to his guns and demonstrated that one could not only lose weight with a high-protein and high-fat diet, but that diabetes would improve and frequently, lipids would improve.

We got past these two crazes and then began to understand that trans-fats—largely these partially hydrolyzed vegetable oils—were even a greater evil than sugar and fat put together. These things never go away! What you ingest, you likely take to your grave, as there is absolutely no metabolic pathway to handle trans-fatty acids, especially the variety that comes about from frying foods with partially hydrogenated vegetable oil. They attach to the phospholipid membrane covering cells and are associated with accelerated coronary heart disease and sudden death. Yet, until recently, this completely flew under the radar. Food manufacturers would label something "low fat" and it could be full of trans-fats! Where is Ralph Nader? This has recently been rectified, at long last, and they now have to list the trans-fat content. However, and this is very important, the restaurants still do not have to list the trans-fat content in the food they serve. The French fries you get are absolutely loaded with them, and they are dedicated killers. They are also very good, and I have to hold onto the table to control myself when the server passes by me with a plate loaded with them. The first batch deep-fried in fresh oil is fairly low in trans-fat; however, the content goes up with each consecutive batch until, at the end of the day, they are the food industry equivalent of a firing squad. Showing our dedicated bent for unhealthy food, in Europe, the trans-fat level in the same type of French fries is lower than in the same franchise stores in America. I am not sure, but I think this is due to the type of vegetable oil they use for frying French fries. Soon, I am told, every store will have to divulge how much trans-fatty acid content is found in each food, and we can then at least choose whether or not we wish to be poisoned.

Olive Oil Can Turn into a Bad Fat

Along these same lines, many of us have been told that olive oil is good for us and raises the good stuff, the HDL. It does. However, if you use it for cooking at high temperatures, it gets converted basically into a type of trans-fat. The same is true for many of the processed oils. As my father used to say to me, "Watch out, son, there's a snake under every rock!" Like so many things he told me, he was entirely correct. However, I didn't learn this olive oil lesson from my father or my mother but from my tour guide in a mountain range in Umbria, Italy. I suspect she was a great cook because she kept talking about food. I'm a great eater, not such a great cook, but I would like to get better. In our discussions, she was horrified that I fried my Egg Beaters omelet in olive oil. She told me that no one in all of Italy would do something so crazy. I slinked off to pout.

Someone Has to Watch the Blood Fats

I think that patients with arteriosclerosis anywhere in their bodies have to watch their treatment protocol very carefully because there are doctors who are really just technicians, capable of opening arteries, but totally unaware of the prevention of the disease. They think that someone else is going to handle that. For example, I recently saw a patient who was an aggressive and very successful 50-year-old trial lawyer who had gone through five separate interventions on his leg vessels in order to salvage his limbs. They had all been expertly performed at a fine medical facility and the care from that standpoint was impeccable. However, he had received absolutely no lipid-lowering therapy, and his lipids were all sky-high. He traveled, and his favorite food in the world was French fries, full of trans-fat. Additionally, he announced proudly that the arteriosclerotic disease had spared his heart. Yet when I did an electron beam tomogram, his score, which should have been about 50, was 3,500! An angiography showed he had a 90% left main coronary blockage and was simply looking for a proper place to die.

Determined that he would not do this on my watch, I promptly submitted him for coronary bypass surgery. He was also counseled about dietary alterations and was started on lipid-lowering therapy. Being what he was, he immediately wanted to sue the previous doctors. I assured him that no one in his right mind would open all of these blood vessels and not start him on a statin. I told him he must have forgotten. He arrived back in my office a month later armed with all of his records and his detailed personal notes from each physician interaction. He was right! No one told him to start a statin. No one had counseled him on dietary modifications. This guy was smart enough to ask most of the hard questions. He just didn't have a resource book and was quite busy. When he returned, armed with all of this stuff, I fell back to my favorite quote from my favorite physician, the esteemed Sir William Osler, a British scholar who published and taught with great passion. It goes like this: "Look wise, say nothing, and grunt. Speech was given to conceal thought." I merely grunted.

REMINDERS

1. We manufacture over 75% of our blood lipids within our bodies.
2. Each person's lipid profile is as unique as that person's fingerprints.
3. You can influence your lipid profile by exercise, dietary modification, stopping smoking, and watching your weight.
4. We now have a great treatment for an elevated LDL-cholesterol level.
5. We have only modest treatment for a low HDL-cholesterol level. If you have this, you have to do everything right.
6. Help is on the way for those with a low HDL in the form of the "Milan Factor."
7. If you take statin drugs, you must also take CoEnzyme Q10.
8. Don't use olive oil at very high temperatures; it turns into a trans-fat.
9. Olive oil, as one of the main ingredients of the Mediterranean diet, is a monounsaturated fat and will help raise your good (HDL) cholesterol.

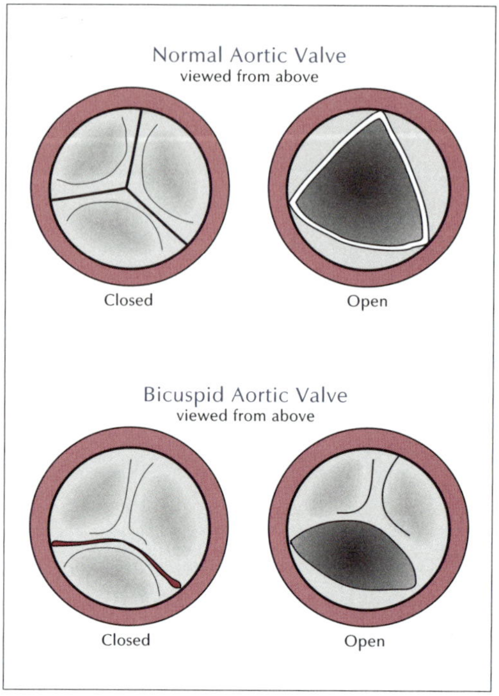

ARTIFICIAL HEART VALVES VERSUS TISSUE VALVES

What Happens When I Need a New Heart Valve?

WHEN A HEART VALVE NEEDS TO BE REPLACED, we must choose which type of replacement valve to use. The cardiologist and cardiac surgeon should interact with the patient regarding this very important choice. As with most things in this world, the choice is often not black and white, but is made gray by the uncertainties of the future. Drawing on our experiences of the past, however, we can make sensible suggestions regarding which valve will work best for you. The following will help you participate in making a sound decision.

Pros and Cons of Mechanical versus Tissue Valve Prostheses

You are better off with the valve you were born with unless it is very significantly diseased. For this reason, we try to watch a diseased valve until we think it has to be treated with surgical measures. We ask the cardiac surgeon to repair any valve that has to be treated with surgical measures. *We ask the cardiac surgeon to repair any valve that is amenable to this approach, as this allows you to keep your own valve.* Frequently, when the problem is a degenerative mitral valve, repair is possible using a variety of techniques. Some surgeons are masters at valve repair; others balk at the idea. Valve repair is generally not an option with the aortic valve. We must presume that, at this point, you are destined for valve replacement.

There are basically two types of heart valve:

1. Mechanical, known as artificial, since they are made with a manufactured material.
2. Tissue, also known as a bioprosthetic valve, which is harvested from an animal.

The essential differences between these two general types of valves have to do with durability and the need for anticoagulation. We want your valve to perform flawlessly for the duration of your expected life. On the other hand, we know that a certain percentage of patients will need to stop their anticoagulant therapy at some point in their lives. This interruption may be very brief to allow for an operation or possibly to help manage a gastrointestinal bleeding problem. It might conceivably be a permanent discontinuation because of an uncontrollable problem with blood loss from diffuse lesions within the entire colon. These considerations are paramount when selecting a valve. The crux of the decision about valve choices has to do with whether or not you are a candidate for chronic anticoagulation. A secondary factor is life expectancy.

Anticoagulation, in its chronic day-to-day form, consists of taking Coumadin. It ties up the clotting factors manufactured in the liver. The dose you take today generally exerts its major effect tomorrow. These two pertinent points underscore just why this decision is so difficult. Anticoagulation is difficult to control and poses an increased risk of bleeding. The dosage of Coumadin has to be tightly regulated. This is easy in some, a virtual nightmare in others. We utilize a standardized measurement, which thankfully, is internationalized as well. The test for measurement of the Coumadin effect is called a prothrombin time, which we abbreviate to Protime. In my view, 75% of the bleeding complications we see from Coumadin have to do with gross deviations of the Protime from the established range. Of these, 50% are due to miscommunications about dosage changes, inadequate knowledge of which medications will affect the Protime, and inadequate follow-up Protime checks. The other bleeding problems are pretty much unavoidable due to underlying pathology, usually in the gastrointestinal tract.

Thankfully, the dreaded hemorrhage into the brain is rare. The neurosurgeons in a large tertiary care hospital probably think it is common, as they see all of them. It is *not* common, especially if the Protime is tightly regulated. In reality, the major bleeding complication we see from Coumadin is gastrointestinal bleeding. It seems these days that every other person is taking some sort of medication for joint pain. These all greatly increase the risk of bleeding from the gut. Any slow blood loss has to be considered as gastrointestinal in origin. Trauma, including frequent hip fracture from falls in the elderly, constitutes another risk of Coumadin usage. For this reason, habits must be considered. I am obviously emphasizing the anticoagulation risk aspect of valve selection because, in my view, everything else is secondary. If there were no bleeding risk, everyone would receive a mechanical valve for replacement therapy.

A. Mechanical Valve

The most durable valve prosthesis is the mechanical valve. Utilizing our current mechanical valves, we very seldom have to replace one due to some intrinsic structural failure within the valve. If it malfunctions, it is because of a thrombus (clot) that has formed on the valve, usually due to a lapse in anticoagulation or because a stitch has come out creating a para-valvular leak around the valve. The mechanical valves that we currently use are absolutely great valves, showing very little deterioration with age.

The drawback to having a mechanical valve is that you must receive lifelong anticoagulation with Coumadin to prevent clot formation within the valve. Whenever Coumadin is stopped for some reason, a looming threat of clot formation within the mechanical valve always exists. We can usually prevent this through use of temporary measures. However, should the clot form, there are two major problems: It can hamper appropriate function of the valve and it can potentially shed fragments of emboli to the brain or elsewhere. This is no small consideration because, when a mechanical valve is implanted, you are basically committed to lifelong treatment with Coumadin.

There is always some risk of bleeding with anticoagulant therapy, no matter how carefully the Protime is controlled. This is especially true in the patient population that receives the greatest percentage of heart valve replacements—those over 60. These bleeds form a wide spectrum—from protracted bleeding from a nick while shaving legs or face to a life-threatening hemorrhage into the brain tissue. In order to prevent catastrophic bleeding problems, the anticoagulation profile has to be rigidly controlled, and this is sometimes an arduous affair.

There are other considerations. From 60 on up, it is extremely common for a patient to have degenerative joint disease; some to the point where the joint is destroyed. This is what orthopedists refer to rather graphically as "bone on bone." This is a more serious problem in those with a mechanical heart valve. These patients have to face the risk of taking non-steroidal anti-inflammatory drugs (NSAIDs) to control the pain or to have a joint replacement. It's a tough decision. The risk of bleeding from gastric irritation due to NSAIDs is substantial because the clotting factors are tied up by Coumadin anticoagulation therapy. Gastritis that would ordinarily be well tolerated if the clotting mechanism were intact might develop into a hemorrhagic gastritis (multiple little bleeding points in the stomach) when on Coumadin. On the other hand, if one stops anticoagulation in preparation for surgery, there is a risk of clot formation on the valve and possible embolism to the brain during this vulnerable period.

While this sounds like a terrible Catch-22 situation without hope or help, it isn't always. In fact, we usually prefer that you go ahead and get the joint replaced if you are miserable. This way, at least we can usually get you off the dreadful NSAIDs. Fortunately, we usually get by with these surgeries without a catastrophe. The way we pull this off is by making Lovenox injections into the subcutaneous tissue to provide anticoagulation while we wait for the Coumadin effect to wear off. Then we stop the Lovenox, wait a few hours, and perform the operation. We restart Coumadin as soon as it is safe following the operation, using low-dosage Lovenox for protection against valvular thrombosis until the Protime is therapeutic once again.

B. Tissue (Bioprosthetic) Valve

The tissue valve's major claim to fame, which is a huge plus, is that it does not require anticoagulant therapy. Usually a pig valve is used. However, increasingly, a pericardial valve—frequently obtained from a cow source—is used. The major drawback to these valves has to do with gradual degeneration of the tissue matrix with thickening, scarring, and calcification. It seems that the younger the recipient, the more aggressively the valve degenerates. For this reason, we try to avoid using a bioprosthetic valve in younger people. The exception is the young woman who might want to have children, as there is increased fetal mortality with Coumadin use. In such a case, we usually recommend a pericardial tissue valve, and allow her to go ahead with her childbearing plans; then when that valve has deteriorated, replace it with a mechanical valve.

Tissue valve degeneration frequently proceeds to the point where a decision has to be made about a repeat valve replacement. Fortunately, in the older population of 60 and above, this doesn't usually develop for 10 to 15 years. Still, this can be a difficult situation.

Let's say, for example, that an individual received a valve replacement at age 60. The pros and cons were discussed in full and a decision was made to use a tissue valve prosthesis. At the time the patient made the decision, it seemed fine with him or her that the valve would likely last about 15 years. That seemed a long way off. Time passes quickly. Fast forward 15 years. Now, the patient is 75 years of age and is possibly looking at another valve replacement because of bioprothesis degeneration. A redo operation is much harder on anyone at age 75. Not only that, but a redo heart operation always carries an increased mortality and morbidity risk over the initial operation. Therefore, at a more advanced age, this sometimes becomes a very big decision, especially if a number of additional health problems have surfaced in the meantime.

This is the main reason we're flexible. For example, if you are 60 and extremely vigorous and robust and looking forward to your next 40 years with eager anticipation, we might well suggest a mechanical valve, especially if you've had no health problems. On the other hand, if you are 60 but have had repeated bouts of bleeding from the colon, drink like a fish, or have generally had a tough life making you an old 60, a tissue valve is for you.

C. The Role of Destiny and Imponderables

Sometimes the decision regarding the type of valve to use is easy. For example, many people are destined for anticoagulation therapy no matter which type valve you put in. Folks with chronic atrial fibrillation should receive a mechanical valve, as they are going to be committed to lifelong anticoagulation therapy anyway. This is because of the risk of clot formation in the heart with subsequent systemic embolus (a clot that forms in the fibrillating left atrial appendage, breaks loose from its mooring, and travels to the brain or elsewhere), an always-present risk with atrial fibrillation. Additionally, many mitral valve replacement recipients will predictably develop recurrent atrial fibrillation due to a large left atrium from their underlying mitral valvular disorder, and it seems unlikely they will ever be able to discontinue Coumadin therapy completely. These patients should probably receive a mechanical valve. It is more durable and in this case, the main advantage of a tissue valve is lost, as they are going to require anticoagulation on a different basis.

On the other hand, if you developed an overwhelming problem with a gastrointestinal bleed because of some intractable or inoperable disorder, it would be much simpler to treat if we could simply take you off Coumadin therapy altogether. We would *never* think of doing that with a mechanical mitral valve unless we simply couldn't control the problem otherwise because the mechanical mitral valve would almost certainly eventually clot. On the other hand, we would stop Coumadin readily if the mitral valve prothesis were a tissue valve. We also feel safer stopping Coumadin if the mechanical prosthetic valve under consideration is an *aortic* valve rather than a mitral, since the pressure is much higher at the aortic valvular level and it seems to "wash" the valve more effectively, preventing clot formation. The filling pressure washing the mitral valve is quite low by comparison. Given our choice, however, we would never interrupt Coumadin anticoagulation therapy when any mechanical prosthetic valve is in place.

I do think that a young person should receive a mechanical heart valve if at all possible. But there are exceptions. Occasionally we see a young person with aortic stenosis (a narrowing in the aortic valve between the left ventricular pumping chamber and the large blood tube, the aorta) who also has a very small annulus, the ring within the valvular structure. In this case, because a mechanical valve is bulkier than a tissue valve, we might have to implant such a small-sized mechanical valve that it would leave behind a large gradient, a pressure drop from the left ventricle to the aorta. This situation is exactly the same one that we set out to treat in the first place and thus it makes no sense. What is usually done, instead, is to perform a procedure on the valve annulus and, if this renders the orifice size sufficient, proceed with implantation of a mechanical prosthesis. If not, we place a stentless tissue valve within this small annulus in order to reduce the gradient to as low a level as possible. A zero gradient is what we are after.

Another unique group of valve replacement recipients are those who, by virtue of habits or other health problems, are statistically destined to bleed if they are chronically anticoagulated. These are sometimes more difficult to determine but chronic alcoholics and those with recurrent gastrointestinal bleeding come to mind.

The Ross Procedure

No treatise on valve replacement would be complete without a nod to the wonderful innovations of Dr. Donald Ross, who explained to the world how a revolutionary operation could be performed on young patients who had clinically significant abnormal aortic valves. Despite the fact that he described this procedure many years ago, it is still performed in only a few medical centers even today. It is a truly wonderful operation, especially for young people who want to remain active, perhaps continue aggressive physical exercise and habits, and remain off anticoagulation therapy.

Remember, the aortic valve is supposed to consist of three leaflets. The most common congenital anomaly is a bicuspid valve—made up of only two leaflets. This will degenerate and will ultimately block flow.

Instead of replacing the defective aortic valve with a pig valve (which would degenerate rapidly in a young person) or a mechanical valve (which would require anti-coagulant therapy), the aortic valve is, instead, replaced with the person's own *pulmonary* valve. The aortic and pulmonary valves are similar in design and function. However, the pulmonary valve is much less important. When it is removed and sewn into the aortic annulus, it is replaced by a cryo-preserved cadaver valve (a frozen preserved human tissue valve). In the proper hands, and there aren't that many, this is the preferential surgery for a bicuspid aortic valve replacement in a young person. The patient's own pulmonary valve, transplanted to the aortic valve position to replace the faulty valve from birth, will actually grow as the individual grows. It must be performed by someone who has great experience with this technique. There have been problems with this complex operation so you must discuss the pros and cons with your surgeon to see if it is for you.

Summary of Valve Recommendations

In general then, with unique exceptions, we make the following recommendations:

1. Patients who are less than 60 years old should generally receive mechanical valve prostheses.
2. However, for patients who are under 60 but have had gastrointestinal bleeding, are alcoholic, have intractable risky habits or hobbies, have a condition that mandates NSAID usage, or have had previous hemorrhagic episodes, we also implant a tissue valve. Obviously, we cannot always accurately predict who will bleed on anticoagulant therapy. We do know, however, that patients comprising this short list are at high risk of bleeding.
3. If the patient is older than 60, we usually recommend a tissue valve.
4. If the patient is in "fixed" atrial fibrillation and will require Coumadin anticoagulation anyway, we tend toward implanting a mechanical prosthesis.
5. Also, we occasionally become involved with a patient who never, ever wants another heart operation performed. These people receive a mechanical valve.

As you can tell, these situations are as unique as the individual and his or her idiosyncrasies. Therefore, it is extremely important that the cardiac surgeon (who has to implant the valve), the cardiologist (who has to follow the valve), the patient (who has to live with the valve), and the family (who has to live with the patient) all participate in the decision-making process.

Life Long Coumadin Therapy? Personal Protime Machine

One point should be emphasized. If you are committed to lifelong anticoagulation therapy, you should acquire your own Protime machine. You can prick your finger, run the test, and adjust your Coumadin dosage depending on a schedule your physician has provided you. If you are lucky, you'll require only monthly Protimes. Many people have to do this weekly. If you go to a physician's office or an anticoagulation laboratory, you will be reliant on phone calls and subject to mistakes that can occur whenever numbers are handled repeatedly. It is just too cumbersome for the long run, especially if you are one of those persons who needs frequent Protime measurements.

An Individual Choice

This information constitutes a rough guideline for valve replacement and selection of prosthetic material. There are too many variables out there to prescribe for each conceivable circumstance in this chapter. However, we do individualize this process in real-life situations. We always try to balance the likelihood of bleeding against the possible necessity of replacing the prosthesis at some later point, perhaps when the individual is not as strong or capable of withstanding another operation. The thing that makes this more difficult as I get older is the realization that people age at incredibly different rates. This makes risk categorization based on age alone nearly meaningless. However, we have to generate guidelines. Those I have provided for you have been developed over the 30 years I have interacted with patients making this choice. Follow-up, watching the course of such valve recipients, seeing complications resulting from either decision, and studying the nuances of disease processes have factored greatly into my recommendations to you. I have been very impressed, for example, that gastrointestinal bleeding complications increase almost logarithmically in the over-60 group. This is frequently exacerbated greatly by Coumadin. We know that if you have valve replacement for aortic stenosis, a thickening of the aortic valve, you are also at higher risk of having small vascular lesions in your colon called *angiodysplasia*. If you have such a thing and are on Coumadin for a mechanical valve, you may be destined to a perpetual threat of bleeding. For this reason, I frequently ask the gastroenterologists to perform a colonoscopy on individuals who are borderline when we are having a very difficult time choosing which valve replacement modality is best. As the patient, you must also have input. As always, it is my hope that this book will provide you with the tools you need to interact in the management of your care.

REMINDERS

1. Tissue valves frequently do not require anticoagulation therapy.
2. Mechanical valves always require anticoagulation therapy.
3. If you receive a mechanical heart valve prosthesis and will require lifelong anticoagulation with Coumadin, you should purchase a Protime machine that will allow you to make personalized Protime checks without multiple trips to the anticoagulation clinic and recurrent phone calls to and from the physician's office.
4. If you are young and were born with a congenital bicuspid aortic valve that has degenerated rapidly, you might well consider the Ross procedure—replacement of your faulty aortic valve with your own pulmonic valve, then replacement of the pulmonic valve with a frozen human tissue valve. This provides the best of both worlds: You have the benefit of a tissue valve, yet you do not have to take Coumadin.

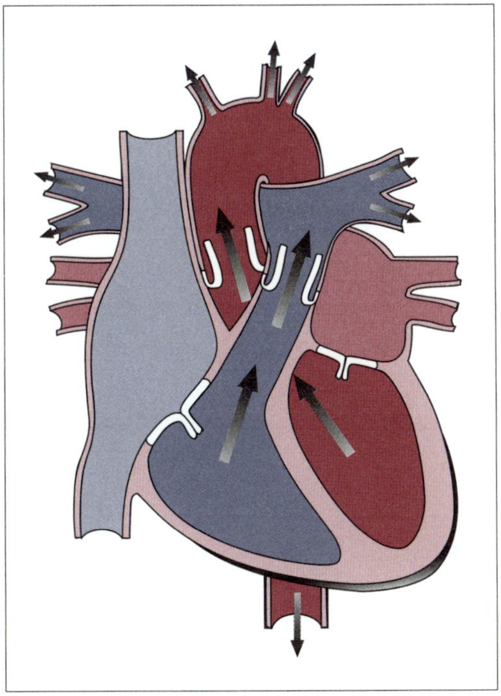

25 MITRAL VALVE PROLAPSE

A Click, a Murmur, Some Pain, and Some Extra Beats

MITRAL VALVE PROLAPSE (MVP) IS ONE OF THE MOST over-diagnosed cardiologic processes in the world! It is so over-diagnosed that I do not agree with the previously formulated diagnosis in about half of the people who come to see me with this diagnosis already firmly in place. While there is no doubt that this problem exists and that it is capable of causing great distress, it needs to be emphasized that a huge number of people have been scared and are laboring under the belief that they have something wrong with their mitral valve when they really don't. That out of the way, there is a large population of individuals who really *do* have this problem and, for some, it hinders their happiness. Fortunately, there is only a small minority that has serious problems with this disorder.

Anatomy of the Mitral Valve

If we were to remove the mitral valve and spread it out on the table, it would be about three to four times larger in surface area than the area of the annulus, or ring, of the orifice in which it fits. It is basically comprised of two large leaflets, tethered by just over 30 thin, string-like structures that extend down from the valve to their insertion into the protruding muscle of the ventricle, the papillary muscles. These strings are called *chordae tendinae*. The valve with the chordae closely resembles a parachute. Since this valve was first examined by very early scientists who were often involved with the church as well, it was likened to the miter's cap worn by bishops and senior abbots within the church. Hence, the name "mitral valve." It is by far the most complex of the four valves of the heart.

When the pumping chamber, the left ventricle, is relaxed, the valve is open, the chordae are slack, and the chamber fills with in-coming red blood from the lungs. As the electrical current activates ventricular muscle and it begins to contract, the mitral valve closes and the chordae become tensed, holding the valve leaflets in place to prevent leakage. Obviously, in this miraculously choreographed repetitive act, everything has to fit just right for the proper sequence to occur.

Any significant elongation of the chordae, or redundancy of the valve tissue, will result in leakage. However, since the valve closes by a process of coaptation, the wrinkling up of tissue—one part snugged up against its neighbor so that the excess material is all contained—there can easily be an over-diagnosis of mitral valve prolapse.

Symptoms and Findings of Mitral Valve Prolapse

People who have MVP will frequently complain of one or more of the following symptoms: palpitations, atypical chest pain (usually sharp), intermittent shortness of breath, or fatigue. Of these, by far the most common complaints are palpitations and atypical chest pain. Frequently, these symptoms are made worse by caffeine. These individuals are often very susceptible to the effects of any stimulant and to monosodium glutamate (MSG), a taste-enhancer salt.

The palpitations are frequently caused by an increased number of premature beats from both the upper and the lower chambers. However, I believe that the anatomy of the chest, and the heart within it, are as responsible for this awareness of cardiac action as the premature beats themselves. Individuals with MVP are most typically somewhat thin and stretchy, with a straight back, an *ectomorphic* body habitus. Many will have some degree of concavity of the sternum (the bone in the very center of the front of the chest), a situation known as pectus excavatum, where the sternum is "scooped out" and in the most striking cases, this can be very dramatic. In these instances, the heart is very close to the sternum. In extreme examples of pectus excavatum, the heart may be somewhat compressed between the sternum and the vertebral column, a so-called "pancake heart."

If I see a rather short, stocky individual (*mesomorphic* body habitus) with the previous diagnosis of MVP, I am immediately suspicious of the diagnosis as it is rare in such patients. It can occur; it is just rare. On the other hand, tall, thin people don't have to have it either. They are just more likely to. In my view, the proximity of the heart to the sternum in these individuals is one of the most prominent causes of awareness of heart action.

We all have premature atrial contractions (PACs) and premature ventricular contractions (PVCs). These become more frequent with advancing age and are increased by alcohol, tobacco, stress, and caffeine. While the mean number of such PACs and PVCs is increased in individuals with MVP, as opposed to those without the diagnosis, the complaint of palpitations is usually far out of proportion to this increase in number.

This prototype is also more likely to have one of the clinical standards of MVP: the mitral click. This is a prominent clicking sound usually near the end of the first third of systole or in the middle of systole, when the ventricle has just begun to contract. This click is probably generated from the tensing of the chordae or the coaptation of the mitral leaflets with part of the structure elongated (frequently the thin support tendrils are too long) or redundant (in some, there is just too much valve tissue for the job and it has to go somewhere when the valve closes—it may billow out). As this choreography progresses, the click is generated and frequently followed by a late blowing systolic murmur generated from the escape of blood across the segment of the valve that is not in exact juxtaposition (tight joining) with its neighbor.

The above finding, coupled with an echocardiogram showing prolapse (tongue-like protrusion) of tissue beyond the line of closure, allowing for some mitral regurgitation, makes the diagnosis of MVP. It took us a long time to get here, but now you have the definition. These patients warrant further investigation.

We have no idea why such individuals have atypical chest pain beyond what the non-MVP population has. By atypical chest pain, we refer to pain that is unlike that which occurs with narrowing of a coronary artery (angina). This is typically brought on by exertion. On the other hand, atypical chest pain commonly occurs at rest, particularly at night or at a time when the patient is performing no strenuous activity. It frequently lasts for hours. If chest pain is due to oxygen-deprivation from a narrowed coronary artery, there will be damage to the heart muscle if the pain persists relentlessly for two or three hours. This type of duration is common in those with MVP and atypical chest pain, perhaps due to increased nutritional needs of the MV apparatus. The difference is they don't have heart damage as a consequence. My suspicion is that it is at least partially related to the proximity of the heart to the chest wall, the same mechanism that I believe is responsible for the awareness of cardiac activity. There also seems to be, in some instances, a problem with the mitral valve apparatus receiving enough oxygen and nutrients. I suspect we do not have the full story on why some people with mitral valve prolapse have this atypical chest pain, which is sometimes sharp and very frightening to the individual.

Individuals with MVP who are symptomatic should all have a treadmill exercise test. There is an uncommon individual with MVP who will develop *ventricular tachycardia* as a response to the increased level of circulating catecholamines (epinephrine and norepinephrine) brought on with exercise. This is a potentially dangerous arrhythmia, important to recognize, as we can almost always block this response with a beta-blocker, such as Inderal. It is important to repeat the treadmill test after treatment with Inderal to be sure this response is truly blocked. It makes no sense to recognize a threatening process, treat it, and then not make sure that it is, indeed, effectively blocked.

We should also make sure that these individuals don't have something more menacing than MVP, such as occult coronary artery disease. Many of these patients come to us as young adults and the possibility of occult coronary artery disease is unlikely. Others come in at age 40 or beyond and are, indeed, in the coronary age group. And, of course, there is no biological rule that prevents the two from occurring together.

Medical Treatment of MVP

In this immense population with MVP, who should be treated? Not very many actually need to be treated with drugs at all. In my view, the only ones who should be treated are those with exercise-precipitated ventricular tachycardia and those with life-changing palpitations or chest pain. The treatment is nearly always a beta-blocker.

Should antibiotic prophylaxis be given to those patients with MVP? Only a fraction is the proper answer. I have seen thousands of people who dutifully took their penicillin prior to, during, or following dental procedures. Most of them didn't need it. Someone with a loud click and murmur, coupled with an echo that demonstrates violent prolapse, should receive antibiotic prophylaxis for dental and surgical maneuvers. However, if the click is quiet or intermittent or the valve looks only slightly deranged on echo, I think the risk of antibiotic prophylaxis outweighs the potential good. In 30 years of doing this, I have seen only two or three patients with endocarditis (an infection of the mitral valve) that I thought was due to bacterial invasion of the prolapsing valve as a result of a dental procedure. You will need to determine which group your doctor feels you belong in regarding need for antibiotics for dental and surgical procedures. In general, the ones with thickened valves are the ones we worry about.

Severe Problems with MVP

What about other potential calamities of the valve in individuals with MVP? Some of these valves degenerate with time. They are the ones that were probably not normal from birth and, with the wear and tear of the years, thicken and degenerate. These valves may well possess an intrinsic abnormality of the tissue matrix, a situation we call *myxomatous degeneration*. Another term you might hear is *pseudo-mucinous degeneration*.

At any rate, the chordae in these situations are more apt to become rigid and fracture at some point. This rather dramatic occurrence, somewhat rare, is quite obvious. Basically, all of these chordal structures are needed to act in concert with the papillary muscle and the valve tissue to maintain a reliable barrier to leakage across the valve back into the left atrium. With 32 chordae tendinae involved, one might logically think that the loss of only one strand would result in a trivial problem. It is, however, akin to a puppet show. If one single string is out of commission, the whole show ceases to "work." In this instance, if one of the chordae pops, a segment of mitral tissue will protrude, and significant leakage will occur. The patient usually experiences the abrupt onset of shortness of breath and usually has a pronounced murmur of mitral regurgitation. An echo will promptly confirm the diagnosis.

Such patients with myxomatous valvular abnormalities should be followed more closely than other patients with simple MVP. I have seen patient after patient with a normal-looking mitral valve, or mild MVP, who had received an echocardiogram each year for the last ten. This is not only unnecessary, but it is taking an unethical advantage of the patient's fears. Such valves almost never disrupt. On the other hand, the patient with a very thick mitral valve due to a myxomatous process should be looked at every year with an echo.

Surgical Treatment for a Ruptured or Degenerative Mitral Valve

In the event of disruption of the valve apparatus, usually due to the fracture of a chordal structure, an attempt at valve repair should be carried out. A good "garden variety" cardiac surgeon can *replace* a valve. However, the mitral valve should always be repaired rather than replaced whenever feasible. You do better with the one that "comes from the factory." In such instances, I always search for a surgeon who is confident he or she can perform mitral valve repair with predictable success.

Also, in the last few years we have come to realize that these moderately leaking myxomatous valves need to be treated with more respect than we previously thought. We used to wait until the left ventricle had dilated considerably before we operated on them. Sometimes the outlook is not good following valve surgery if we wait this long and, infrequently, the individual with substantial mitral regurgitation will die suddenly. We must presume that the left ventricular muscles were laboring more than we thought and caused a reentrant and very malignant arrhythmia as a result. Therefore, we feel that it is better to proceed on with mitral valve surgery if the valve is leaking significantly—repairing it if the individual is less than 60 and usually replacing it with a bioprosthetic (tissue) valve if over 60.

REMINDERS

1. **MVP is due to overlapping mitral valve tissue or an elongation of the support structures, the chordae tendinae.**
2. **Symptoms of atypical chest pain or palpitations are seldom more than a nuisance. But sometimes this sharp pain is so bothersome it should be treated. Likewise, "skipped beats" can be enough of a bother to warrant treatment. Both symptoms are treated with a beta-blocker such as Inderal.**
3. **A person with MVP may have a tendency to develop exercise-induced ventricular tachycardia. This can almost always be blocked with Inderal or some other beta-blocker.**
4. **Only those with violent MVP or degenerative mitral valves require antibiotic prophylaxis.**
5. **Mitral valve repair, rather than replacement, should be performed if a chordal structure ruptures, especially in the younger patient.**

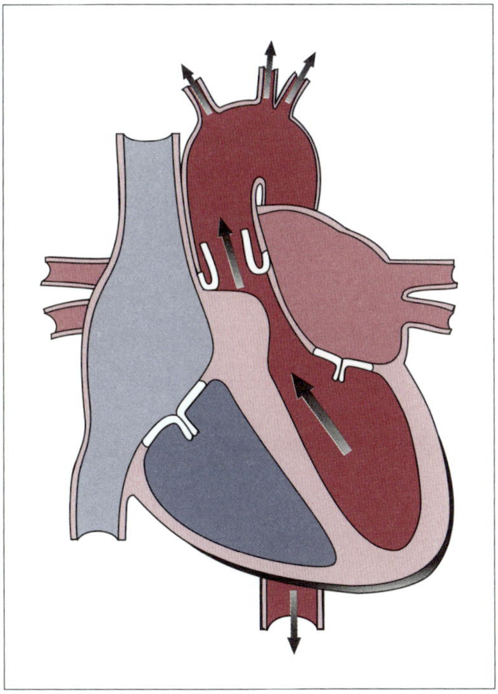

27 HYPERTROPHIC CARDIOMYOPATHY

Too Much Heart, Muscle That Is

MY MOM AND DAD USED TO DESCRIBE people who are so charitable that others are always taking advantage of them as having "too much heart." Yet my father, a rancher, described his best horse as having "a lot of heart." I suppose I grew up conflicted. Now I truly know that too much heart can be dangerous to your health.

Incidence

Hypertrophic cardiomyopathy is not common, but it is not really all that rare either. Its prevalence is about one out of every 500 people. This statistic means that a mid-sized city of one million people would contain 2,000 with this disease. There are well over a half million people with this disease across the United States!

Definition and Pathology

Hypertrophic cardiomyopathy is due to a genetically endowed, inappropriate proliferation of heart muscle tissue in a specific area of the left ventricle. Some will have only a large muscle bulge just below the aortic valve in the area of the left ventricle we call the outflow tract. This is the area to which oxygenated blood is funneled just prior to its being pumped into the giant blood tube, the aorta. This is a discreet muscle

Figure 24 Idiopathic Hypertrophic Subaortic Stenosis

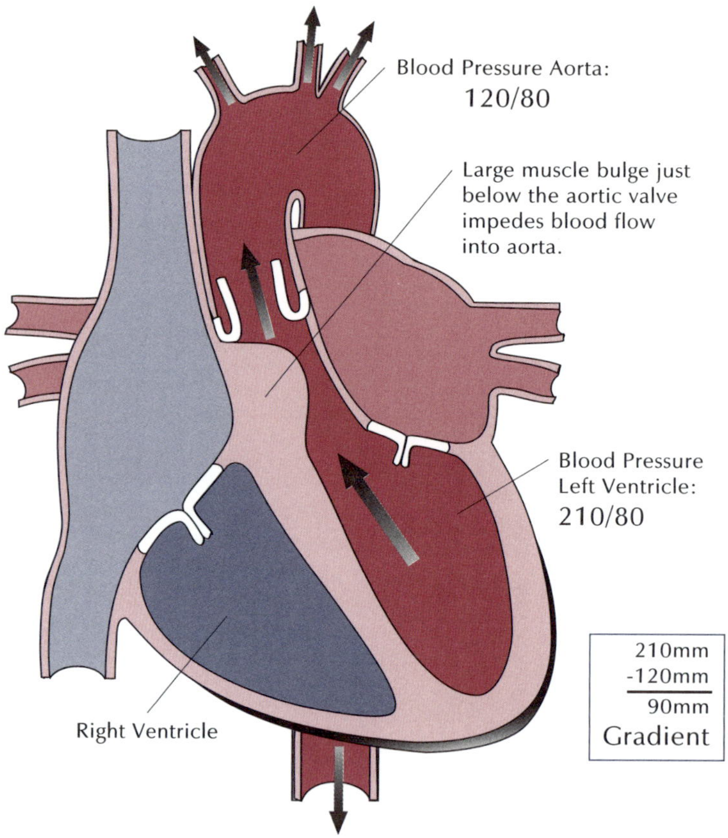

bulge. This situation is referred to as *Idiopathic Hypertrophic Subaortic Stenosis* (IHSS), representing the most dangerous form of hypertrophic cardiomyopathy and also the most common. (Figure 24)

Other individuals will have a much more generalized proliferation of heart muscle cells throughout the left ventricle, and there is yet another group of people who will have muscle proliferation near the tip of the left ventricle. These are all genetically determined and each pattern poses its own set of problems.

Currently a great deal of work is going into determining exactly which chromosomal factor has mandated each type of abnormal pattern. With this delineation, hopefully, genetic correction is just around the corner. Until that time, we must deal with this pile-up of muscle fibers using the tools available.

This abnormal cell proliferation and enlargement frequently occurs in a chaotic fashion. Heart muscle fibers should lie in neat, organized rows, one beside the other. In so doing, they form a unique network, with each fiber working in concert with its neighbors. This is the world's best example of organized labor.

In the *hypertrophic cardiomyopathies*, the medical term that indicates this sort of problem, cells within the abnormal zones frequently exist within a pattern of spatial disarray, growing in bundles of disorganized fibers. These fibers are abnormal in size and orientation, especially in the IHSS variety.

These various types of hypertrophic cardiomyopathy are mostly inherited patterns. Therefore, if one person is identified as having hypertrophic cardiomyopathy, others in the family should be examined. This can be done efficiently with a simple echocardiogram. With many of these forms, the family tree can be traced back for generations, with certain family members dying suddenly along the way. In such families, a full genetic evaluation should be carried out in a center where such studies are being actively done. Frequently, these medical centers will curtail much of the cost in order to be allowed to study this condition.

Tests to Determine Risks and Treatment

There are two or three tests that should be done in each patient in whom the diagnosis of hypertrophic cardiomyopathy is made. The first, which usually corroborates the diagnosis, is the echocardiogram. In addition to giving a name to the process, it will allow the doctor to establish if there is a pressure drop across the muscle bulge, a so-called "gradient." The amount of this gradient, and any increase with provocative measures, such as exercise or a valsalva maneuver (from straining down hard), is important in counseling patients as to how strenuous they can be in daily activities and sports. It can also serve as a guideline to therapy.

The next most important test is a Holter monitor—a 24-hour electromagnetic tape recording of the heart rhythm. If individuals have a great number of extra beats from the lower chamber, ventricular premature beats, and especially if some of these are repetitive in nature, they should undergo an electrophysiology test to determine if they are at high risk for development of ventricular tachycardia and potential sudden death. Ventricular tachycardia, remember, is a very rapid repetitive heart beat coming from the lower chamber, the ventricle. It is usually life-threatening. The electrophysiology test should be done straightaway without delay if the patient has symptoms of blackout, dizziness, or rapid palpitations.

The tendency to develop this potentially lethal arrhythmia is frequently related to the severity of the pressure drop across the muscle bulge in the outflow tract. For instance, a gradient of 20 mmHg would be a low number and usually not very dangerous. However, if one had a gradient of 60 mmHg at rest and it rose to 110 mmHg with provocation, this is in a worrisome range for development of cardiac sudden death from an arrhythmia. In this case, the blood pressure with an arm cuff measurement might be 120 mmHg, perfectly normal. A 60 mm gradient would mean that the left ventricular pressure becomes 120 plus 60 or 180 mmHg. This is pretty high, placing undue strain upon the left ventricular muscle. With provocation, the pressure in the left ventricle rises to 120 plus 110 or a total of 230 mmHg! This is an alarming pressure, putting incredible strain on the left ventricular muscle and taxing its blood supply limitations. It is not difficult to imagine how a fatal arrhythmia could be triggered in such a setting.

The other possibility with this same provocation is that the muscle bulge so obstructs the passage of blood through the outflow tract that the pressure within the aorta, and consequently the arm cuff pressure, falls substantially, say to 80 mmHg. The individual will get dizzy and if this low blood pressure persists for very long, he or she might pass out. This is a dangerous situation.

Sudden death is the common method of departure for some who have IHSS. Ventricular ectopy (extra beats originating from the left ventricle) and blackout spells can, in most instances, be prevented through drug therapy and the implantation of an Automatic Implantable Cardiac Defibrillator (AICD). Such patients—with dizziness, blackout spells, palpitations, and a high gradient, or the provocation of a high gradient—should be promptly evaluated and treated. However, since the development of a life-ending arrhythmia is well correlated with the degree of obstruction across the muscle bulge, AICD implantation should be withheld until it can be determined exactly what relief either surgical or catheter intervention has brought about. If a dramatic decrease in the pressure gradient has been effected, the risk of sudden cardiac death from an arrhythmia usually falls correspondingly. Frequently, a good result from intervention obviates the need for an AICD unless another process, usually coronary artery disease, is also present and has created left ventricular dysfunction from previous heart damage.

Drug Treatment

The major drug group we use in these individuals with IHSS is a beta-blocker. This type of drug blocks the initial phase of muscle contractility and can sharply reduce the gradient across the muscular zone in the outflow tract. There are a number of other drugs that can also drop the pressure gradient across the muscular obstruction. Fine-tuning the drug therapy is often required in order to achieve the needed result.

Interventional Treatment

Surgical resection of the muscle bulge has been performed for 30 years. From statistical studies, it provides significant relief from the obstruction.

In the past, we would sometimes place a right ventricular pacemaker in order to pull the inter-ventricular septum away from the left ventricle and enlarge the region in the outflow tract. This produced a good result in some, but is not a uniformly effective therapy. I have resorted to this only after placing a catheter within the left ventricle, measuring the gradient, then pacing the right ventricle and repeating the measurements. If the gradient dropped dramatically, I would implant a permanent pacemaker. I think this procedure has largely fallen by the wayside.

A relatively new technique has been that of cannulating the septal artery that feeds the hypertrophied, bulging muscle zone so that pure alcohol can be introduced via the catheter with the purpose of destroying some of this culprit heart muscle. In doing this, we are producing a "therapeutic heart attack" of the septal muscle bulge. This should be done only by someone who is experienced in this technique, as it is tricky. In the proper hands, this procedure results in a dramatic reduction in the pressure gradient in many of these patients, as the damaged muscle shrinks and scars down. (Figure 25, page 326) This is currently the technique of choice in those individuals with extremely high gradients, at least in those past the teenage years.

Current Therapy for Severe Obstruction: Surgical Resection of the Muscle Bulge Versus Alcohol Ablation

In the past we have asked the cardiac surgeons to perform a septal myectomy on the muscle bulge in extreme instances. After all, the problem is due to a pathologic accumulation of muscle blocking the easy transit of blood from the pump into the aorta. This procedure consists of surgically removing this abnormal muscle bulge. It

Figure 25 Alcohol Ablation of IHSS

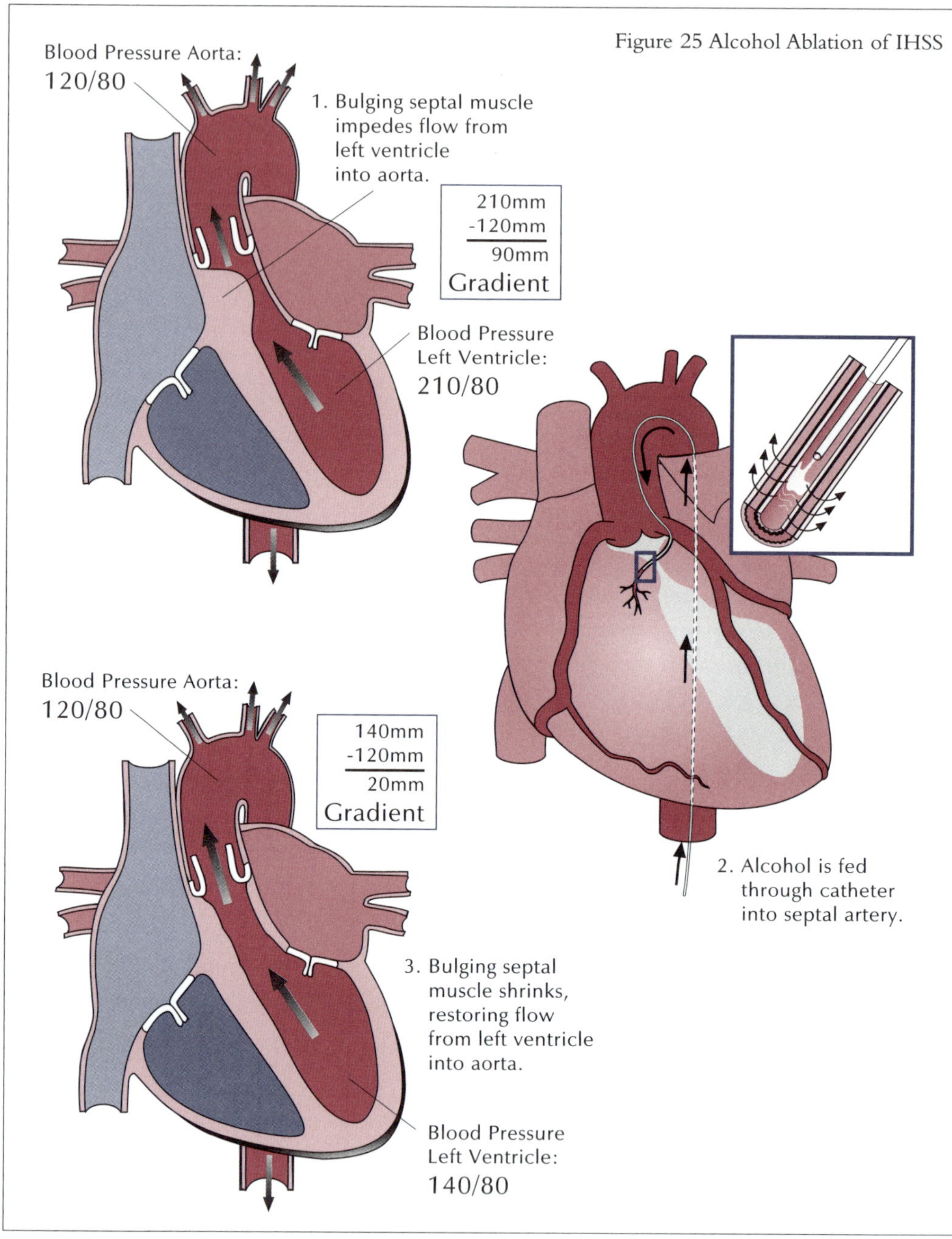

sounds as though this should do the job nicely, doesn't it? However, there is no signal to notify the surgeon when enough tissue has been removed. Furthermore, IHSS is an incredibly dynamic process. I have never personally had a totally satisfying result from this intervention. I realize this is supposed to be the "gold standard" of treatment for this condition. It has been used for years. I've just never had a good result from this operation in any of my patients.

I'm sure my experience is colored by my first patient with such an intervention. It turned out badly. Likewise, every one of the five patients I have sent for this surgery has had problems. All have come back with substantial pressure gradients requiring large amounts of beta adrenergic-blocking drugs for control. Perhaps I've just had a bad sampling. I don't think so, as these were all done in different institutions by seasoned, name-brand cardiac surgeons. It's soured my view on the surgery. One of the reasons for only a moderate result is that part of this disease is due to the incredibly hypercontractile state of the left ventricle, especially in the region of the septum. The force of contractility of the heart muscle in these individuals is, in many instances, simply enormous. It is frequently impossible to completely block this hyperaggressive squeeze of the heart muscle, leading to a high gradient yet again.

In my view, the alcohol septal ablation therapy has been a real Godsend. I have great respect for the physicians who stuck with this technique and perfected it. After all, it sounded kind of crazy when it was first proposed as therapy. That's the way it has been throughout history when a totally new procedure was proposed for a perplexing problem. The driving force for this particular intervention has been, and continues to be, Dr. William H. Spencer III.

In the right hands, this produces marvelous results. Like every other procedure, it is not without risks. Since the electrical conduction system runs right through the septum, occasional patients have developed complete heart block due to destruction of enough of the electrical conduit that it is simply inept in carrying current to the lower chambers. These individuals obviously require a pacemaker. The symptomatic results have generally been good for this group as well, however, as the obstruction to left ventricular emptying was dramatically relieved. Just as you would expect, the results are proportionately related to relief of the obstructive gradient. Because of this, about 10% of all patients need a second go-around to obtain the needed drop in pressure gradient. However, we're not talking about a second open-heart procedure with a three-month healing time; we're talking about a two-day hospital stay with only a sore groin where the catheter was inserted.

When I first heard about this alcohol ablation technique, I was concerned that the scar from the therapeutic heart attack would cause fatal arrhythmias down the line. This hasn't proven to be the case. Indeed, in these very high-risk individuals, the mortality rate has been well less than 1% per year.

I think very young people, symptomatic from high resting or provocable gradients across the left ventricular outflow tract should still receive an operation, a myectomy, at an medical facility where they do a large number of them. However, I feel that alcohol septal ablation is clearly the procedure of choice in patients over age 21 with this form of hypertrophic cardiomyopathy in which the collection of muscle fibers form a huge obstructive bulge of tissue in the outflow tract.

REMINDERS

1. If you have had a family member with any form of hypertrophic cardiomyopathy or unexplained sudden death, have an echocardiogram to make sure you do not have a familial form of this process.
2. Initial treatment of IHSS is usually a beta-blocker. This may be exceptionally effective, especially for those who have the problem in modest form.
3. If the gradient is high, alcohol obliteration of septal tissue is a very effective and safe therapy, but should only be done by someone who has learned this technique from the masters. This is not for everyone and is not to be done by just anyone.
4. Certain individuals with IHSS are at reasonably high risk for sudden cardiac death. This can be prevented by drug therapy, coupled with either surgery to remove the muscle bulge or alcohol injection in the septal artery. In most cases, the decrease in risk of sudden cardiac death is directly proportional to the relief of the gradient across the muscle bulge.
5. Certain people, usually those with very thick hearts, those with damage from a previous extensive heart attack, or those with other cardiac problems, will retain a risk of sudden cardiac death after the gradient has been relieved. They deserve an AICD as added protection against sudden death.

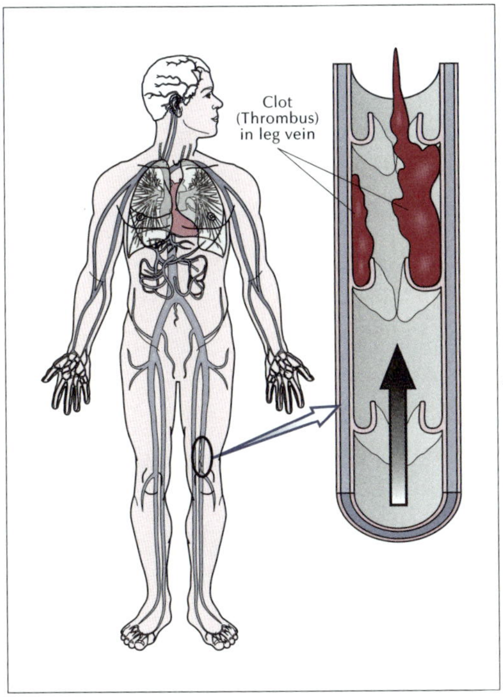

ANTICOAGULATION AND PLATELET DRUGS

Blood Thinners and Platelet Greasers

AS PUT SO ELOQUENTLY IN AN ARTICLE in the *New York Times* by Abraham Verghese, "The secret in the care of the patient is caring for the patient." I wish I had come up with this phrase but, in lieu of that, I will just borrow it, with due respect to the author. I am afraid that, when it comes to caring for the patient who requires Coumadin anticoagulation, the system is woefully inadequate. More people are damaged through inadequate monitoring of this drug—in some fashion—than by any other medication. I hope to help change that.

First, I want to make one thing clear. Patients love to refer to their Coumadin as a "blood-thinner." It doesn't thin the blood; it's just as thick on Coumadin as before. I see where they get that, as it seems thinner because it doesn't clot as well if you cut yourself. They also like to refer to their platelet drugs as "greasers." Maybe I'm just giving in to West Texas–speak, as I subtitled this chapter according to common parlance. Oh well, if you can't beat 'em, join 'em.

Acute Anticoagulation

Acute anticoagulation is performed when you are in urgent need of protection from clot proliferation. We are all forming clots—and we are also breaking down clots continuously. These two should be in balance, what we call homeostasis. Clot, or thrombus, formation can be life-saving especially at the time of trauma. If I had an auto accident that resulted in the rupture of my spleen, I wouldn't stand a chance if my clotting mechanisms didn't rev up and cause clot formation. On the other hand, we sometimes form clots when it is clearly a pathologic process, and one that threatens our life at that. This has to be interrupted if we are to survive the ordeal. And this is accomplished by the acute administration of anticoagulation therapy.

Frequently, an individual will enter the hospital with a problem that warrants the use of acute anticoagulant therapy. As such, we choose a drug that prevents clot formation and, hopefully, if the clot is not too well formed, will also erode and disperse a previously formed clot to some degree. This pathologic process can range from a blood clot that is forming in the leg veins all the way to a heart attack, where a clot forms in an artery supplying the heart muscle. If we wish to acutely interrupt a pathologic clotting process, we use one of two drugs. The drug that has been used for many, many years is Heparin. It is still a good drug. It is given intravenously for this task, though it can be given under the skin, subcutaneously, in smaller doses as a preventive measure. Nowadays, we frequently use a purified derivative of Heparin called Lovenox. It is more effective plus we do not have to measure its effect by drawing blood every few hours. Additionally, we can give it subcutaneously, even for the big problems. We can use one of these drugs for days or weeks if necessary.

Heparin and Lovenox are the only drugs used for acute anticoagulation. Sometimes, if the pathologic clot is life-threatening, we may wish to employ a thombolytic drug. This drug, which I call a clot-buster, is in an entirely different category than Heparin. These drugs are exceptionally powerful in tearing down a previously formed clot. Such a drug dramatically increases the risk of a catastrophic bleeding problem so we only use it when we think the risk of the clot is greater than the risk of precipitating a bleed. Such a pathologic clot is one in a coronary artery; another is a huge clot in the large vein draining the leg, especially if it has already resulted in embolism to the lungs. Thrombolytic therapy is on a totally different level of intervention than our more commonly administered anticoagulation drugs, the Heparin family.

Obviously, if we are interrupting a clotting process with any drug, we may cause bleeding as a side effect. This is especially true in the elderly. This inappropriate bleeding can result in just a nuisance issue, such as blood in the urine, all the way to a life-threatening process, such as an intracranial bleed, a disastrous hemorrhage into the brain. This potential for bleeding complications, always looming, causes us to attempt very tight control over the administration of these drugs.

Heparin-Induced Thrombocytopenia

No commentary on these drugs would be complete if a word of caution was not mentioned about an unpredictable complication that might occur. Anyone who receives Heparin can form antibodies against it. Antibodies are the defense structures that form constantly in our bodies in response to antigens that we might come into contact with. Some of these antigens (proteins that are foreign to us) cause us to form antibodies that save us from destruction by the offending antigen, if it happens to be a virus or a bacterium. This is the way vaccines work, too. Sometimes, however, antibodies can hurt us.

If you have had previous exposure to Heparin and have formed antibodies to it because it is a foreign protein, the next Heparin administration may lead to a much more aggressive formation of antibodies and, ultimately, to the development of *Heparin-Induced Thrombocytopenia* (HIT). This is marked by a sudden and progressive drop in the platelet population in the bloodstream. HIT, in its most malignant form, can be life-threatening, and it is up to the physician to check a platelet count to be sure it is not dropping precipitously. As a macabre component of the most aggressive form of this situation, much more intense thrombosis can occur, right along with this precipitous fall in the platelet count, sometimes causing loss of limb, stroke, or even death.

This issue of antibody formation against Heparin has emerged as a particularly important problem in the interventional laboratory where someone with generalized arteriosclerotic disease might need to be recurrently treated with a balloon or a stent, utilizing Heparin. With the serious form of HIT, the use of Heparin can be counterproductive and even very dangerous. We now have a good drug, acting by a totally different route that inhibits thrombin, called Bivalirudin. It can be safely used in such circumstances. We have even used it for off-pump aortocoronary bypass in one patient who demonstrated profound HIT—a potential for disaster if the conventional Heparin protocol had been followed.

Interestingly, the incidence of Heparin antibodies in those who have been exposed to Heparin is fairly high. The occurrence of the malignant form of HIT is low.

Despite these anecdotal problems, Heparin and Lovenox provide us with wonderful tools to use for acute anticoagulation. We have fortunately learned how to watch for the unusual side effects of HIT.

Chronic Anticoagulation

Frequently, if your acute anticoagulation was performed for something like atrial fibrillation, or a clot in the leg veins—maybe a clot that traveled to the lungs—you will be discharged on chronic anticoagulation. Or perhaps you had a new heart valve implanted. At any rate, you now require chronic anticoagulation, quite different from the acute treatment protocol.

Chronic anticoagulation basically translates into Coumadin usage, which requires active participation by the patient. At this time, while there is promise on the horizon, we have no other drug for chronic anticoagulation. In the hospital setting and during acute anticoagulation, you don't have to make decisions. At home, however, you are now faced with this new task of participation. With sometimes weekly adjustment of dosage, consideration of foods and medications that might alter the effectiveness of the Coumadin, and worries that something might go awry, this becomes a tedious drug to use. To make this seamless, you must form a tight affiliation with whomever is regulating your Coumadin dosage. You must be proactive in letting the person treating you know that this is new to you and you want to do it right.

Coumadin works by tying up clotting factors manufactured in the liver. This is a terribly difficult drug to regulate, at least in 50% of the population taking it. One of the reasons is that the dosage you take today really only starts to show up on the clotting test we perform, called a prothrombin time (Protime), tomorrow or even the next day. Similarly, if your blood gets over-anticoagulated, it will remain that way for several days unless you are given Vitamin K to reverse it. Vitamin K may well reverse it *too* effectively, making your anticoagulation less than effective, a situation that can itself be disastrous if you are taking the Coumadin for artificial heart valve protection, for example.

Every person has unique liver metabolism and manufacturing efficiency. This is affected by diet, drugs, alcohol, and your general level of health. Therefore, everyone has a unique Coumadin dose requirement. We can "guestimate" it, based on body surface area, liver enzymes, and experience. However, we have to check a Protime every couple of days at the beginning of treatment until we get it just right and then, subsequently, at variable intervals. The particular interval necessary in your case has to do largely with how stable your Protime remains on a certain dose of Coumadin. I have people in my practice who haven't changed their Coumadin dosage for 15 years. I have others, equally conscientious, who get it changed every week or so.

Our criteria for the degree of anticoagulation vary with the disease state for which the drug is being given. For example, a common cause for Coumadin anticoagulation is clot formation within the veins of the legs. For this, after you have been anticoagulated with Heparin for a period of several days, we may keep the Protime derivative INR (the International Ratio) in the range of 2–2.5. On the other hand, if you have a mechanical mitral valve prosthesis implanted, we might well shoot for an INR of 2.5–3.5. Since these are logarithmic, this is a big difference. If someone has a bleeding problem or a previous stroke but still needs Coumadin, we may straddle the fence and keep that patient's INR at a very low level, say 1.5 to 2.

My plea for those of you who are committed to chronic anticoagulation with Coumadin is to get a prescription from your doctor so you can purchase your own Protime machine. Most insurance plans will pay at least part of the cost. You can then perform your own tests in the comfort of your home without traveling to your doctor's office or to an anticoagulation monitoring clinic. If, for example, you get your blood checked at an anticoagulation clinic, you still have to rely on proper interpretation and phone calls or email for a change in dosage. This is the very best circumstance. I have seen the nurses frantically attempting to reach someone who has a frightfully out-of-whack Protime, but that person is blithely going about his or her life—shopping, mowing the lawn or whatever—unaware that the phone is ringing and the nurse and doctor are beside themselves. It is no wonder that so many bleeding complications occur with Coumadin administration. I think it has become so commonplace to put someone on Coumadin therapy today that we inappropriately educate them. Almost everyone wants desperately to take care of themselves if they only are told how.

Along these lines, if you eat leafy green vegetables, eat the same amount every day. They are very difficult to keep constant, as the fresh ones are powerful in negating the effects of Coumadin, while the frozen variety is much weaker. You can't gorge on vegetables from your garden in the summertime, and you can't go out on Saturday night and load up on alcohol. You don't have to stop either one; however, your intake of leafy green vegetables needs to be kept constant, the same each day, and generally not in large amounts. Likewise, if you drink, keep your alcohol intake small and constant. You need to be aware that many drugs will affect your Protime. We see patients every day who are given a prescription that will profoundly affect their Protime without any mention of it to the patient. This "ain't" great medicine; however, you must take on a lot of responsibility when you start Coumadin. You must assume that every new drug has the capacity to hurt you, therefore, quiz your doctor about every new prescription. One of my doctor friends who has a strange sense of humor but may be right since he himself takes Coumadin and should know, has commented that, "you have to assume that everyone is trying to kill you when they hand you a new prescription." Make sure that you receive a pamphlet outlining drug interactions.

While you are taking Coumadin, check for inappropriate bleeding, such as blood in your urine or stool. Your greatest risk, by far, while on Coumadin therapy is blood loss in the stool. Blood entering the upper gastrointestinal (G.I.) tract will be acted on and will turn your stools tar-black. Blood entering the lower G.I. tract will remain red. The kicker in this surveillance plan is that you can lose blood so slowly that you don't even know it and can't recognize it. For example, my healthy 40-year-old friend recently stopped and talked to me while I was on my walk. I thought she looked a bit pale and was less chatty than usual. It was hot, she was working very hard in her yard, and I just dismissed it. I was embarrassed to learn a couple of days later that she had gotten her blood checked because she was dizzy in the sun and was found to have a hemoglobin of 5.5 gm% (normal is about 15). She had an active ulcer in the stomach. This G.I. blood loss can be extremely insidious. If you get weak, dizzy, or if you notice that you are extremely pale, get your blood checked and make sure that you have not experienced inappropriate blood loss. This can be hidden, such as a bleed into the retroperitoneum (the space behind the abdomen), but it is usually G.I.

Platelet-Active Drugs

Patients seem to regularly confuse anticoagulant drugs with platelet-active drugs. The latter do not require any type of routine testing of the blood, and the most common one is aspirin. Another much stronger drug is Plavix. This drug is used when we want to render the platelets in the blood stream ineffective.

Platelets, the tiny elements in the blood stream that initiate the clotting process, are microscopic. There are about 2 million of these in a teaspoon of blood. If you rupture your spleen in an automobile accident, platelets are the first to go to the site of injury and start to clot off bleeders. They save your life more times that you realize. We could never make it through even a trivial operation if the platelets didn't do their thing. When activated, they come together and form a clump initiating clot formation. This is later bolstered by the laying down of fibrin, creating a more mature clot.

Not to get on their bad side, but these platelets are dumb. They don't know whether you have turned your motorcycle over and have sustained extreme injury or have ruptured an arteriosclerotic plaque in your coronary artery. They just know how to recognize an injury as any process that interrupts the integrity of a blood vessel, whether it's the inside or the outside of the artery. If you do rupture a coronary artery plaque, the platelets start to swarm to that area, attracted to one another to form a clump, and this is the beginning of a heart attack. A similar mechanism can cause a stroke if plaque rupture happens in one of the carotid arteries leading to the brain. A leg vessel could close off in similar fashion.

To interrupt this mechanism which could take your life, we administer Plavix orally along with other drugs, such as Heparin. Plavix is administered for several months following implantation of a coronary or carotid stent or, in the event of severe arteriosclerotic disease in the lower extremities or in a carotid, it will sometimes be given lifelong.

We usually administer 75 milligrams of Plavix daily. However, just as most drugs require adjustment for size, this drug should be similarly adjusted. For example, a 300-pound man with a huge frame will likely require twice as much as a 120-pound woman with a small frame. This is frequently overlooked and I have personally seen coronary stent thrombosis as a result of inadequate dosing with Plavix. The metabolism of this drug also dictates that a loading dose is given, usually 300–600 milligrams, as the initial dosage.

Another drug that is a fairly good platelet-inhibitor is aspirin. We always urge our patients to chew a couple of aspirin if they believe they are having a heart attack. Some people are relatively aspirin-resistant. This can be measured and is likely of significant clinical importance especially if you have a disease process that mandates long-term platelet inactivation to prevent a catastrophic vascular clot.

Obviously, these platelet drugs can cause bleeding from the G.I. tract. Indeed, this is their major side effect.

There are other platelet drugs. But aspirin and Plavix are the best.

Almost everyone who has to take Coumadin would like to substitute it for a drug that does not require constant monitoring. We are always being asked if aspirin and Plavix are effective for these measures. Apirin and Plavix are good platelet-active drugs and work to prevent platelet activation and aggregation in the arterial circulation. They are effective and protect against clot formation in areas where a cholesterol plaque may undergo erosion, with rupture of the fibrous cap, whether it's the coronary, the carotid, or a leg artery. They also protect against platelet accumulation in areas where foreign material has been introduced, such as a stent in any one of these arteries. They are *not* effective in protecting against clot formation on an artificial heart valve or within a leg vein. Therefore, they will not replace Coumadin when it is used for its intended purpose.

REMINDERS

1. Plain old aspirin is a decent platelet-active drug. If you suspect you might be having a heart attack, chew two of them immediately.
2. Plavix is a very effective platelet drug. If you are over 250 pounds, ask your doctor if you should take two Plavix instead of one.
3. Chronic anticoagulation is carried out with Coumadin. This requires close attention to dosing amounts, dietary adjustment, interaction with other medication, and a good education regarding signs and symptoms of bleeding. Most blood loss from Coumadin happens in the gastrointestinal tract.
4. If you have a problem that requires lifelong anticoagulation with Coumadin, you should purchase a Protime machine so that you can perform your own testing at home. This eliminates multiple handling at your doctor's office or anticoagulation clinic, decreasing the chances of a mistake. No one cares as much as you do!

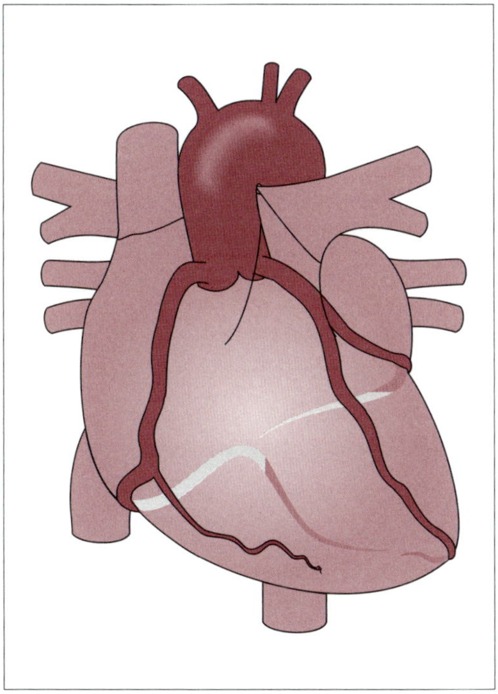

PERICARDITIS

Inflammation in the Sac Surrounding the Heart

PERICARDITIS IS ALMOST ALWAYS FRIGHTENING due to the symptom complex it produces; however, many times it is not due to a serious etiology. Pericarditis is frequently very painful. Moreover, since it can be part of a dangerous disease, it always warrants some degree of investigation and certainly always demands treatment of the inflammatory insult.

Bob Dylan, the famous poet and musician, was diagnosed with pericarditis caused by histoplasmosis (a fungal infection) in 1997. It must have been very painful because as he was leaving the hospital, he reportedly commented, "I really thought I'd be seeing Elvis soon." However, with pericarditis, its "growl is often worse than its bite" and he performed before the Pope in Bologna, Italy just a few short months later.

Function of the Pericardium

The heart is surrounded by two layers of a thin but protective connective tissue membrane called the pericardium. The evolutionary purpose for its existence is threefold:

1. It keeps the heart in a stable position when an extreme impact is exerted to the chest wall, a near-daily event as we are jerked, bounced, and tossed about during routine daily life. For example, a heavy blow to the chest, or the violence of the body being thrown to the ground in a football tackle might otherwise cause the heart attachments to be torn.
2. The pericardium protects the heart from the spread of infection from contiguous structures, such as pneumonia in the lungs.
3. The sac layers are greased by a lubricant (about 30 ccs or approximately six teaspoons) which lies within the pericardial sac to allow for painless contractility of the heart. Without the pericardium, there would be no lubricant and the heart, endowed with millions of nerve fibers, would be subject to all sorts of painful stimuli each minute.

The Pain of Pericarditis

Inflammation, created within the pericardial sac when it is invaded with a virus or some other process, causes an excruciating *pleuritic* pain (increased pain upon breathing) in the front of the chest. This pain frequently radiates straight into the back, directly between the scapulae (shoulder blades). This is usually a very sharp, stabbing type of discomfort.

There is a good reason why the pain is more severe during breathing. The heart rests upon the diaphragm, the leaflets of which dome up, separating the chest from the abdomen. These leaflets act just like the billows one uses to start a fire in the fireplace. When the diaphragm, triggered by signals from the phrenic nerve, retracts downward, the lungs pull in air. When they push upward, they force air out through the airways. This mechanism acts as our main method of getting air into and out of the lungs.

Since the pericardium, the double-layered heart sac, extends onto the diaphragm, the heart is tethered in place. Therefore, since the heart is gently pulled downward when the billows pull in air, the pericardium tenses. If there is any inflammation within the pericardial sac, this motion of breathing in produces intense pain.

Individuals who experience this quickly learn how to breathe in very shallow breaths in order to avoid wide excursions that accentuate the pain. I have even seen individuals, usually young ones, who rest on all fours, as this position releases the tension on the heart sac and relieves the pain. Many will just lean over, which does the same thing.

Frequently, the examiner can detect a pericardial rub, a three-component sound over the heart detectable with a stethoscope. This noise is similar to taking a Kleenex and rubbing it together as you hold it close to your ear. This rub is generated by the layers of the inflamed pericardium rubbing against each other as the heart contracts.

Causes and Treatment of Pericarditis

The most common type of pericardial disease, by far, is that of viral invasion of the heart sac. All viruses have tropism, or affinity, for certain cells in different body structures. Some of these viruses, otherwise of nuisance importance only, can invade the pericardium and wreak havoc. The most common are those of the Coxsackie family.

Invasion of the pericardium with bacteria can also occur but, fortunately, this is fairly rare, especially in the adult population. In adults, at least, this occurrence almost always is secondary to contiguous pneumonia, or a lung abscess, or it occurs in an immunologically compromised patient.

Since there are other more serious causes of pericarditis, such as myocardial infarction (heart attack from an occluded coronary artery) or aortic dissection (tearing of the walls of the aorta), we need to determine expediently if one of these potential causes is the culprit. Fortunately, post-viral inflammatory pericarditis most frequently occurs in a young person who is at exceptionally low risk for these two more serious diseases. However, occasionally a viral pericarditis does occur in someone in the coronary or hypertensive age category. Since it would be disastrous to miss either one of these diagnoses, they have to be promptly excluded before one can comfortably state the diagnosis of inflammatory pericarditis, likely secondary to a virus.

Since we can't find the virus, we must make a diagnosis by exclusion of anything else. Pericardial inflammation secondary to a previous, perhaps silent, heart attack can be ruled out with cardiac enzymes from a blood test, coupled with an electrocardiogram. If still in question, an echocardiogram to look at structure and function of the left ventricle will usually solve this issue. We will obtain an echo anyway, so it is really not redundant. If a silent heart attack has occurred, we should see a zone of heart muscle that doesn't move as well as its neighbors. If the cause is plain old viral pericarditis, we may or may not be able to detect a pericardial effusion, a collection of fluid in the pericardial sac secondary to the inflammation. Actually, when an effusion ultimately develops, the pain will usually diminish as the layers of inflamed pericardium are forced away from each other by the fluid. An aortic dissection can be ruled out readily by a CT scan of the chest.

Inflammatory, post-viral pericarditis can be quickly treated with an intravenous bolus of steroids. This will offer relief very promptly. This is followed by a tapering schedule of steroids over the next ten days, but with a warning to the patient that the process may well recur at least once and perhaps several times. I always give at least two refills to cover this eventuality, as it is simply cruel to treat the initial process and have the patients think that they have completely recovered only to have a sudden recurrence a couple of weeks later.

The alternative treatment is to use is a non-steroidal anti-inflammatory drug such as Ibuprofen. Indocin, another anti-inflammatory drug, works well also. I usually prescribe a non-steroidal anti-inflammatory drug in diabetic individuals because steroids will dramatically raise the blood sugar in many diabetic patients.

Patients with a recurrence almost always have to go through the entire emergency room routine once again. These recurrences seemingly never develop during the daytime or during nights when their cardiologist is on call, so they face an interaction with a brand new doctor who doesn't know them. If the physician tells these individuals, at the first meeting, that the pericarditis may recur and informs them how to deal with it, they can do so without being frightened to death when the pain recurs and can merely start the steroid regimen over again.

Fortunately, these recurrences will stop. It may take as long as six months of intermittent treatment but usually not. This is a benign process, painful but of no lasting importance. If the patient has recurrences, I always routinely make sure that they do not have some other situation such as lupus, rheumatoid arthritis, or scleroderma, more serious inflammatory diseases that are important to know about. They almost never do, but it is sloppy to let one of these go along without knowing about it.

Additionally, if there are recurrences, I repeat the echocardiogram at some point. We would have already performed one upon initial presentation since this is the best way to look at the pericardium, as well as the heart wall. I repeat the echo just to make sure there is nothing developing that might not have been obvious on the first exam.

Other causes of pericarditis are not so benign. The most noteworthy are those secondary to heart attack, aortic dissection, or tumor spread from a contiguous structure.

When I was an intern, we frequently saw pericarditis as a complication of a heart attack. At that time we had no way of interrupting a heart attack, and it destroyed the heart muscle all the way through the heart wall. The inflammation on the outside of the heart, the pericardial side, caused typical pericardial pain. We do not frequently see this now, as we have multiple means of interrupting the heart attack, thereby attenuating its course. And since injury begins in the inside portion of the heart muscle, we infrequently hear a pericardial rub in a heart attack patient.

Likewise, aortic dissections are, thankfully, rare and this is an uncommon cause of pericarditis. When the layers of the aorta tear, it is extremely painful and these patients also have quite severe high blood pressure. It is not too difficult to determine that something life-threatening is happening.

Sometimes, especially in connective tissue abnormalities (these are congenital abnormalities, not to be confused with *connective tissue diseases*, which are acquired), such as *Marfan's Syndrome*, the dissection is much less painful. In this process, the patient is born with an abnormality in the connective tissue matrix, or network, in the aortic wall. This makes it more likely to tear under the daily duress from blood pressure stresses, and the looseness of this poor-quality matrix makes it more likely to dissect without the overwhelming pain that a dissection brings about in the non-Marfan population.

When a malignancy spreads to the pericardial sac, it may cause extreme pain at first. However, as this implant settles in and grows, a sizable pericardial effusion consisting of a collection of malignant cells with fluid accumulation usually develops rapidly. Since a large pericardial effusion is uncommon with plain old viral pericarditis, its presence signals the probability that something else is occurring.

The so-called connective tissue diseases, such as lupus erythematosis and scleroderma, can also produce pericarditis. In the course of the last 35 years, I have seen several patients with these diseases who literally came in with the initial symptom of pericardial pain or a large pericardial effusion. If one digs a bit deeper, one can find other symptoms and signs. A diagnostic test from a blood sample will usually make the diagnosis quickly. These are readily treatable with steroids, which are usually given for the underlying disease as well.

REMINDERS

1. The most common cause of pericarditis is a viral process, painful but harmless.
2. The pain of pericarditis, accentuated by breathing and located in the center of the chest with radiation into the back, will usually resolve with steroids or non-steroidal anti-inflammatory drugs.
3. Pericardial pain associated with a viral invasion may recur several times. Do not worry. Each recurrence will promptly respond to a course of steroids.
4. If you have more than one recurrence, a battery of tests should be performed to be sure that you do not have one of the connective tissue disorders. A repeat echocardiogram should also be performed.

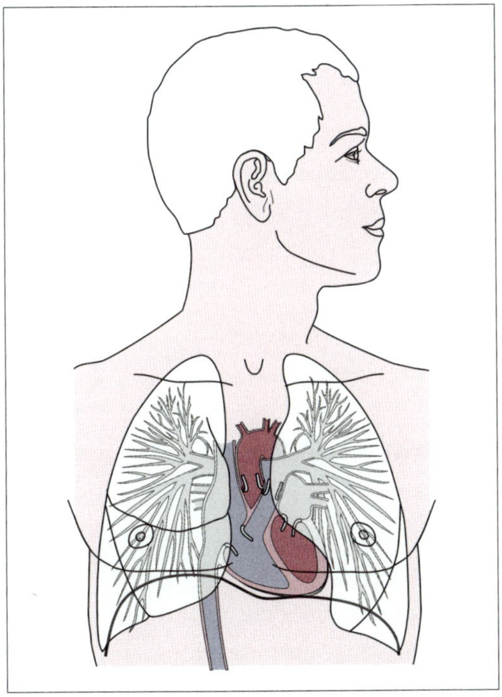

32 PERICARDIAL EFFUSION AND TAMPONADE

Problems with Fluid Around the Heart

A *PERICARDIAL EFFUSION* REFERS TO A collection of fluid within the pericardial sac surrounding the heart. The sac is a double-layered connective tissue membrane that is present to protect the heart from trauma and invasion by bacteria and other culprits. If a tumor or a virus invades the pericardial sac, or if any other disturbance to the tranquil, lubricated pericardium develops, a collection of fluid will form between the layers of the pericardium within the sac. If it gets large enough to choke off the action of the heart, if the collection of fluid is tense enough that it prevents the heart from relaxing and accepting the proper amount of blood within its chambers, this is called *cardiac tamponade*.

About 30 ccs of fluid, six teaspoons, is always present. It is an oily substance that serves as a lubricant so the layers of the pericardial sac will slide smoothly, one surface upon another, without pain. Without this lubricant, each beat of the heart and each breath pulling the heart downward with the diaphragm would cause pain. Using an echocardiogram, one can barely detect these six teaspoons of pericardial fluid. Any demonstrable amount beyond that represents some sort of pathologic process and is usually serious enough to deserve an investigation.

When the heart is choked, unable to relax, it becomes relatively empty. This is soundless; however, its results are not. As William Shakespeare wrote, "I did never know so full a voice issue from so empty a heart." The saying is true: 'The empty vessel makes the greatest sound.'

Causes of Pericardial Effusion (Fluid Around the Heart)

There are many causes of pericardial effusion. We will discuss the common ones. For practical purposes these can be divided into those that are basically harmless—just a worry and a nuisance—and those that are of great concern and usually reflect some very serious situation somewhere within the body. A pericardial effusion is not a common event; therefore, each one deserves an explanation. Any pericardial effusion represents a pathologic process. It is not something that just develops and can be shrugged off.

There are many causes of a so-called benign pericardial effusion. These are fluid accumulations that are not due to cancer or any other life-threatening process. The fluid accumulates because of some insult to the integrity of the pericardium or some generalized overall process going on in the individual. One develops sometimes when a virus invades the heart sac. Every virus has an affinity (called tropism) for certain tissues. This explains why some infections with a virus cause sore throat, cough, and nasal congestion while another might cause nausea, vomiting and diarrhea. Others attack the liver, still others the brain. Certain viruses, common within each community, have affinity for the sac surrounding the heart. These tend to occur in little epidemics, several people developing this complaint within days of each other. When such an infection occurs, inflammation develops within the sac and pain with respiration becomes a prominent symptom. Generally, only a small collection of fluid accumulates in response to this infection. Sizable pericardial effusions can occasionally develop with viral invasion of the pericardium, but these are unusual especially if the problem has been aggressively treated.

It is uncommon for an adult to develop a bacterial invasion of the heart sac. It can occur but is almost always due to a lung abscess close to the heart or, more commonly, develops in an individual who is immunologically compromised by either drugs or an infection, such as HIV. These latter individuals are more prone to develop unusual pericardial infections, too, such as tuberculous involvement.

A sizable pericardial effusion frequently alerts us that this person has something serious, in need of immediate investigation. Large pericardial effusions do not always mean that something ominous is occurring. But since large effusions are much more apt to develop in response to something serious, they have to be treated with great respect. In such circumstances, we must rule out a neoplasm (cancer) contiguous to the heart. Since these most commonly spread from a tumor in very close proximity to the heart, the usual suspects are primary breast or lung involvement. These tumors are usually quite obvious. While remote tumors may spread to the pericardial sac, they are distinctly uncommon. These malignant effusions are almost always bloody, as contrasted to non-malignant ones, which are seldom bloody.

Connective tissue diseases, such as lupus and scleroderma, can cause either small or large effusions and are found by examining markers within the blood stream. While we sometimes see pericardial effusion as the initial warning of such a process, characteristically there are other signs, such as rash, arthritis, pleurisy, or evidence of kidney disease. I remember one 40-year-old lady who came to the emergency room with a feeling that she would pass out. She had no other symptoms and her examination was normal with the exception of low blood pressure. Thinking that she was volume-contracted from dehydration, I administered some normal saline intravenously. This did nothing. By this point, I suspected a pericardial effusion, as her neck veins were elevated, suggesting that she was either volume overloaded or that her heart could not handle extra water. I obtained an echocardiogram and it showed a huge pericardial effusion. She later turned out to have an aggressive form of scleroderma and required a kidney transplant within four years.

One situation that causes pericardial effusion deserves special comment, as it is often not considered. In a person who has had a large operation with a protracted recovery or trauma or serious illness, anything that requires a massive caloric intake while not able to ingest it, the protein level in the blood stream will fall. This occurs even if we are administering large amounts of calories by intravenous feeding. Protein is not manufactured the way it should be because the patient is malnourished. This protein content in the blood stream, made up largely of albumin, is the main way we hold water within the blood stream. Otherwise, the force of the blood pressure would push all of the water into the tissues. If this protein level falls significantly, which it does in most serious illnesses, water is, indeed, pushed into the tissues. Such a person will frequently develop collections of fluid within the pleural spaces surrounding the lungs. They will also frequently develop small pericardial effusions. These should be left alone unless there is some compelling reason to obtain fluid.

We frequently used to see large pericardial effusions in those individuals with renal failure. Now, with aggressive dialysis techniques and regimens, we usually see only small effusions at most. In those who have ignored their problem or have refused dialysis, we continue to see occasional large *uremic* effusions.

Withdrawal of Fluid from the Heart Sac: Pericardiocentesis

Sometimes if the effusion is large enough, we will perform a pericardiocentesis, the placement of a catheter from the skin into the sac in order to remove fluid. Analysis and culture of the fluid will very frequently yield a diagnosis. However, we always send along instructions for cell analysis, cytology, and cell block so we will not miss a malignant tumor. This should be done in every pericardiocentesis, no matter if the doctor is pretty sure that the underlying cause is known.

A word about percardiocentesis is in order. When there is a sizable accumulation of fluid, performing a percardiocentesis is safe, even though it sounds terrible. It is when the effusion is borderline that it poses a significant risk, the most common of which is the needle entering the heart muscle or even worse, the tearing of a coronary artery. This can be dangerous. As with everything else, judgment is of paramount importance. If your doctor suggests a pericardiocentesis, ask about the size of the effusion and the relative safety.

Sometimes such a withdrawal of fluid is done for the singular purpose of establishing a diagnosis as to what exactly is causing the effusion. Others are performed in order to remove pressure on the heart because the fluid in large quantity or even modest quantity, if loaded with blood or protein, will choke the heart. In other words, if the effusion is extensive enough, it will compress the heart chambers so much that they are incapable of expanding to receive blood. This development is called *cardiac tamponade*. In this circumstance, we often remove fluid both for a diagnosis of the cause, as well as to relieve the pressure on the heart.

I once accepted a stowaway on a container ship arriving in the Puget Sound harbor as a patient. I was a cardiologist and it was just my luck that this very emaciated young woman had a "huge heart on chest x-ray," as the ER physician put it. It was obvious that this lady needed someone with a lot more knowledge about tropical diseases than I possessed and I tried to get the ER doctors to admit her to someone with that specific knowledge. However, the poor young woman was in shock with a blood pressure about the same as her weight, about 60 mmHg systolic (normal is twice that), and I took her as my patient.

When I examined her, she had a palpable pulse during exhalation, but not during inhalation. In other words, I could obtain a pulse when she breathed out but I could not feel one when she took a breath. This is the most important clinical finding in cardiac tamponade so I had a strong suspicion that the "huge heart" actually represented a large accumulation of fluid around the heart. A quick echocardiogram, a sound wave test, confirmed this. In other words, a massive amount of fluid had accumulated between the layers of the pericardial sac. For this to occur to such a degree meant that it had been going on for a long, long time and the pericardium had ample time to stretch and accommodate it. Such a large amount of fluid, had it accumulated over a short time, would have resulted in tamponade and death, as it would have strangulated the heart.

I performed a pericardiocentesis, leaving a large bore catheter within the pericardial sac. I instructed the nurse at 6 a.m. to remove 200 cc of fluid per hour from the sac and to give the young lady 200 cc of normal saline intravenously per hour. I went back around 2 p.m. and the nurse, God bless her, was still at it! We obtained 1,600 ccs of pericardial fluid from this young lady. This may be a world record. I trained at a large referral center and the only thing I had ever seen that caused this was tuberculous pericarditis. I got some help from infectious disease experts (she also had every parasite endemic to the region from which she came) and started her on tuberculosis therapy. I had a cardiac surgeon cut a pericardial window into the pericardium through a small chest incision and this allowed further accumulation of fluid to drain into the more accommodating chest cavity so we wouldn't have to keep draining the pericardium with needle entry through the skin. She recovered from what indeed turned out to be tuberculous pericarditis.

This story describes the course of action in cardiac tamponade. Frequently, drainage is an emergency and without it, the patient will die. In this instance, the patient had survived this long only because she was young and her pericardium was yielding. The elasticity of the pericardial sac has a lot to do with how much fluid can accumulate, at what rate, before it chokes the heart and drops the blood pressure to levels below that needed to sustain viability of vital organs. For instance, if whatever causes the fluid accumulation also causes enough inflammation in the connective tissue sac, it may lose elasticity. We call this a restrictive/effusive pericardial process—the thick, unyielding sac being restrictive, therefore unable to accommodate the effusion.

Trauma to the chest wall, especially if the ribs or sternum are cracked, can result in pericardial effusion. These may well be bloody effusions and, as such, are loaded with protein. The pericardium will not tolerate large accumulations of bloody or protein-laden effusions in contrast to the more "watery" effusions. In such instances, we need to look at performance of the heart chambers and draw cardiac markers in order to quantify the degree of cardiac contusion, or damage. Occasionally the blunt trauma will impact a coronary artery and, especially if it strikes an area where an atheromatous plaque is present, a coronary occlusion with heart attack can result. This is thankfully quite rare. In 30 years, having seen an awful lot of cardiac contusion, I have infrequently seen this problem. One particular person developed a pericardial effusion and it was impossible to determine how much of this was due to the impact of the injury and how much was due to the through-and-through infarction (heart attack) from the vessel closure.

The role of the echocardiogram cannot be overemphasized in all of these instances of pericardial effusion and cardiac tamponade. The echo will give you an immediate rough quantification of the amount of fluid that is present within the pericardial sac. It will also tell an accomplished reader if tamponade is imminent or even threatening. Occasionally we see a tumor implant within the pericardium, growing directly into the heart structure. Sometimes we will see strands of proteinaceous material within the pericardial effusion. Commonly, we see an area of heart muscle that does not work properly; if so, we suspect that a silent heart attack occurred at some previous time and the effusion developed in response to it. The echo is the most valuable tool (and the quickest, as it can be done at the bedside) in the evaluation and follow-up of this disorder.

Occasionally a pericardial effusion can be secondary to an underlying disorder and we overlook it for a while, as it may be completely silent. The good news is that, if silent, it usually is not due to something terrible. The most embarrassing one of these for me was in a cardiac transplant patient. This young man had received his heart in Houston and I had never seen him before. I noticed when I first saw him that he had a rather unusual voice but he had only recently been transplanted, and I thought it was due to the endotracheal tube used during his operation, as these injuries sometimes take a long while to heal. His face was puffy but all such patients, on large doses of steroids, are puffy.

He was on schedule for his endomyocardial biopsy, a sampling of muscle done periodically so that we can be sure that the patient is properly immunosuppressed and not silently rejecting the transplanted heart. We do these once a month immediately after transplantation, less frequently after some time has passed. I put him in the hospital for this, ran a bioptome up from the groin and took a few samples from the lower septum of the heart. We watch such patients for three or four hours and, at least for the first several biopsies, obtain a post-biopsy echocardiogram. Much to my surprise, this showed a very large pericardial effusion, probably at least 600ccs of fluid. I thought I had inadvertently biopsied all the way through the heart muscle and caused blood to accumulate within the pericardium. However, that didn't really fit, as this much blood should have choked off his blood pressure, resulting in tamponade. He was clinically stable, though his blood pressure was low.

I remember being bone-tired, not wanting more work, and I was talking to him, preparing to do a pericardiocentesis, when a nurse entered. When the nurse and I left the room, she asked if he had always talked "like a bullfrog." Suddenly it hit me that he was low on thyroid hormones. I stopped in mid-stride, turned around and told him that I thought a very astute comment from his nurse had saved him from another procedure. He did, indeed, have barely detectable levels of thyroid hormones. He responded to thyroid medication.

This illustrates how doctors can get so wrapped up in the little world they work in that other possibilities may be missed. This is the reason for this book. Of course, you should not serve as your own doctor. But it won't hurt to participate fully in the process!

This example should also re-emphasize that not all pericardial effusions need to be analyzed by fluid withdrawal. The smaller the effusion, the more dangerous it is to try to withdraw fluid. I have personally followed many effusions over time, determining whether or not they increased in volume or diminished and went away. Sometimes the cause is simple and responds to treatment of the underlying disease. The large effusion in the transplant patient completely resolved with thyroid replacement.

Treatment of Pericardial Effusion

Treatment of pericardial effusion is directed toward the cause of the effusion. If it is secondary to a virus, there is no treatment directed toward eliminating the virus. This "benign" invasion by the virus causes intense pleuritic pain, discomfort exaggerated by breathing. We treat it with either non-steroidal anti-inflammatory drugs or steroids. When the inflammatory process is effectively treated, formation of the effusion will usually be attenuated. The culprit virus clears out on its own, usually well in advance of the major symptoms of its invasion.

Similarly, the effusion secondary to some sort of connective tissue disease, such as lupus erythematosis, scleroderma, or rheumatoid arthritis is treated within the treatment framework for the primary process. This is almost always a steroid bolus followed by a maintenance dose.

Effusions secondary to a malignancy are treated by drainage of the fluid from the pericardial sac, usually ultimately diverting it into the left chest so that persistent formation of the malignant effusion will not choke off the action of the heart. The primary malignancy is treated in the same manner that it would be treated if there were no effusion.

Effusions due to insufficient thyroid hormone are obviously treated with replacement supplements. The effusions that develop because of depletion of blood stream protein will resolve spontaneously when the serum albumin comes up to normal levels.

REMINDERS

1. There are many causes of pericardial effusion.
2. Not all of these have to be analyzed.
3. The safety of placing a needle into the pericardium is related to the size of the effusion. The larger the effusion, the safer the procedure.
4. In the event of an effusion, if the doctors are stumped, ask if they have checked the thyroid.

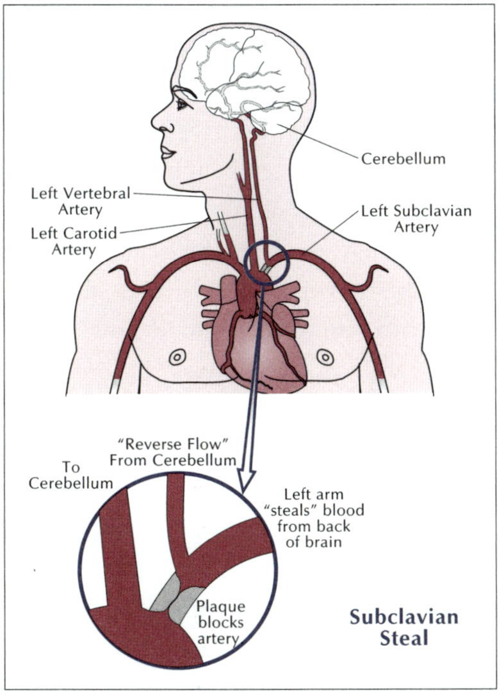

SUBCLAVIAN STENOSIS AND SUBCLAVIAN/ VERTEBRAL STEAL

Blockage of an Arm Vessel Can Lead to Dizziness

THE ARTERIES SUPPLYING THE ARMS ALSO PROVIDE blood to the arteries supplying the part of the brain that controls our stance, posture, and equilibrium. Blockage of one of these arteries can cause a lot of trouble. As with all parts of the body, this comes from the factory with a fall-back system to provide blood to the arm should the arterial supply completely block off. However, that fall-back system can bring with it a new set of problems.

The Anatomy

The subclavian arteries originate from the aortic arch and supply arterial blood to the arms. Each subclavian also gives off an arterial branch that supplies the base of the brain. These are the vertebral arteries, and they supply the hind brain, that portion that sits in the recession at the back of the skull known as the posterior fossa. This part of the brain, the cerebellum, is responsible for balance and spatial orientation. We take it for granted. As we go through our day, perhaps carefully walking between paint buckets on the floor, maneuvering down the aisle of a supermarket as we drive our carts close to others, we are incorporating the complex function of the cerebellum constantly. If it malfunctions, our world is badly compromised. The blood supply to this important structure, the cerebellum, is principally via the vertebral artery. The vertebral artery may become involved in some primary process within its own structure that limits its flow. However, by far the most important event that compromises blood flow up the vertebral artery to the base of the brain has to do with a primary disease process in its *parent* artery, the subclavian artery.

Predisposition of the Left Subclavian Artery to Arteriosclerosis and Obstruction

The subclavian arteries are also susceptible to the nemesis of the modern world, cholesterol deposits within the wall of the artery (arteriosclerosis) or hardening of the arteries. Women seem somewhat more susceptible than men to isolated subclavian stenosis. In other words, women may develop this problem without having much coronary artery disease. If a man develops subclavian disease, it is almost always in conjunction with severe coronary artery disease. A stenosis is a blockage in a blood vessel, and the stenosis in the subclavian artery is almost always discreetly within the mouth of the artery.

The left subclavian artery is much more commonly involved than the right, likely because of the angle from which it branches from the aorta. This causes it to receive more hemodynamic stress than the right from turbulent blood flow. The left subclavian artery originates from that portion of the aortic arch as it completes its curve to send blood to the abdomen and lower extremities. The force of turbulence within the aorta at that point involves the take-off of the left subclavian and therefore renders it more susceptible to the build-up of plaque material as this washing machine–like turbulence goes on for every minute of your life.

Over the course of five or six decades, in the presence of risk factors such as high cholesterol, diabetes, hypertension, or tobacco usage, an arteriosclerotic plaque commonly forms. This can remain dormant for many years, causing no symptoms. In fact, unless one aggressively exercises the arm supplied by the culprit artery, there will generally be no symptoms until the subclavian becomes much greater than 75% blocked. Indeed, a sedentary individual can block off the left subclavian very quietly, with almost no symptoms until the artery is almost completely closed off, only a faint spurt of blood squeaking past this high-grade blockage. The singular problem in this design is that there is no way to get blood to the arm except by "stealing" it from the cerebellum via the vertebral artery. Thus, the name for this complex situation: *subclavian stenosis with vertebral steal.*

How does one determine that the subclavian artery is closing? One of the duties of a good doctor is to check for the equality of wrist pulses. Let's say that the left subclavian artery is closing slowly. In this instance, the left radial pulse will be weaker than the right and there will be a right-to-left pulse lag between arms. A vascular sound, called a *bruit* (pronounced *brew-e*), will frequently be heard over the subclavian artery just below the medial collar bone.

Hazards and Symptoms with Subclavian Artery Blockage

If and when left subclavian stenosis becomes so tight that it significantly blocks flow to the left arm, the arm will begin to steal blood from the base of the brain. This will be especially pronounced with repetitive exercises involving the left hand and arm. Exercise increases the blood and nutrient needs of the muscle and the only way to get more blood to the left arm is via the left vertebral artery. The arm muscle doesn't much care where the blood comes from; it just wants more! This demand will bring about a *reversal* of blood flow in the vertebral artery, stealing blood away from the cerebellum. (Figure 26) This may, in turn, cause extreme dizziness and disequilibrium as the cerebellum is robbed of its blood supply.

Figure 26 Subclavian Stenosis

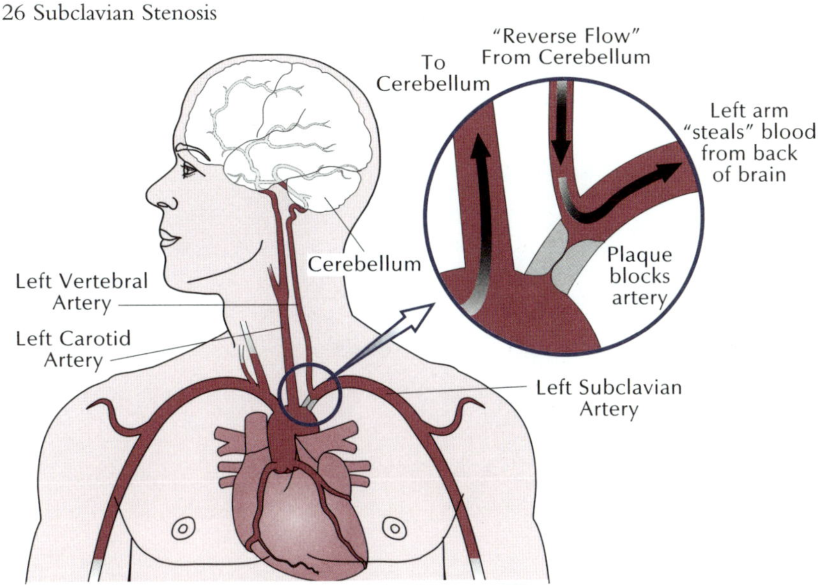

Additionally, if the exercise is prolonged, the vertebral is seldom large enough to provide that needed extra blood flow and the arm will become starved for oxygen-rich blood. Therefore, the combined symptoms of dizziness or vertigo along with arm pain and weakness associated with repetitive arm exercises constitutes a good case for subclavian stenosis with vertebral steal.

A prompt and reliable diagnosis can usually be made through the use of a Doppler test, a sound wave test which should show increased velocities past the obstruction and, frequently, evidence of vertebral artery flow reversal.

Treatment of Subclavian Stenosis with a Stent

If corroborated, a good interventional cardiologist or radiologist can advance a small wire down the artery and insert a stainless steel stent. These are high-tension mesh devices that look somewhat like a miniature slinky. The stent is crimped onto a balloon and is deployed under high pressure within the plaque material. (Figure 27) In the usual

Figure 27 Repaired Subclavian Stenosis

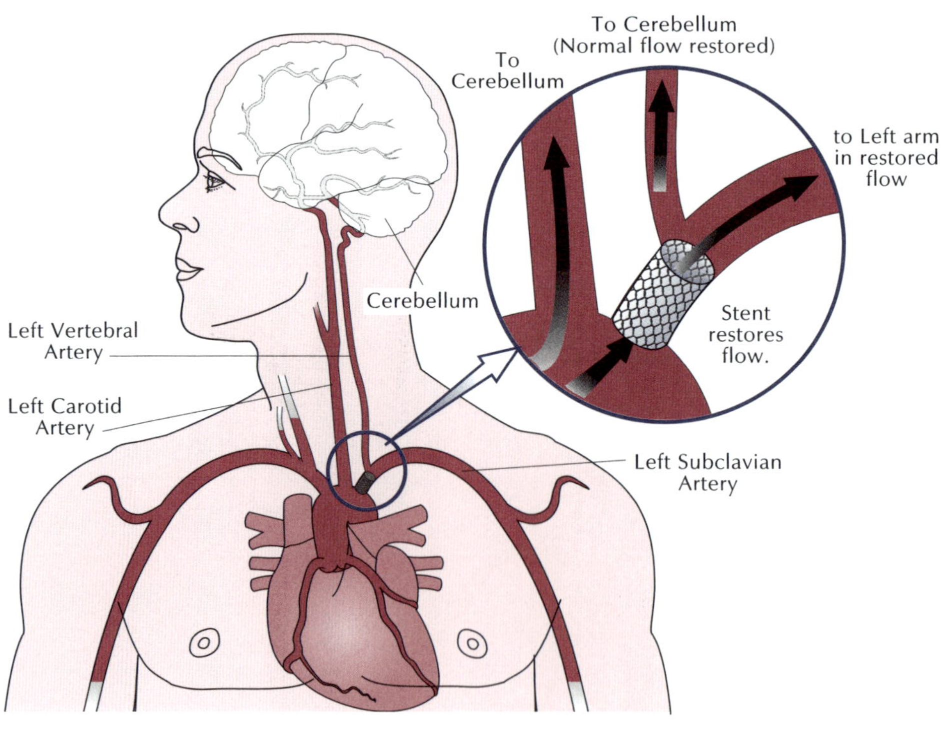

subclavian stenosis, we use simple stents, as the artery is frequently large enough to accommodate some degree of restenosis. In other words, as with all arteries, the deployment of such a device under high pressure incurs some degree of injury to the inside of the artery. Some individuals respond to this with minimal change; others will respond with intense and aggressive proliferation of smooth muscle and fibrous tissue. If the artery and the stent that is used within it are large enough, even fairly aggressive growth of tissue within the stent will fail to obstruct flow and this will be a good long-term result.

Petite Subclavian Arterial Blockage: A Challenge

If the artery is small, which is often the case with petite women, an aggressive restenosis might well return these individuals to exactly the same predicament they were in before intervention: almost total blockage of the subclavian artery with its attendant symptoms and risks. These small subclavian arteries are usually found in petite women, frequently smokers, who are exactly the ones prone to get this problem in the first place. Traditionally, if this restenosis results in high-grade blockage within the stent, we go back in with a catheter and utilize a cutting balloon, one with blades within its balloon material. This actually cuts the scar tissue, allowing the artery to expand. This frequently is quite durable, whereas simple repeat balloon angioplasty, merely stretching out the wall of the artery, quickly returns to a high-grade blockage.

Carotid-Subclavian Bypass

Traditionally, if this second intervention did not result in a good long-term result, we would have little recourse but to recommend a carotid-subclavian bypass. This entails connecting the subclavian artery to the carotid artery. In this case, we are actually taking some of the blood that would normally be sent to the cerebrum (the motor strip of the brain) and diverting it to the arm. This is not very satisfactory when you start thinking about it. The good news is that it frequently works. The bad news is that the carotid has to become involved in this complex event, and any surgical interaction that utilizes the carotid artery poses the threat of potential stroke. Thankfully, in the selection process, we offer this only to those individuals who have a nice wide-open carotid artery. Nonetheless, it is not a very savory option.

In my view, in the future we will be using the same drug-eluting stents that we now use almost exclusively in coronary circulation. These are coated or impregnated with a cancer drug, either taxol or sirolimus, which inhibits cell replication. There have been recent reports about late closure in *coronary* arteries treated with drug-eluting stents. This is because they do not cover over with tissue like the bare metal stents do. Many of us have argued from the beginning that individuals receiving drug-eluting stents should remain on aspirin and Plavix as platelet-inhibitors indefinitely to prevent this problem.

Due to the slow release of the drug from the drug-eluting stent during the first three months after it is installed, the surrounding tissue is inhibited from growth within the stent even though the same damage has been incurred. Therefore, this would allow these petite arteries to be stented with a much better long-term result than if a bare metal stent were utilized. I think it is going to be only through such extension from one successful use (drug-eluting coronary stents) to another utility (subclavian and renal drug-eluting stents) that we solve some of these issues in women with small arteries.

Men are not exempt from being born with small subclavian arteries either. We have seen an occasional man who has this same problem. However, this issue with very small arteries to work on is primarily a woman's issue and I don't think it has been properly addressed. On the one hand, we have taken great pride in the fact that we are able to open these almost totally blocked arteries with a stent. On the other hand, we know when we work on such a diminutive vessel there is probably at least a 25% chance that we will have to go back in and work on it again. This is not very satisfying so I believe the fast track to get a drug-eluting stent for this task, to be used in diminutive vessels, is the correct answer. (Again, if this is done, the patient should be instructed that he or she will need to take platelet drugs indefinitely. This *still* beats the surgical approach.)

The same logic applies to an effort to try to get these arteries adequately opened prior to a total occlusion, even if the individual is not very symptomatic. I mentioned that some of these are almost totally silent until they reach a greater than 90% blockage. This is because a great percentage of people do not use their arms very much in repetitive exercises. Therefore, an occasional steal from the cerebellum doesn't result in crippling symptoms. However, if we wait until the subclavian artery is totally blocked, usually symptoms emerge suddenly as prominent features. We then see the full-blown process:

1. Any exercise, such as writing or cooking, will bring about pain in the arm because the only blood the arm is receiving has to be stolen from the cerebellum via the vertebral artery.
2. When this blood is drained off from the cerebellum to the arm, the cerebellum doesn't get enough blood and you get dizzy and lose equilibrium.

These are crippling symptoms, frequently preventing these people from driving, for example, because they are not sure that they will not develop pain in the arm. Most people could simply grit their teeth and live with pain in the arm. Many, however, are incapacitated when they cannot focus well, get dizzy, and lose their ability to control the automobile. In short, the selfish demands of a bloodthirsty arm can rob enough blood from the brain to make ordinary arm exercises unthinkable.

With a totally blocked subclavian artery, we are on the horns of a dilemma: We can seldom get through this total blockage with a wire in order to open it and deploy a stent. Additionally, the only way to restore blood flow to the arm is to divert it from the carotid on the same side, the carotid-subclavian bypass. These do not always remain open, as the bypass results in a right-angle diversion. Now we have an individual who has closed off the subclavian artery, is very symptomatic, and receives a carotid-subclavian bypass; it fails, with closure of the subclavian once again, and we are back in the same situation we were initially in, only we are now three procedures or so down the road. These are among the unhappiest patients we see, and for good reason. Who wants to go through three procedures, with their attendant risks, and be back where they started? And yet, in each case, they were likely receiving state-of-the-art care from a competent interventionalist and surgeon.

REMINDERS

1. **Pain in the arm and hand with exercise, especially if coupled with vertigo and dizziness, may be symptoms of subclavian/vertebral steal due to subclavian stenosis.**
2. **Ask your physician to check for equality of pulses in the wrists.**
3. **Early detection is vastly superior to late recognition because a partially blocked vessel can be readily opened via a catheter. A completely closed artery usually requires surgical intervention—with some risk of stroke and closure—as this surgical procedure calls for the formation of a communication between the carotid and subclavian arteries.**
4. **Women are slightly more predisposed to develop subclavian stenosis than men. However, the small arterial size in many women brings about a higher failure rate with stent deployment than with**

larger arteries. This is because there is some degree of tissue growth within the stent due to damage to the inside of the artery. We need drug-eluting stents for use in the small peripheral vessels in women. However, if used, these individuals should be on platelet agents indefinitely.

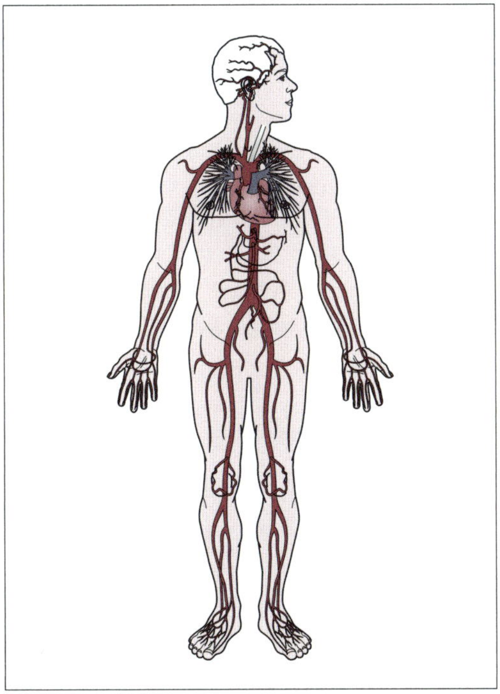

32 HEART DISEASE AND DEATH IN ATHLETES

You Can Run Fast, but Still be in Trouble

SELDOM DOES A MONTH GO BY THAT we don't read of the tragic death of an athlete, whether a teenager playing for his or her high school basketball team or a professional athlete, playing football for $5 million a year. They are equally tragic, snatching away a young person with so much of life ahead. The tragedy is that it's not just a death but, in many cases, a needless death. This problem seems small when seen in the context of the vast numbers who play competitive sports in the U.S.—only about 100–150 kids and young adults per year. But it's an enormous problem if one of them is your kid.

Since the beginning of recorded history and myth, even the strongest have had points of vulnerability. The mighty Achilles was felled by an arrow shot into his heel by Paris. We need to protect our youth from their Achilles' Heel!

Screening Athletes in America

Screening for risks is not a worldwide omission. In Italy, athletes undergo a number of screening tests before they can play. For example, everyone has an electrocardiogram (ECG), which is not required in the U.S. It's true that Italians have a more homogeneous population and, therefore, have a higher incidence of some electrical problems that make the risk of sudden death with strenuous activity more likely. One of their particular concerns has to do with a higher-than-expected incidence of *arrhythmogenic right ventricular dysplasia* (ARVD), a condition that predisposes its owner to sudden death from an arrhythmia. It only affects about 40 out of every 10,000 youth. However, if you live in Italy and you have this, you don't play competitive sports. By adopting this posture, they have reduced their incidence of sudden death in athletes dramatically.

In the United States, while we don't see much ARVD, we have substantial risks in our population also and we're basically ignoring them. For example, the incidence of hypertrophic cardiomyopathy, a situation marked by inappropriate muscle growth in certain areas in the left ventricle, is 1 in 500. This situation can result in death from an arrhythmia and is one of the most common causes of death in our young athletes. This means that if you attend a football game and there are 50,000 people in the stands, 100 of them have hypertrophic cardiomyopathy. A mid-size city of one million people will contain 2,000 people with this problem. That's a lot. Yet, we don't screen for it in our athlete population, even though we know that most fatalities from this disease occur during times of extreme exertion. The reason given is that it's simply too expensive. We are currently doing quite a few things in this country that are very expensive; so this excuse doesn't hold water. It has been shown that an ECG will discover about 95% with this disorder. Those with positive results should go on to the next stage, the echocardiogram.

Screening for Risk: What Should Be Done?

What should we do to evaluate an athlete? First and foremost, a complete medical history should be filled out, with particular emphasis on family members who died suddenly of unexplained causes. *Rarely does an athlete die of cerebral hemorrhage or a pulmonary condition, such as intractable asthma, but over 90% of sudden death cases in athletes are due to some sort of cardiac involvement.* Frequently, a positive family history will sound a warning of a potentially inherited problem.

Every person entering athletic competition should have a blood pressure check, a cardiac exam, and an ECG. Theoretically, an echocardiogram (echo) should be performed on everyone, but it would be prohibitively expensive and would be too unwieldy. Or is it? This test will discover those with hypertrophic cardiomyopathy, which is responsible for 36% of cardiovascular deaths in athletes. Expensive? Yes. However, echocardiograms have been performed on all athletes in Italy since 1985. Some athletes—based on family history, an exam, or ECG—should *clearly* have a treadmill stress test or an echo. The echo is the most sophisticated and takes about 30 minutes to complete. It consists of bouncing sound waves off the cardiac structures and recording them when they return to the transducer. This, coupled with Doppler analysis (a measurement of the velocity of blood flow showing us pressures within structures), gives us ample information about the heart structures and function, the valves, and the pressures within the heart.

How does this translate into protection? The most common causes of sudden cardiac death in athletes are hypertrophic cardiomyopathy, dilated cardiomyopathy, valvular heart disease, congenital heart disease, coronary artery anomalies, electrical abnormalities within the conduction system, and the syndrome of obesity/dehydration/deconditioning. Of these, many can be detected by an exam and an ECG; others require an echo. The obesity/dehydration/deconditioning syndrome, more prevalent today than previously, can only be prevented by good old common sense. Someone who shows up for August training camp 100 pounds overweight, who gets short of breath with only modest exertion, is at high risk of a calamity if pushed hard.

If we detect a potentially serious electrical abnormality, we should determine whether or not the athlete has an intrinsic tendency to develop a potentially life-ending arrhythmia with exertion. Blood levels of epinephrine rise significantly in response to strenuous exercise, especially in the young. At extreme levels of performance, the heart rate is sky-high. There is almost always an oxygen debt and some degree of acidosis from tissue accumulation of lactic acid. If we determine that this mix triggers a malignant arrhythmia, drug therapy coupled with the implantation of an Automatic Implantable Cardiac Defibrillator (AICD) should be used. The major question is whether or not these individuals should be allowed to compete. I seriously doubt that any responsible cardiologist would allow it, especially if they are involved in activities that could result in blunt trauma to the device. Additionally, competitive athletes are not like me. They frequently perform at more than 100% capacity and, under the physiologic circumstances outlined, an implantable defibrillator just might not convert them from a life-ending arrhythmia, especially if there is profound accumulation of lactic acid. But let's not wait until that young athlete has dropped dead on the basketball floor! Only an occasional survivor will get a second chance to go on to become a candidate for an AICD.

Take a history. Is there any family history of unexplained sudden death? Does anyone in the family have a heart problem other than coronary artery disease? Is there any ECG evidence of an electrical problem?

Inherited Sudden Cardiac Death Syndromes with Structurally Normal Hearts

Most frightening to us as doctors are the hidden electrical problems that can end a life. These people have normal hearts structurally, so they don't get unduly short of breath, don't have chest pain, or other cardiac symptoms—except perhaps dizziness and blackout spells—if they're lucky. Fortunately, these are pretty rare and are mostly inherited, though they can show up out of the blue as well. These—the Long QT Interval Syndrome and the Brugada Syndrome—constitute just two of the so-called "channel-opathies."

There are others, marked by abnormal movement of sodium, potassium, or calcium ions through "channels" within the cell. There is almost always a family history of sudden cardiac death with either one of these. This is the reason why knowing the family history is so important. The ECG features are subtle but frequently diagnostic. Whenever one of these is found, these people should receive an AICD if they are to remain active, especially if they've had a blackout spell. The Brugada Syndrome has the distinction of causing sudden cardiac death at rest or while asleep, so these people should be treated with an AICD if they have had a blackout spell no matter what their level of activity.

Tendency to Have Arrhythmias with Structural Abnormalities

Other electrical problems accompany a structurally abnormal heart, such as mitral valve prolapse, which may be associated with exercise-stimulated ventricular tachycardia. Another is ARVD, mentioned previously. This is usually seen in people between 15 and 40 years of age and is marked by an abnormal electrocardiogram, as well as a well-performed echocardiogram. However, either condition may cause no symptoms to notify its owner of its existence.

There may be no good way of predicting an anomalous coronary artery, such as the one that resulted in the death of a well-known professional basketball player a number of years ago. To recap, we should be born with right and left coronary arteries that feed the heart. The left divides into two branches; therefore, we should all have three coronary arteries. Well, "Pistol" Pete Maravich was born with only one. Is it likely that this could be detected by an echocardiogram? It would be unrealistic to think that a man could be playing aggressive basketball with only a single coronary artery and have a totally normal echo. I think a yearly echo would have discovered his condition by demonstrating some segment of abnormal left ventricular wall motion from long-standing and repeated bouts of oxygen deprivation. Certainly, a treadmill test would have turned it up.

I have always worried about missing the anomalous coronary artery that is commonly referred to as the "Tunnel of Death." This occurs when the left main coronary artery originates from the right coronary cusp instead of the left, traversing the space between the pulmonary artery and the aorta to reach its intended distribution. When these very large vessels (the aorta and pulmonary artery) are distended with blood, they may compress the coronary artery between them, decreasing blood flow to enough heart muscle to precipitate a fatal arrhythmia. There is usually a history of exertional chest pain with this, hopefully enough to result in a treadmill test, then an angiogram. Actually, an anomalous (misplaced) coronary artery accounts for 13% of all cardiovascular deaths in athletes.

While one could make a valid argument against performing a treadmill test and an echocardiogram on high school and college players unless directed to this avenue of testing, it is inexcusable that professional players don't have these tests on a yearly basis. Fortunately, one of my most valued mentors, Dr. Robert Vogel, is now working with the NFL on fitness, risks and especially, obesity. I have a feeling he will change things.

Obesity, even in seasoned athletes, is a cardiovascular risk factor. Very few people are equipped with a frame suited to carrying over 300 pounds. Excess weight puts inordinate strain on the pumping capacity of the heart. The major risk in some of the hugely obese players may well be that of occult coronary disease. A coronary calcium score can be obtained for $100–$200 and takes 15 minutes. It's a valid test in males over 35 years of age and is frequently positive in those as young as 25.

Will an External Defibrillator Save Them?

Great attention has to be given to the obesity/dehydration/deconditioning syndrome. This seems to be common. I first became aware of it years ago when it was my tradition to go down into the Grand Canyon on my birthday, and then come back out on the same day. Part of hiking down and back up in a day was probably machismo, part had to do with the fact that lodging is sparse down there and I hate to share my sleeping bag with rattlesnakes. I went down one day with a physician who was one of the team charged with caring for the sick and injured in the Grand

Canyon. It probably comes as no surprise that there are 25–30 deaths each year in the Grand Canyon. A frequent cause is that of dehydration and acidosis (build-up of lactic acid in the blood stream) coupled with hyperthermia (markedly elevated body temperature). Many of these individuals are young but significantly overweight and not fit. Many drink only pure water despite the fact that they are losing body fluids like crazy through perspiration. Sweat is not just water. It contains electrolytes. When these hikers collapse with a very high body temperature, dehydration, and electrolyte abnormalities and then have a seizure causing a huge elevation in blood stream lactic acid on top of the level they are already carrying, they cannot be resuscitated.

These are the same elements that occur in a linebacker who shows up at a training field—overweight and deconditioned—in 100° weather. I know that all trainers these days use electrolyte solutions to replace body fluids. I think, however, our society-at-large has a false sense of security when they see an external defibrillator on the sidelines. If you get hot enough, dehydrated enough, and have enough electrolyte abnormality and this precipitates a seizure, it may not be possible to resuscitate you with a defibrillator. For example, we know that a patient in the hospital can generally be defibrillated from ventricular tachycardia/fibrillation—fatal processes—if an external defibrillator is applied promptly. However, if these patients have a large amount of acid in their bloodstream from a poorly functioning heart, complications from surgery, or any number of other problems, it is more difficult to defibrillate them back to a normal rhythm. The same is true with these athletes. If they are playing with a huge oxygen debt, acidotic from the build-up of lactic acid in their tissues, and then if they perchance have a seizure compounding the problem, it can be very difficult, if not impossible, to shock them back into a normal rhythm. Also, there is sometimes a significant time delay. We know that the incidence of getting someone back from one of these fatal electrical events decreases by 10% per minute of delay. If it takes five minutes to get the defibrillator onto the field and activated, the incidence of salvage has already dropped to 50%.

I am a great proponent of having external defibrillators at the ready in all schools and especially in close proximity to athletic events. But to be effective, responsibility has to be relegated to one particular person who is to be in charge of the external defibrillator at all times and is familiar with its prompt deployment. There is no time to read the instructions when a young man or woman is down, and the decision about who is going to deploy it has to be firmly in place.

A Blow to the Chest Can Cause Sudden Cardiac Death

One of the most tragic events in the world is the young baseball player who receives a fastball blow to the chest and falls over dead. Just as a forceful thump on the chest can sometimes convert a life-threatening arrhythmia back to a normal sinus rhythm, an extremely high velocity blow to the chest, usually a ball off a metal bat, can induce a fatal arrhythmia (ventricular tachycardia and ventricular fibrillation) called *Commotio Cordis*. There is no way to screen for this one, unfortunately, but there is something to do. We don't want our children to live their lives in a bubble; however, some things are just too dangerous to allow. For example, the velocity of a well-hit baseball by a metal bat is, on average, 20–30% greater than one hit off a wooden bat. These metal bats should be outlawed in non-professional baseball.

Sudden cardiac death from a blow to the chest can be promptly and effectively treated through use of the external defibrillator. These usually occur in pitchers or shortstops who don't have acidosis or an oxygen debt; therefore, they should promptly be shocked back to a regular rhythm.

The Aging Athlete

Baby boomers are helping to redefine several ideas in today's society and, certainly, one of these is exercise. Any chapter on the problem of heart disease and death in athletes would be incomplete without a discourse on the dangers to the *aging* athlete. I am emphasizing this not to scare the over-50 crowd from exercising—even competitively and aggressively—but so they will know how to get tested to make sure they are okay to excercise safely.

By far the greatest risk to the aging athlete is silent occult coronary artery disease: a partial blockage of one or more coronary arteries that supply the heart muscle. It is not enough to go out and run and feel that you are "cleared" for exercise because you have no symptoms of a blocked artery, such as chest pain. You need a test to be sure you are okay to exercise vigorously—especially if you are over 40 years old and male, or over 50 and female. Let me give you two classic examples:

Jim Fixx was a popular guy in my era. He was the author of the best-selling book *The Complete Book of Running* and almost single-handedly popularized the running craze in 1977. He was no dummy. He wrote for *Life*, the *Saturday Review*, and others and was a member of the high-IQ club Mensa. He also published puzzles for the super-intelligent. He had run 60 miles per week for several years when he died of a massive heart attack at age 52—after his daily run at his home in Vermont. All three coronary arteries were almost completely clogged. As far as anyone knew, he had no chest pain or other symptoms to indicate a problem. His risk factors were a strong family history (his dad died at age 42), high cholesterol, and a previous history of cigarette usage.

Brian Maxwell started the PowerBar company with his girlfriend when he was forced to drop out of a marathon due to inadequate energy to finish. By 1977, he was ranked third among all marathoners in the world. He died at age 51 of an apparent heart attack. As far as I know, there was no prior warning.

I could cover several pages with similar illustrations. Suffice it to say that *silent coronary artery disease* is labeled such for a reason: It is truly silent. In other words, many people have inadequate warning mechanisms to tell them that their heart muscle is not receiving sufficient oxygen-enriched blood to satisfy its extra demands when vigorously exercising. A non-invasive and inexpensive test can be performed on such people and it will largely stratify risks of exercise. It is called a coronary calcium score. We perform this by measuring the amount of calcium within coronary arteries supplying the heart muscle. It is performed by a type of CT scan, measuring pixels of calcium. When plaque forms within the coronary artery, it calcifies. This usually occurs in men to the extent that the calcium score is reliable after age 35, but since women calcify their coronary arteries later and less than men, they must be over 45 for this to be reliable. While we know that one can have a lipid-laden, non-calcified bulging plaque in one of the coronary arteries and therefore have a good test result, the coronary calcium score is still our best screening test. And we know the incidence of heart attacks to be only about 1% a year in those with a zero coronary calcium score.

While there are many cardiac problems that might well be picked up in the aging athlete, silent coronary artery disease is by far the greatest threat. The tragedy of a mishap is that it can be detected for about the same expenditure as a winter jogging outfit.

Dr. Kenneth Cooper at the Cooper Clinic in Dallas has used such a test—an electron beam tomogram or EBT—for many years. He probably sees more famous people than anyone, and is especially well-known by those who are creeping up in years but want to continue exercising. He has cleared a great number of these high-profile people through the results of the coronary calcium score, doubtless coupled with other tests as well. An added benefit—especially for the over-50 crowd—is that it also gives information about the pancreas, the liver, and other intra-abdominal organs and structures. The CT scan used for the coronary calcium score determination is safe (very little radiation), employs no contrast agent such as iodine-based materials, and is statistically reliable enough to make it a superb screening test for silent coronary artery disease.

REMINDERS

1. If you have a family history of unexplained sudden cardiac death, get an echocardiogram, an electrocardiogram, and a treadmill test prior to participating in a sport or ongoing activity that requires extreme exertion.
2. If you or one of your family members develop palpitations, blackout, chest pain, or severe shortness of breath while engaging in athletic activities, see a cardiologist without delay.
3. Don't hide symptoms. We can usually fix it so you can play.
4. Show up for vigorous athletic activity already fit. Drink plenty of electrolyte solution when you are losing lots of body fluids via perspiration.
5. If you are in the coronary age group, over 35 years old if male, over 45 if female, check for silent coronary artery disease with a coronary calcium score before competitively or aggressively exercising.

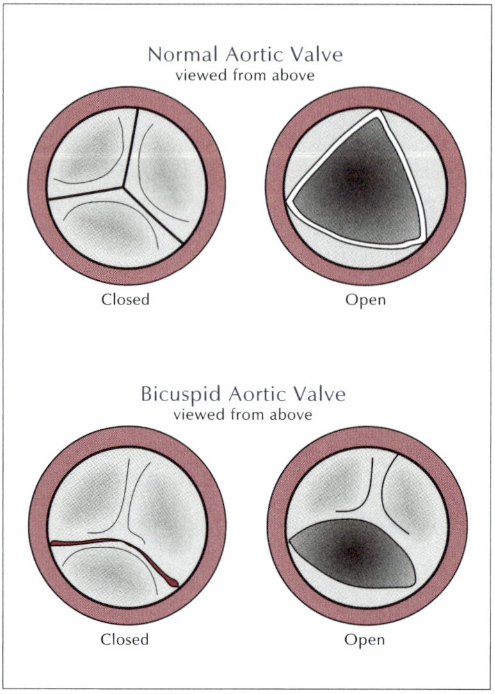

CONGENITAL HEART DISEASE

Silent Heart Problems at Birth May Show Up Years Later

DURING THE LAST 30 YEARS, I HAVE continued to find three or four adult patients a year, most in their 40s or 50s, who were born with defects in their heart or blood vessels and yet knew nothing about it.

These defects had either not caused symptoms or the individual had just learned to live with them. After all, if you grow up with a particular problem, it is sometimes amazing how nicely you compensate for it and frequently live a normal life. *Normal* is defined within our own minds. Some congenital heart defects can be lived with. Others can be responsible for life-changing events. It's important to know all we can about ourselves and be aware of our own unique process.

Bicuspid Aortic Valve

Possibly the most common congenital defect that is detected in an adult cardiology office is that of a congenitally bicuspid aortic valve. The aortic valve should be comprised of three leaflets in order to function as it should for a lifetime. This allows the leaflets to open fully, and to close with a nice close fit with slight overlap. The result is a valve that neither obstructs flow during systole when the left ventricle is pumping blood into the aorta nor leaks blood back into the left ventricle during diastole when that chamber is relaxed.

In a small percentage of people, the aortic valve at birth is not tricuspid but bicuspid, consisting of only two leaflets. Usually, one leaflet is larger and one is smaller. These may go totally undetected in adolescent life and even young adulthood, as the leaflets are still pliable. Sometimes these are not detected until the 30s, 40s or even 50s, at which time the leaflets have become a bit more thickened and perhaps even partially calcified. This develops from the wear and tear of blood flow for all of those years through a valve that is not operating the way it should.

The earliest detection possible is important because these valves are predisposed to bacterial infection during simple procedures such as dental cleaning. Dental antibiotic prophylaxis can protect the individual from an early valve replacement. We routinely watch these valves until they create some form of hemodynamic impairment that we deem important enough to warrant valve surgery.

Coarctation of the Aorta

There is an uncanny association of a bicuspid aortic valve with another congenital abnormality consisting of a fibrous band constricting the descending aorta just below the take-off of the subclavian artery to the left arm. This is called *coarctation of the aorta.* These seldom miss early detection, but I have seen the combination in a previously undiagnosed individual as old as 50 years of age. The coarctation may exist as a singular entity as well.

Atrial Septal Defect (ASD)

It is actually somewhat common to find a previously undiagnosed hole in the septum separating the upper heart chambers. Remember: The right and left sides of the heart should be completely separate from each other. We call such an opening a *communication* because it allows for "sharing" of blood between the chambers. The medical term for such a problem in this part of the heart is an *atrial septal defect* (ASD). This may not make much noise as a youth and can be easily passed over as an innocent murmur related only to the normal flow of blood as it is handled by the heart. However, as the left ventricle becomes less elastic and stretchy with age, the left atrial pressure required to fill it increases. With this increase in left atrial pressure as a natural consequence of aging and not accompanied by a corresponding increase in right atrial pressure, the left-to-right shunt may increase significantly. In other words, it now makes the ASD an important problem, sometimes with voluminous flow from the left to the right atrium. This becomes worse with any problem that will raise the left ventricular filling pressure, such as diabetes, a heart attack, or just high blood pressure. Closure of the hole should be considered in this instance.

Ventricular Septal Defect (VSD)

A communication between the lower chambers, a *ventricular septal defect* (VSD), is less commonly found, at least as a surprise, as these are usually noisy from birth. One is the so-called *Bruit de Roger* (pronounced *brew-e, d, Row-Jay*), due to a tiny membranous VSD. The smaller the hole, the higher the velocity of the blood going across the hole—the blood pressure is high in the left ventricle but low in the right—creating a significant gradient. So, while this thing may make a horrific noise, it is frequently due to a tiny hole that does not cause enough abnormal flow for serious volume overload problems. Some people have chosen to leave these alone. I think that is a mistake, as the blood velocity is so great where it strikes the other side that it creates thickening of the tissue. This damaged zone is very susceptible to becoming infected when bacteria enter the blood stream.

Bacteria in the Blood Stream Can be Dangerous if You Have a Congenital Defect

As it turns out, such bacteremia is not uncommon. It happens more than we would suspect. For example, if blood cultures are drawn from individuals leaving the dentist's office after dental cleaning, there is a substantial number that grow bacteria. These have entered the blood stream during the dental procedure, as there are millions of bacteria surrounding the teeth. Normally, the spleen and other structures filter the bacteria out of the blood stream and get rid of them. If you have a structure in your heart that literally begs for bacteria to alight on it and start a family, it should be treated.

Complex Congenital Problems Can Escape Detection for Many Years

Occasionally we will see something in an adult that is very complex and so unexpected that we can hardly believe it. I recently saw such a problem in a physician's wife. The hole or fault in the heart wasn't creating much noise at all, and had gone undetected until she developed chest pain that was secondary to a partially blocked coronary artery. In examining her, I found enough abnormalities to make me suspicious that she had an undiscovered congenital problem. It was corroborated at the time of cardiac catheterization. She had an unusual form of ASD, associated with abnormal pulmonary venous drainage of blood from the lungs, and there was a significant shunt across the ASD because her left ventricle had become stiff. This particular anomaly is also commonly associated with a cleft in the mitral valve. Hers was of this variety. When we looked at the catheterization anatomy and hemodynamics, we were amazed that an individual had accommodated this situation for over 50 years without significant symptoms. The answer is, of course, that she grew up with it.

Anomalous Left Main Coronary: Silent but Dangerous

Probably the most important congenital anomaly of the heart and blood vessels that goes hidden and is potentially fatal is that of an *anomalous left main coronary artery*. This artery, the left main, supplies branches to 75% of the heart. It should originate from the left coronary cusp of the aortic root. If it arises, instead, from the right coronary cusp, there are three potential pathways it can take in order to get over to the left side where it delivers its branches to the heart muscle. The course between the aorta and pulmonary artery is the life-threatening one, as vigorous exercise will fill these large vessels with blood and compress the anomalous left main coronary artery. This renders much of the heart oxygen-starved, and sudden death can occur due to a disturbance of heart rhythm. This is the result of an electrical aberration provoked by the afflicted muscle cells. This anomaly has been given the dramatic moniker of "Tunnel of Death" and needs to be treated with surgical revascularization without delay.

A *single* coronary artery can also cause sudden death. Several years ago, the hard-charging basketball player "Pistol" Pete Maravich died of this problem. This situation is very difficult to detect without angiography.

Innocent Vascular Anomalies

Other vascular abnormalities also show up from time to time. Most of these are of academic interest only. One such is a *coronary-kameral fistula*, a communication between a coronary artery and a heart chamber or the pulmonary artery. These almost never need to be repaired. If someone suggests surgery, be sure you know exactly why it has been recommended and get a second opinion if you need it for a sense of security.

Diagnosis

Almost all of the problems we have discussed can be diagnosed with a well-performed echocardiogram. With this test in such vogue as it is today, it seems unlikely that a well-trained cardiologist will miss any of these shunt or valvular abnormalities. But anomalous arteries have been missed in the past, and some of these will continue to escape detection. I have performed angiography on some fairly young individuals who were complaining of typical anginal pain—brought on by exertion, relieved by rest, usually due to a blocked artery from arteriosclerosis—just so I won't miss something like the anomalous left main traveling between the aorta and the main pulmonary artery.

I suppose I was influenced by a patient I saw early in my cardiology training in Denver. A ten-year-old boy scout was playing with his friend in a drainage system not far from the university hospital. He was running full out, suddenly stopped, grabbed his chest, and slumped over unconscious. His friend gave him closed chest massage and waved down a passing car. The boy survived, probably only because he was very young and was wise enough to have chosen a boy scout as his playmate. He had an anomalous left main coronary artery; its course was between the aorta and the pulmonary artery. I remember being shaken by the fact that this young boy had previously complained of mild chest pain when he ran hard. He had great parents. I'm sure they just thought he had "growing pains."

It is amazing how events shape our lives. I have never seen another young child with this problem. I have, however, seen young adults with it. Over the years, I have seen three or four of these patients. Their coronary arteries were otherwise normal. They were just born with their plumbing slightly wrong. I have heard over and over, "What you don't know won't kill you." However, with these abnormal conduits, that's not true!

Because of these situations, I've taken chest pain complaints seriously in every single person who ever came to the hospital or my office with this complaint. I figure *something* is causing discomfort. It's not enough to just blow it off and tell these patients they have nothing wrong with their heart or blood vessels. If they come to a cardiologist for it and it's bothering them, they deserve an answer. After a thorough investigation if we're not smart enough to find a reason, we should just tell them so. Generally, the individual will appreciate the doctor's candor and will also appreciate the fact that a dangerous cause for the pain doesn't exist.

These days, with the advent of the 64-slice CT angiogram, many more people will be angiogrammed because it is an outpatient procedure. This test is very safe, requires 30 minutes to an hour of the individual's time, and can give us a good, non-invasive look at the vascular system. This is so much different than putting a patient on a catheterization table, introducing a catheter from the groin to the aorta, and taking an angiogram! With this less invasive procedure, we should miss fewer and fewer of these vascular problems.

What needs to be done when a congenital process is found? Not all congenital defects need to be repaired. In many instances the individual has lived in harmony with it for a long time. Many of these congenital lesions, however, do require repair and it will add quality, if not quantity, to the last several years of a person's life.

As physicians, we need to keep in mind Mark Twain's witticism. To paraphrase, "If you're the guy with the hammer, every nail looks like it needs driving." That can certainly be true for us. This is one reason I have tried to approach all patients as though they were members of my family. I don't want something done to my patient that I would not want done to my sister if she had the same situation. Your doctor should be able to balance the pros and cons of repair of an anomaly and give you a very honest opinion of what to do.

REMINDERS

1. **A congenital anomaly can exist completely undetected until a person is 40 or 50 years of age.**
2. **Just finding a congenital anomaly doesn't necessarily mean that it needs to be repaired. Get prognostic guesstimates regarding leaving it alone versus repair.**
3. **Most congenital anomalies, at least valves and shunts, should receive dental and surgical antibiotic prophylaxis.**
4. **The most dangerous congenital anomaly of the blood vessels—an**

anomalous left main coronary artery making its course between the aorta and the pulmonary artery—should almost always be repaired surgically.

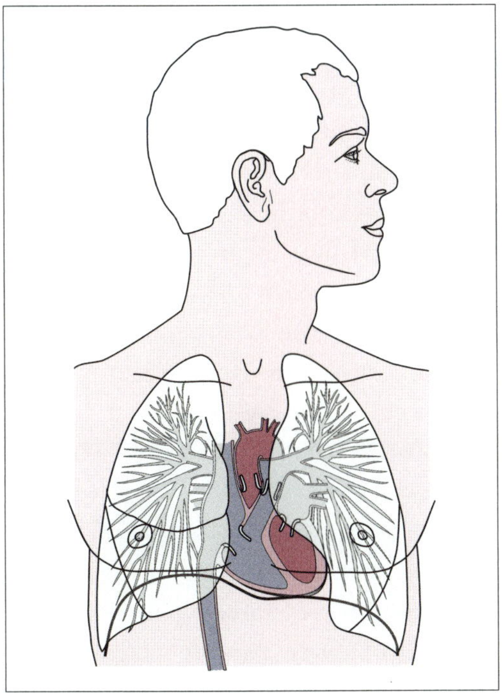

PULMONARY ARTERY HYPERTENSION

High Blood Pressure Can Occur in the Lung Artery Too

ONE OF THE MOST FRUSTRATING DISEASES to have or to treat has been *pulmonary arterial hypertension* (PAH). The main pulmonary artery is the large vascular conduit carrying blue blood, from which oxygen has been removed by the tissues, to the lungs where it will pick up more oxygen. The systolic pressure within it should be less than 30 mmHg. We have identified many causes that will elevate it. We also know that an elevated pulmonary artery pressure is sometimes idiopathic (Latin for "we don't know the cause"). This is the most frustrating of all. However, we now have some therapeutic responses for this strange disease.

Normal Pulmonary Circulation and Response

If you take a contrast angiogram of the pulmonary circulation, it will look like a tree, going from a large trunk to two large branches, then many slightly smaller ones, smaller and smaller branches the farther out the blood travels. The large pulmonary arteries carrying blood to the lungs possess a great deal of elastic within the walls that stretches and rebounds at low pressures. At a transition to much smaller arteries—small branches—the elastic is lost and the middle layer of these smaller arteries is comprised more of muscle. The upper limits of normal systolic pressure in the pulmonary artery is about 25 mmHg (millimeters mercury, the standard unit of measurement of the pressure within any blood vessel in the body) and the upper mean pressure is 20 mmHg. Above these levels, the person is said to have pulmonary arterial hypertension. PAH can vary all the way from mild elevation to a level identical to the systemic pressure, that pressure within the arteries supplying the brain, limbs, kidneys, and gut.

These are the normal levels at sea level. We know that hypoxia, a drop in the normal oxygen level in the blood, elicits what we call pulmonary vasoconstriction, whereby the pulmonary arteries get smaller. The converse to this is pulmonary vasodilatation, whereby they get larger. At higher altitudes, such as Leadville, Colorado which is about 8,000 feet above sea level, pulmonary pressures will be considerably higher in normal people. If someone residing in Leadville goes down to Denver, about 3,000 feet lower, his pulmonary pressure will fall. If he goes on to Miami, at sea level, it will fall even more. Such is the vasoregulatory mechanism in the pulmonary arterial circulation. This change is basically regulated by the state of contraction of the muscular components within the pulmonary arteries.

There are many vasoregulatory compounds that help maintain just the right pulmonary artery pressure no matter what you are doing or where you are living at the moment. Prostaglandins are substances manufactured in the lung tissue and play a role in vascular resistance, the pressure against which the heart has to pump. Nitric oxide is manufactured in the endothelium, the inside of the pulmonary artery, and is a vaso-relaxing substance. Endothelin is a potent vasoconstrictor peptide that plays an important role in maintaining proper tone and resistance. Serotonin causes release of nitric oxide, thereby relaxing the tone of the artery. Angiotensin I is a potent vasoconstrictor. All of these chemicals (plus several more undiscovered) in conjunction with the blood oxygen level, regulate the pulmonary artery pressure. When any of these get seriously out of whack, you can develop pulmonary hypertension.

Pulmonary Arterial Hypertension Secondary to Mechanical Causes

There are many mechanical causes of pulmonary arterial hypertension. In a day and age of prevalent cigarette smoking, the development of emphysema (loss of functioning lung tissue, replaced by large bullae or non-functioning large air pockets) is one of the most common. We commonly refer to the large collection of people with emphysema and bronchitis, a narrowed airway, as having *chronic obstructive pulmonary disease* (COPD). This is always about the fourth leading cause of death in the United States—and the incidence is rising, not falling. Cigarette smoking accounts for at least 90% of all cases. With loss of functioning alveoli, where oxygen is exchanged for carbon dioxide, the blood oxygen level falls, the muscular arteries vasoconstrict, and the pulmonary artery pressure rises.

Another important mechanical cause of PAH is pulmonary embolism, the passage of clots from the leg veins through the heart into the pulmonary arteries, wedging in the arteries that are the same size as the clot. If these clots are silent and become rigid due to lack of diagnosis and treatment, they will acutely raise the pulmonary artery pressure. They then become casts within the pulmonary circulation—rigid clots molded to the wall of the pulmonary artery—and will chronically raise the pulmonary pressures.

Interstitial lung disease, or pulmonary fibrosis, is the destruction of lung tissue from scar tissue. Most of this is due to an unknown cause. However, the end result is a dramatic reduction in the number of functioning alveoli, a drop in the blood oxygen level, and a rise in pulmonary pressure.

PAH Secondary to a Chronically Elevated Left Atrial Pressure

Probably the next major category are those folks who, because of increased stiffness of the left ventricle from aging, hypertension, diabetes, previous heart attack, or anything that damages the ability of the heart muscle to contract and relax properly, have an elevated left atrial pressure. This is called the filling pressure because the left atrium fills the ventricle with blood, and if the pressure within the left ventricle is elevated during the time it is filling, this pressure is transmitted back into the left atrium and into the pulmonary veins. With time, the muscular pulmonary arteries will adjust, increasing the pulmonary artery pressure.

This will also be brought about by a leaking mitral or aortic valve, or by a shunt (a hole in the heart from birth) between the right and left chambers of the heart. One of the main contributors during the rheumatic fever era was mitral stenosis, a scarring of the mitral valve obstructing inflow of blood into the left ventricle.

Idiopathic (Primary) Pulmonary Arterial Hypertension

This is the diagnosis given to the group of patients who develop PAH for no obvious reason. Instead of it being secondary to some other process, it is sometimes called "primary." Several hypotheses, ever changing, have been cited as causes. The most likely has to do with altered endothelial function. The endothelium is the single layer of flat cells that lines any artery. As recently as 20 years ago, we thought these cells did very little except to interface with the blood flowing through the artery. We have come to realize that our lives depend on these guys, as they basically serve as the regulatory mechanism in promoting health of the artery or conversely, disease of the artery.

Remember, nitric oxide is a potent vaso-relaxant agent. It is manufactured within the endothelium, dependent on an amino acid, L-arginine, for its production. The endothelium is truly the arbitrator of health for the arterial system. In people with primary pulmonary hypertension, there is a proliferation of smooth muscle within the smaller vessels, sometimes completely obliterating the lumen of the artery. Relaxation of the artery is lost, too.

Dr. Paul Wood, a revered cardiologist who discovered and taught many of the principles we hold dear today, noted back in the 1950s that there was an element of vasoconstriction in idiopathic PAH. In some forms of this disease there is a genetic predisposition to getting it. We used to think that people who developed primary PAH just had bad luck. The only bad luck may have been in their bloodline, just as with developing coronary artery disease. We used to think also that the pulmonary arterial circulation behaved quite differently from the systemic arterial bed (the one supplying the legs, for example). That is probably only partially true, as they share more similarities than not. One of these shared similarities is that, if you are genetically predisposed, a triggering stimulus (probably having to do with the endothelium) starts the process of vasoconstriction, smooth muscle proliferation, and the inflammation that will eventually result in dramatic increases in pulmonary pressure.

This inherited predisposition probably also explains a couple of things that have been mysteries in the past. One is why, with a large shunt (because of a hole in the heart) from one chamber to the other, certain people would develop fixed pulmonary hypertension, equal to the systemic pressure in the arm (called Eisenmenger's physiology) and why some would not. Another is why two people could set out to climb Mount Everest and one would develop severe high-altitude pulmonary edema (water in the lungs) and one would go on to the summit. When I was in Denver, we routinely saw people who lived in Leadville and developed severe PAH. When we sent them to Miami, it would reverse, frequently coming down to normal. Dr. Jack Vogel, who formulated and proved many of the principles related to high-altitude pulmonary hypertension and edema, showed us that when he was at the University of Colorado. One of these individuals was a competitive skier who wanted to make the Olympic team. Since the snow skiing is poor in Miami, she was not pleased. However, I believe it saved her life, as I think she was on her way to fixed pulmonary hypertension. I believe these differences are due to individual and unique characteristics within the endothelium of the pulmonary vascular bed, influencing tone of the artery at the very least, and probably much more. These differences are endowed by one's own unique genome, inherited from a combination of one's parent's contributions in the roll of the dice that constitutes the formation of human life.

Collagen Vascular Diseases Associated with PAH

Scleroderma is a collagen vascular disease marked by loss of subcutaneous tissue around the mouth and in the fingers, esophageal motility disorders, and a variety of other features. Lupus is different but it is also a collagen disease. Both may cause pulmonary hypertension, though it is more common with scleroderma. In fact, it looks and behaves a lot like idiopathic PAH. Vaso-reactivity is a major component.

Sleep Apnea as a Cause of PAH

We've actually gotten to the point where we really like to find sleep apnea when we are seeing someone with PAH, for it is at least partially amenable to treatment. (There seem to be so many instances whereby PAH is not very treatable.) There are basically two forms (at least in a cardiologist's world) of sleep apnea: central and obstructive. The central variety is due to water entering the lungs during sleep due to a sick left ventricle. The person's blood oxygen level drops, he or she over-breathes, then the respiratory center shuts off and a lapse in breathing—apnea—occurs. We treat it by increasing the drugs to keep the lungs dry. The obstructive form occurs when there is enough adipose (fat) tissue within the oropharynx to drop down and obstruct the airways during deep slumber. We treat this, along with the central form, with CPAP (continuous positive airways pressure). While either form may develop PAH, the obstructive variety develops a much worse pressure, and it is readily reversed, at least in part, with CPAP.

Pulmonary Artery Hypertension and Pregnancy

It is important to include a word of caution to those who have PAH and might become pregnant. In this situation—vascular remodeling, elevation of endothelin levels coupled with low nitric oxide and prostacyclin levels, all of which cause increased tone in the muscular pulmonary arteries—pregnancy is just too risky. These factors, as well as limited capacity for the volume expansion necessary in pregnancy, produce a high risk of becoming very ill or even dying if you have moderately severe pulmonary hypertension.

I must have spent an hour or more with the last young lady with this disorder who decided to become pregnant. She really wanted a baby! I warned her as gently as I could, then more forcefully, and finally in desperation, I came on pretty strong. She decided to go ahead with a pregnancy after another cardiologist told her she would "be just fine."

Her pre-pregnancy mean pulmonary artery pressure was not terrible (about 25, normal is up to 20) but it had been higher, and this pressure was obtained while she was on an endothelin-antagonist. She had to stop this drug because of risks of inducing deformities, and she proceeded to become pregnant. As she entered the final trimester of pregnancy, when the volume expansion of fetal demand is becoming greatest, she started getting into trouble. We managed it, after restarting her endothelin-antagonist and getting her some prostacyclin treatments.

Then a few weeks shy of her due date, her blood pressure dropped. This is the usual cause of death in these women, as pregnancy causes the systemic vascular resistance (in the legs, for example) to fall, just as the pulmonary vascular resistance is rising. The heart then fails from the increased pressure placed upon it and the left ventricle is volume-starved, since the right ventricle can't get enough blood to it. Only through the grace of God, coupled with everything at our disposal, did we get her and the baby through this terrifying out-of-control spiral of events. We used endothelin-antagonists, blood pressure support, and intravenous prostacyclin. After this escapade, she smiled up at me and said, "I knew you could do it." I appreciated the vote of confidence; however, this is not a reproducible act. Now I just plant my foot and say, *"No Way!"* The risk of death of the mother in the case of pregnancy in the face of established PAH is roughly 50%. Death of the mother almost always results in death of the fetus too, as there is so little time to remove the baby surgically when a fatal spiral of decompensation occurs. Therefore, I now advise my patients who have significant PAH to avoid pregnancy. The danger is just too great.

Diagnosis

A quick and effective way of making the diagnosis is with an echocardiogram, utilizing Doppler analysis to give us the pressure within the pulmonary artery. We can also use this test to monitor those with this disease, to determine if a particular drug is working, and to evaluate the status of the right ventricle.

Treatment and Clinical Course

This is a difficult disease to have, partially because we can never tell you for sure that we can cure it. If you have it, you are stuck with a chronic disease. However, we can favorably alter its course and we are learning more every day about this strange and frustrating problem.

The most effective treatment, especially for those in the COPD group, is continuous oxygen administration. We noted that hypoxia, a low blood stream oxygen level, is a vasoconstrictor. If we correct the oxygen impairment, we can positively influence the arterial bed, vasodilating it. This will sometimes drop the pressure markedly. Anyone with pulmonary hypertension should receive continuous oxygen in proper amounts to maintain a normal blood oxygen level. These patients must stop smoking, as it destroys more lung tissue and also is a vasoconstrictor substance.

Obviously, if the cause of the PAH is thought to be due to a primary cardiac problem, we need to address it. By unloading the left ventricle, we may positively affect the pulmonary pressure.

If there is evidence of pulmonary embolic casts (rigid clots) within the pulmonary bed (especially if they are extensive and proximal), surgical retrieval of these casts in the larger vessels will sometimes result in a dramatic improvement. This is complex surgery and should only be done in a center where they've had a series of good outcomes.

This leaves the idiopathic variety. Most of the forms of treatment are directed toward dilating the vasoconstricted pulmonary vascular bed. This is done with hydralazine, ACE-I drugs, ARB drugs, endothelin antagonists, and prostaglandins. If the primary problem was only vasoconstriction, this would be effective therapy. However, we now know that this is only one small piece of the puzzle. It appears that much of this obliterative process has to do with endothelial dysfunction and other undiscovered mechanisms. We have tried steroids and other immunosuppressants with mixed success.

So, if you have idiopathic PAH and it steadily gets worse, what are the problems that develop? One of the most significant and threatening is pressure overload of the right ventricle. This chamber was built to pump against a pressure of only up to 30 mmHg. As such, it contains a scant amount of muscle and has a limited ability to thicken the muscle. When it is faced with a pressure double or even triple its expected load limit, it starts to falter. The right ventricle dilates, muscle contraction weakens and soon blood dams up behind the right ventricle, a process called *cor* (Latin for heart) *pulmonale*. This was the term introduced in 1931 by Dr. Paul Wood to imply right heart overload due to a lung condition. With this situation, water is pushed into the tissues causing swelling of the abdominal girth and the legs. As this gets worse, requiring more diuretics, the blood pressure feeding the brain and kidneys falls because the left ventricle becomes volume-starved. This is the beginning of the end of this vicious cycle.

Centers of Excellence

One of the hardest decisions a doctor has to make is when to send an unusual patient to a super-specialized center that studies a particular unusual disease. In my view, the patient with idiopathic primary PAH fits into this category. This is a rare disease. The only way we are going to lick it is to study enough people at a specialty center until someone discovers the treatment. In my part of the world, the National Jewish Hospital in Denver, Colorado is recognized for its compassion, dedication, and expertise, as well as its ongoing research into this and many other rare pulmonary diseases. I send all of my patients with primary PAH to the National Jewish Hospital and am always impressed with the level of care and consideration that is extended to each of them. I am sure there are other centers across the United States with similar interests and levels of commitment. If you need the name of a facility in your area, your pulmonary doctor or National Jewish Hospital can provide you with information.

Before I send someone to them, I make sure I have adequately done my job and have determined beyond any shadow of doubt that this patient's PAH is not due to any fixable process within the heart or blood vessels. We actually see more of these patients in this area than our population would suggest. I believe this is due to some of the environmental influences that are prevalent here. For example, a great deal of cotton is raised in this area in Texas. I have seen at least three patients who developed their first symptoms during cotton harvest. Each year, it seemed to be exacerbated during harvest time. I am becoming convinced that there is some sort of reactive, perhaps inflammatory, component in some of these patients.

REMINDERS

1. There are many potentially treatable causes of pulmonary hypertension. The largest group is comprised of those with COPD, the fourth leading cause of death in the United States. Treatment is first and foremost discontinuation of cigarettes. Continuous oxygen administration is a must, as hypoxia (low blood oxygen level) causes vasoconstriction of the pulmonary arteries.
2. Before someone receives the diagnosis of idiopathic pulmonary arterial hypertension, they must be shown not to have any of the potentially reversible or more treatable causes of PAH.
3. If you are diagnosed with idiopathic PAH, ask your doctor about referral to a specialized treatment center where they see many patients with this disorder.

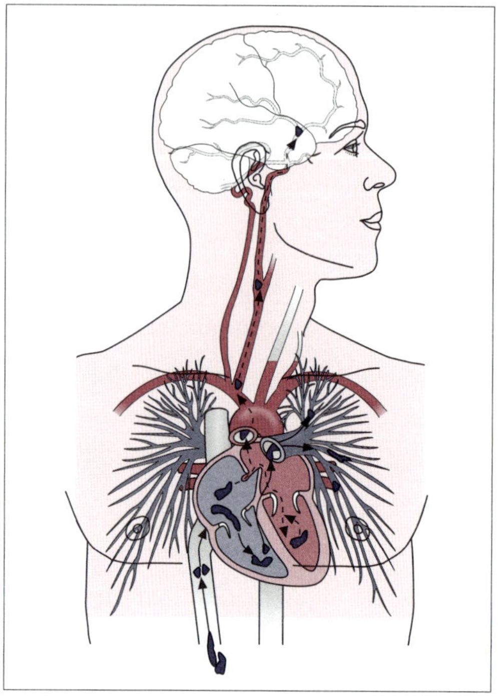

35 PATENT FORAMEN OVALE

A Silent Hole in the Heart from Birth Can Cause a Stroke

AS WE DEVELOP WITHIN THE WOMB, we all have an ovoid opening between the top two chambers of the heart, a *foramen* (Latin for "hole") *ovale*. Upon taking the first breath, the pressure in the left atrium will force a small flap of tissue against this opening, effectively closing it. This produces a barrier between the right atrium, carrying spent blue blood, and the left atrium, carrying oxygenated red blood. In a normal heart and for proper function, there should be no connection whatsoever between the right and left chambers.

If we had our druthers, we would rather have this flap of tissue tacked down, growing to the edges of the foramen, permanently sealing it and preventing it from opening at some point. This is what occurs in the majority of individuals. However, in a large postmortem study done in London years ago, it was found that approximately 20% of individuals have an identifiable connection, though it is tiny and tortuous in many. Most of these cause no mischief whatsoever and these people never know they have such a thing. However, in about 2%, the flap covering the foramen ovale is somewhat active, widely opening intermittently with any pressure stimulus. This is known as a *patent* (open) *foramen ovale* (PFO).

Physiologic Factors Influencing the Status of a PFO

If the right atrial pressures are normal, the PFO is closed by the flap most, if not all, of the time since the left atrial pressure is just slightly higher than the right atrial pressure. This difference in pressure keeps the flap firmly pressed to the edges of the hole, closing off the right and left sides of the circulation. However, with any maneuver that raises right atrial pressure, such as blowing up a balloon, the flap will release its firm covering and blood can then flow right to left across the PFO for a few seconds. This means that many people have an opening between the right and left upper heart chambers several times during the day, as this bearing down maneuver is common in our daily routine.

The occasional opening of the PFO in such circumstances would be of no importance if a pathologic process didn't develop elsewhere; the minute amount of right-to-left blood flow would not even be noticed. However, if you develop a blood clot somewhere in a vein, it can spell trouble. Since pathologic blood clots don't usually start to form until our 30s or 40s, this is the age when we usually detect most PFOs complicated by stroke. The risk dramatically climbs after age 50, as the incidence of pathologic blood clots in the leg and pelvic veins increases with age.

Paradoxical Embolus Through a PFO

Consider for a moment the development of *deep venous thrombophlebitis* (DVT), the pathologic formation of a clot within the veins draining the legs or pelvis. Under normal circumstances, when such a clot breaks loose from its tether to the vessel wall, it travels to the right heart and then on to the lungs, wedging in one of the small branches. Whenever this happens, there is frequently an increase in the pulmonary artery pressure and this is reflected back into the right atrium, raising the right atrial pressure as well.

Usually, the larger the clot, the more the pulmonary pressure will rise. This increase in right atrial pressure can cause the flap covering a PFO to lift away, much like a door on a hinge. It is no longer prohibiting flow across the opening between the two chambers. A second clot can then readily cross the PFO, move into the left heart, and on to the brain or elsewhere. (Figure 28) A dislodged clot traveling within the blood stream to another site is called an embolus. In this instance, since it goes

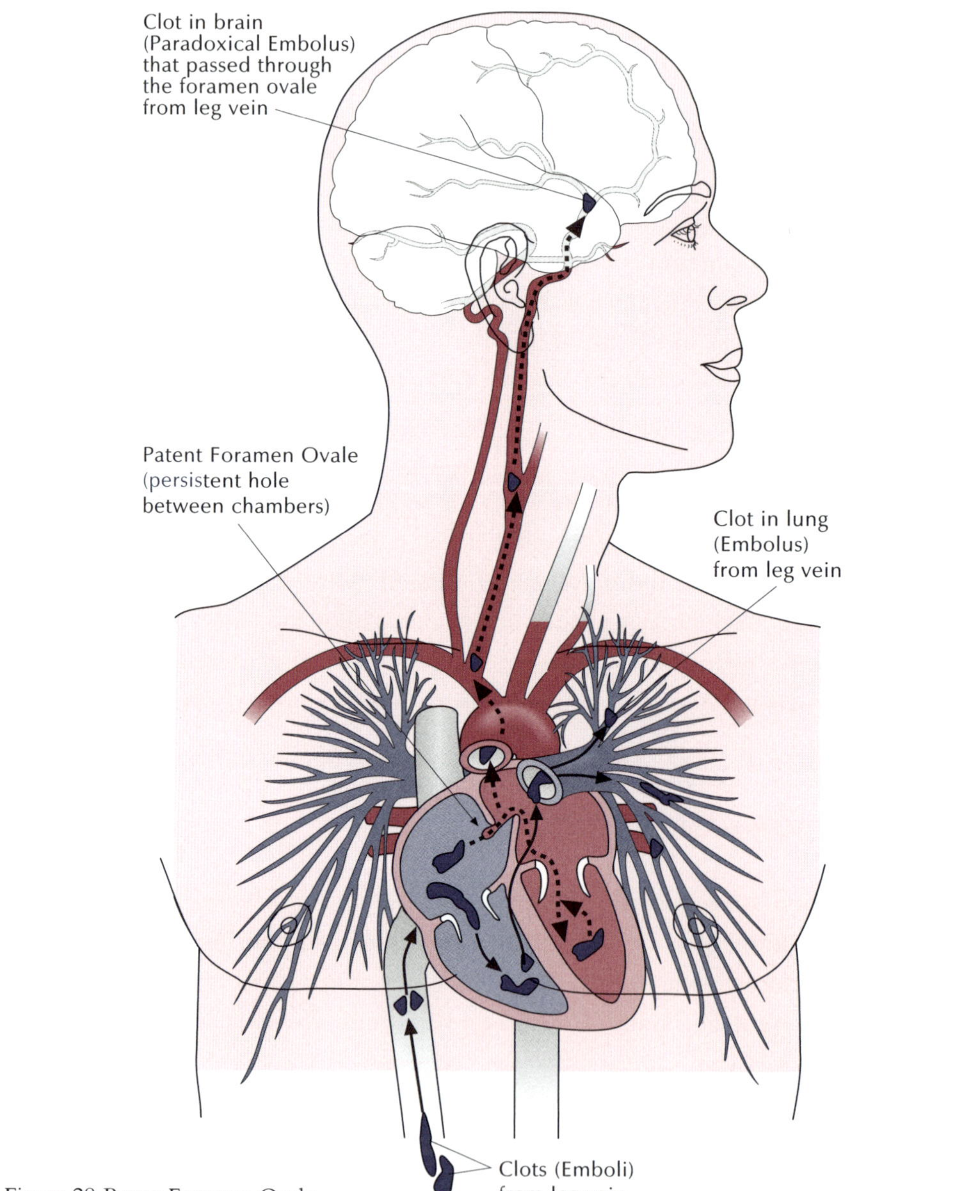

Figure 28 Patent Foramen Ovale

someplace it would not be expected to go, crossing from the venous to the arterial circulation, it is called a *paradoxical embolus.* Therefore, whenever anyone has a stroke or a reversible neurologic deficit without an obvious explanation, a PFO with paradoxical embolization should be looked for. We also refer to a stroke with no apparent cause as a *cryptogenic stroke*. We know that the incidence of cryptogenic strokes is much higher in individuals who have PFOs. If someone has a cryptogenic stroke and then we find a PFO, the stroke is no longer cryptogenic; it is usually presumed to be secondary to the PFO.

In some individuals, the situation is made murky by finding more than one potential cause. For example, we recently took care of a 55-year-old man who had a limited stroke. He was found, by transesophageal echo, to have a sizable PFO. However, he also had thick plaque within the aortic arch. We know that the arch will embolize predominantly to the left brain, and that was the side of his stroke. To make it even more confusing, he had an ulcerated plaque in the left carotid artery. There were three potential causes for the stroke! This stroke wasn't cryptogenic, we just didn't know for sure which of these three possible causes was the culprit. We closed his PFO and then treated him with a platelet drug.

Another set-up for similar havoc is someone who has a PFO with a chronically elevated right atrial pressure. This could be someone with sleep apnea because these individuals routinely raise their right atrial pressures when they have long episodes without breathing. This elevation in pressure persists if the sleep apnea is not effectively treated. Any person with a PFO who also has lung disease causing an elevated pressure in the pulmonary artery is at risk. Since DVT is more likely to develop in such patients, this group of individuals is at particular risk for the occurrence of a paradoxic embolus.

Indeed, you don't have to have any of these mechanisms at the time of paradoxic embolism. The only necessary ingredients are pathologic clot formation in the leg or pelvic veins plus an open PFO. Since we all strain down many times during our day, and since that straining maneuver raises the right atrial pressure temporarily, we just need to dislodge a tiny clot at the same time we strain and, presto, it can readily be diverted across the hole in the atrial septum and it's on its way to the brain.

Not to create more fear, but the formation of small amounts of pathologic clot is likely more common than we know. The one thing we know for certain is that we have no reliable way of determining which people will and who won't form a pathologic clot at some point in their life.

Diagnosis of a PFO

A diagnosis of PFO is actually quite easy, but usually involves a procedure. A routine echocardiogram performed by placing the transducer on the chest wall will miss at least 50% of these structures, or at least those that are not blatantly obvious due to their size and inappropriate right-to-left flow because of high pressures. If, by chance, we clearly detect a PFO with a regular transthoracic echocardiogram, this is great. Frequently, however, we have to sedate the patient, pass a transesophageal echo (TEE) probe down the esophagus to a position behind the heart, and then inject agitated saline solution containing microbubbles into an intravenous port. We then press against the upper abdomen to raise the right atrial pressure. If a PFO is present, bubbles will pass from the right to the left atrium. If bubbles can cross the small hole within the atrial septum, a blood clot can do so as well. A seasoned operator can perform this test quite safely within about 20 minutes.

Treatment to Prevent Recurrent Paradoxical Embolus

If a PFO is found in an individual who has had a small stroke or a transient cerebral ischemic episode, the patient should be anticoagulated immediately with Heparin—a drug used intravenously—or a purified fraction of this drug called Lovenox, which can be given under the skin. This should be followed by ongoing Coumadin therapy. Coumadin is a commonly used oral anticoagulant that works by tying up the clotting factors in the liver. It has to be monitored by a Protime test.

At some point, the doctor should decide if this PFO should be closed. In the past, I felt strongly that the majority of these could be treated with chronic anticoagulant therapy. As the closure procedure becomes more routinely performed, I am rapidly changing my feelings regarding this.

There are two methods of closing a PFO:

1. One is the way we have been doing it for 30 years—open-chest surgery. A good cardiac surgeon can close one of these in about an hour. Of course, there is a recovery period, and there is some discomfort involved. Some are great surgical candidates. On the other hand, the person who is prone to DVT and paradoxical embolus is frequently not the best surgical candidate, usually because of a very high pulmonary artery pressure.
2. The second method of closure, currently much more acceptable, is that of implanting an occluding device via a catheter from the groin, utilizing

transesophageal echocardiography to guide proper placement. If you choose this procedure, make sure you find a cardiologist who has done at least 20 of them because it involves a fairly steep learning curve. I have witnessed a couple of real disasters when this was performed by a cardiologist who was not well trained in this complex maneuver. This is an effective and durable treatment, usually requiring only one day in the hospital—and when performed by someone seasoned in this technique, it can be done safely.

This occlusion device is a double flat button device attached by a stalk. One button goes on either side of the hole, then they are connected to one another by the stalk. When finished, the buttons are both snugged up against either side of the septum, effectively sandwiching the septum between the two buttons. With time, they will eventually become surrounded by the body's intrinsic walling-off mechanisms in response to a foreign substance. This will ultimately cause the entire device to become incorporated within the inter-atrium septum, with the result being nice, smooth walls containing no communicating corridor.

I have seen several individuals who had experienced a small stroke, were subsequently found to have a PFO, with no other explanation for their stroke, and yet no extensive evaluation was carried out to determine just how susceptible they were for a second event. Like anything else, this is a common-sense issue. That clot had to come from somewhere! It is the ultimate responsibility of the physician to determine the likelihood of a potentially catastrophic second embolus.

Another Major Question: How Extensive is the Clotting Process?

Just how aggressive is the pathologic clotting process and what triggered it to become activated? This question deserves an answer. In a conservative environment, it also helps decide whether or not to close the PFO. Also, it makes no sense to close the PFO, only to allow a large chunk of clot to subsequently travel to the lungs, perhaps with fatal consequences.

The presence of a clot anywhere in the body reflects a pathologic process. We are all clotting and breaking down clot every second of our lives. The two should be in balance. If we manufacture a clot anywhere except at the site of surgery, it represents a pathologic process.

The usual site of a pathologic clot is in the lower extremity venous system. This system, like all veins, carries blue blood back to the heart. There are a number of v-shaped valves originating from the wall of the larger veins in the legs. (See Figure 6, page 31) Blood is milked back toward the heart by the force exerted by muscle contraction, then that column of blood is held by this system of valves. If you perform a venogram (injecting contrast material that shows up on x-ray) into a foot vein and watch it being carried upwards to the heart, you are impressed by just how slowly venous blood from the legs moves along. Once you have seen this, it never comes as a surprise that someone could form a blood clot in these vessels. This is where over 90% of blood clots are formed; the remainder are formed within the pelvic veins.

Women who form pelvic vein clots have usually borne children or have experienced a serious pelvic infection or pelvic tumor. Men who form pelvic vein clots have usually had prostate cancer. Either sex may form a clot if they have had pelvic trauma, such as a fracture.

Several things can predispose a person to clot formation. The most common one is surgery, which increases overall clotting activity. In this instance, the tissue that was operated on has to clot in order to prevent continued bleeding. When the clotting system becomes activated by surgery, the deep venous system also is susceptible to clot proliferation. In other words, as much as we'd like it, we can't have selective clotting. Another common cause is trauma. Another is long distance travel, legs low and immobile, frequently accompanied by mild dehydration. And occasionally, the cause of abnormal clotting can be an unannounced cancer. There are also a number of thrombophilic disorders, mostly inherited, that cause inappropriate clot formation.

Sometimes the patient is diagnosed with a PFO with paradoxical embolus to the brain or to some other vital organ. Alarmingly, no extensive evaluation is carried out to detect the cause of the pathologic clot formation. We do know that "it just happens" in some people. However, if the clot that broke loose from the leg vein had not crossed the inter-atrial septum, it would have traveled on to the lungs, and it's likely that a different fragment did just that. The decision is usually made at this point to proceed with closure of the PFO. However, in my view, the work-up is not complete until the doctor has determined how much clot is present in the leg veins, whether or not some of it has embolized to the lungs, and whether there is some ominous underlying process that needs to be addressed after the PFO is closed.

For example, take an illustration of a limited CVA from pathologic clot formation in the leg veins, a small piece crossing the PFO. The plan should be to close the PFO as soon as feasible. If you knew there was extensive clot formation in the leg veins, you would want to place an inferior vena cava filter after the PFO is closed to prevent an overwhelming pulmonary embolus. This requires no more than an additional

10 minutes with almost no additional risk, but would afford immense protection against a pulmonary catastrophe.

The Risk of a Calamity with PFO Increases after the Fourth Decade

I have seen major calamities from simple PFOs that appeared after remaining dormant for many years. One was in a patient who was sent to me for cardiac evaluation, as he had experienced shortness of breath with exertion. He was 50 years old, overweight, had a previous cigarette smoking history, and also had a family history with his father's death from a heart attack at about his age. He came to see me with a stress echocardiogram in hand. This is done by performing an echo at rest, looking particularly at wall motion of the left ventricle. The patient is then exercised, usually on a bike or treadmill, and the echo is repeated after vigorous exercise, rechecking wall motion. If a coronary artery is tightly blocked, the segment of heart muscle supplied by that particular artery should become dysfunctional, contracting less vigorously, since it is starved for oxygen-rich blood. I examined him, reviewed his stress echo, and recommended a coronary angiogram. This was entirely normal! I reviewed these findings with him and his family and recommended further tests, including electrophysiologic testing, since he had developed a short run of ventricular tachycardia during his stress test. This is a serious arrhythmia that usually points to some form of heart disease. I also recommended a transesophageal echocardiogram and a lower extremity venous Doppler test. I wanted to be sure he didn't have DVT and hadn't embolized a blood clot from his leg veins to his lungs. I also recommended a sleep study, as I felt he might well have sleep apnea. He looked the part, as he had a large amount of jowl adipose (fat) tissue in the neck. He declined, telling me that he had researched his situation on the Internet and found that a normal coronary angiogram was associated with an overall excellent outlook. I agreed that it usually did, but again discussed with him the fact that we did not have the entire picture with regard to his situation. One week later, he released a blood clot from a leg vein, part of which traversed a large PFO and entered the arterial circulation, a paradoxical embolus. Almost all of these will travel north—a straight shot—to the brain and result in a stroke. This one bounced about in the aortic root and entered the left main coronary artery. He immediately began having the world's biggest heart attack, as the left main gives off branches supplying 90% of the heart muscle. He was taken into the operating room, the clot was removed, and the PFO was repaired. Unfortunately, the man died in cardiogenic shock.

To show you how silent a PFO can be, I never considered that he might have such a thing when I initially evaluated him. I just knew, after the negative coronary angiogram, that he had *something*. I figured it was pulmonary hypertension, perhaps from sleep apnea. I did know that he needed further evaluation; I did not suspect a PFO.

This is not to scare you. Most paradoxical emboli through a PFO are small, causing a warning flag to be hoisted. We can never ignore this. It might never happen again but, on the other hand, it well might, this time with dire results.

No dramatic story regarding these silent communications between the venous and arterial circulation illustrates the danger better than Ariel Sharon's stroke last year. As I understand it, his doctors detected the PFO and were preparing to close it when his large stroke developed. These things have an amazing capacity to remain completely silent for many decades. Then, when something comes along that will raise the right atrial pressure, the flap will hinge-lift off the hole and if there is any clot traversing the right side of the heart, it may well cross the septum on its way to the brain, carrying with it incredible devastation. In an instant, a silent hole in the heart from birth can change a life forever.

More Aggressive Closure Recommended from Newer Studies

In the past, I thought it was absolutely crazy to close these PFOs *before* a major paradoxic embolus had occurred. I have recently had a couple of these, previously silent except for a tiny transient ischemic attack, who went on to have major strokes while on Coumadin. I am changing my mind about how to manage this problem, somewhat influenced by these two patients and also by the fact that the people who routinely perform these closures are getting quite good at them. I subscribe to the eloquent quote by Sir William Osler regarding learning from patients, "To study the phenomenon of disease without books is to sail an uncharted sea, while to study books without patients is not to go to sea at all."

There are increasing numbers of people climbing very high mountains like Everest and some of these have had little strokes probably due to clot through PFOs that they didn't know about. There are more people scuba diving. We have several people who have had small strokes while diving, this time with tiny bubbles crossing the PFO.

There are proponents of closing these, even if the person has had no problem with it whatsoever. The argument is compelling. Why wait until someone has a stroke? After a stroke, your life is changed. If you are lucky, it is minimally changed. But why take that risk?

I've struggled with some of these concepts for years. We know that about 2% of individuals have "dangerous" PFOs—ones that are open all the time. We also know that clot formation in the deep veins of the legs is the world's most silent disease. We know that individuals are much more likely to have leg vein clots after age 40, increasing dramatically after age 50. *DVT plus a PFO can be a deadly duo.*

In large centers that do a lot of them, the closure of a PFO with a device takes less than 30 minutes and is associated with an extremely low complication rate. The patient goes home the same day. I think that if my 17-year-old daughter were found to have one of these perpetually open PFOs, I would want it closed.

The catch is that, in America at least, you must have failed anticoagulation therapy (had a second event while on Coumadin) or have had a complication of anticoagulation in order to receive a closure device. I feel sure this will change—and soon. The data is too good. However, I want to repeat my caveat: If you get this done, make sure it is performed by a seasoned operator.

The Migraine Story

The main reason I have adapted a more aggressive stance regarding closure of asymptomatic PFOs has to do with the dramatic advances in the closure technique. The individual is sedated, the groin is punctured, a catheter is inserted, and the device is deployed. I must also tell you, however, that some of my change of heart has to do with what I refer to as the migraine story. There are a huge number of migraine sufferers. This is frequently a nuisance in the first three or four decades of life, then it becomes associated with a higher incidence of stroke. For years, people have suggested that PFOs might be playing a role, as the incidence of cryptogenic stroke (remember, stroke without apparent cause) increases dramatically just about the time when deep venous thrombophlebitis also starts to become a problem, about age 50 and beyond.

The theory is that many individuals prone to migraines may get tiny clots across their inter-atrial septum due to a PFO, and this triggers the migraine event. It has never been proven; however, the theory has been strengthened by a clinical study that was recently completed. It turns out that if you take all patients who have the combination of migraine syndrome and a PFO, closure of the PFO with a device results in a "cure" from the migraine syndrome in almost 50%, as compared to 20% who received a "sham" procedure, just a little nick in the groin but nothing done to repair the PFO.

This doesn't prove the paradoxic embolus theory in migraine. It *does* buttress its validity, though. It also makes me wonder if far more people don't have little clots crossing a PFO than we had previously thought.

REMINDERS

1. PFOs are present in a substantial percentage of the population. They usually pose no problem and remain asymptomatic.
2. Any stroke or transient cerebral ischemic event without obvious cause should be evaluated with transesophageal echocardiography to determine if a PFO is present. A paradoxical embolus anywhere in the body (heart attack without coronary disease, embolus to the gut, etc.) should also pose a similar challenge.
3. If you have a PFO and paradoxical embolism, you should either be anticoagulated indefinitely, or have the PFO repaired. I am leaning toward recommending closure of the PFO with a device performed in a center where a great number of these are being done.
4. Risk assessment should be carried out in each person with a PFO and a paradoxical embolus. If, for example, the leg veins are full of clot, the spontaneous dislodgement of any of this could be calamitous, especially if a previous blood clot had traveled to the lungs, raising the pressure in the right ventricle.
5. If you decide to get your PFO closed with a device inserted through a catheter introduced from a groin vein, make sure your cardiologist has done at least 20 of them previously. This is not a procedure performed by all cardiologists.
6. If you have migraine syndrome, get screened for the existence of a PFO. There is now fairly compelling evidence that these may be related, at least part of the time.
7. I recommend that every young person have an echocardiogram in his or her teens. The reason would be to screen for an obvious PFO, one open all the time, but any form of congenital structural problem could also be detected.

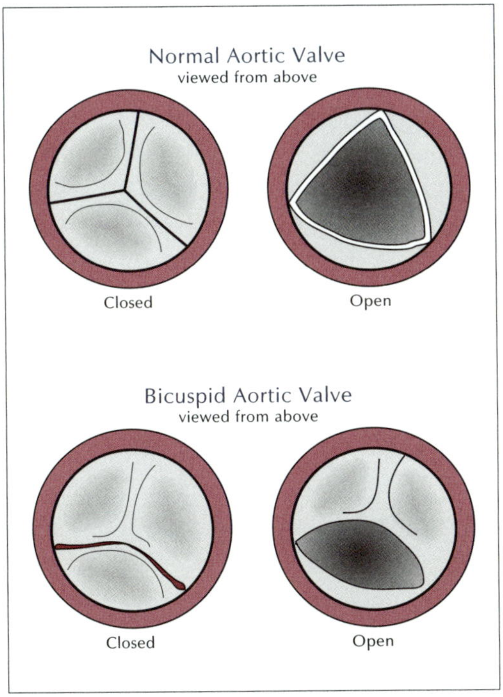

85

VALVULAR HEART DISEASE

Strange Noise in the Heart

A COMMON PROBLEM AT ALL STAGES OF LIFE, but progressively more common from the 50s on, is *valvular heart disease*. Some of these problems are due to a deformed valve from birth with eventual degeneration due to the abnormal structure of the valve. Others are due entirely to wear and tear over the years, usually showing up as substantial issues later in life. Many are a combination of the two. In years past, we wouldn't replace a valve when the individual was quite elderly. Now, with refinement of techniques, not to mention greater expectations and demands, it is common to replace a diseased heart valve up to age 85 and, in certain remarkable instances, beyond.

I. Aortic Valve Disease

Bicuspid Aortic Valve: Anatomy

The aortic valve, the check valve between the left ventricular pump and the giant blood tube, the aorta, should be of three-leaflet construction to allow for easy excursion when the heart pumps, and equally easy and effective closure and competency when the heart is relaxed. A bicuspid valve, comprised of only two leaflets due to a failure of the third leaflet to form as it should in-utero, is a fairly common congenital defect. (Figure 29) This anomaly results in very little trouble in most people until their forties or fifties and, oftentimes, much later. Indeed, there are variations on this theme,

Figure 29 Aortic Valve

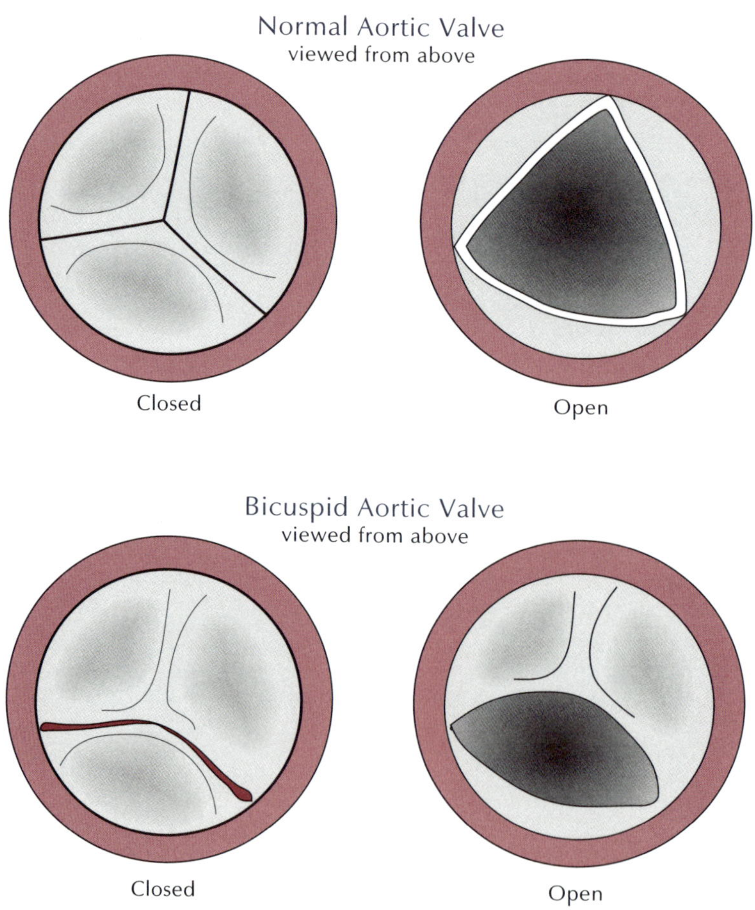

some of these valves being substantially distorted, others performing remarkably well. There is even a difference in orientation of the line of opening and closure between the larger and smaller of the two leaflets. One spatial orientation results in the valve becoming obstructive to flow, referred to as *aortic stenosis*. The other orientation results in predominant leakage of blood back into the left ventricle, a situation known as *aortic insufficiency*. The anatomic orientation of this congenitally malformed valve then, essentially defines the ultimate hemodynamic fault (whether it leaks or causes obstruction to blood flow).

Bicuspid Aortic Valve: Symptoms and Clinical Course

Some of these valves initially make very little noise to announce their malformation. Indeed, we have seen many men who got into the military 20 or 30 years ago, performed well, only to claim our attention when a murmur, a vascular sound produced by turbulence of blood passing through this deformed valve under pressure, became loud.

With time, almost all of these valves will develop enough of an abnormality that they will need replacement. Depending on the degree of distortion, this may occur as early as the third or fourth decade, or as late as the sixth, seventh, or even eighth. The leaflets become thickened, less pliable, and move less readily. This produces either the murmur of aortic stenosis, a harsh murmur, or evidence of profound leakage, aortic insufficiency, also known as aortic regurgitation.

The symptoms presented by the two possibilities are quite different. First, let us consider the symptoms and findings of aortic stenosis. When the aortic valve narrows, limiting more and more the effective emptying of the left ventricle into the aorta, it puts a greater strain on the left ventricular pump. Additionally, since there is obstruction to flow, the pressure will be much lower in the aorta than in the left ventricle during systole, when the aortic valve is open. This pressure drop across the aortic valve is called a gradient. When it exceeds 50 mmHg or with exercise, increases to greater than 60 or so, the valve will need to be watched carefully with an eye toward replacement in the very near future. Such individuals are entering the range where just a slight increase in fusion of the leaflets will markedly increase the gradient. It takes a long time to go from a 10 mmHg gradient up to a 50 mm gradient; however, only a short while is required for this 50 mm gradient to make it to 75 mm. When chest pain, light-headedness, blackout, or profound shortness of breath develop with exertion, the valve should be replaced without delay, as this person has entered a phase marked by sudden death.

If we are seeing someone regularly, we rarely let these valves get tightly stenotic enough to cause such ominous symptoms. Ideally, one could argue, it would be best to wait as long as possible. However, everyone who does this sort of work has at least one remembrance of having waited too long, and the patient skipped an appointment, or some other occurrence happened that caused the valve replacement to be postponed until it was too late. Unfortunately, there is a point where any increase in wall stress imposed on the left ventricle will result in fiber stretch, and "slippage," of the elements necessary for contraction of the muscle cells. When this occurs and the left ventricle begins to lose contractile properties and enlarges, it is becoming too late to replace the valve and expect recovery of pump function. Consider an obstruction posing a 90 mmHg gradient across the aortic valve. If the blood pressure in the arm is 120/80, the pressure in the left ventricle is 120 plus 90, or 210 mmHg. This puts a huge burden on the left ventricle. It can't perform long under this extreme duress.

My one case experience that is imprinted in my mind occurred when I was chief cardiac fellow on the clinical service in Denver. A farmer from western Kansas, who grew a huge acreage of wheat, came into the hospital with severe aortic stenosis. His gradient was 100 mmHg at rest but despite this, his left ventricular function remained quite normal. We recommended aortic valve replacement without delay. He declined, as wheat harvest was about to begin. We discussed the risks of waiting, outlining to him the possibility that the ventricle could dilate to the point of no return due to fiber slippage. He shrugged it off. He returned, not in one month as he promised, but three months later, weighing 50 pounds more, all water. He was in florid congestive heart failure, his left ventricle had almost doubled in size, and contractility had diminished to the point where one could barely discern which was systole and which was diastole on the echocardiogram. He underwent aortic valve replacement, as it was the only maneuver that could possibly save his life. However, he died—by inches—over the next three months. His left ventricle simply couldn't recover function. This underscores the admonition that you can't wait on this problem to cause symptoms. Then, it is frequently too late for the heart to recover.

The findings, changes, and symptoms are entirely different if the aortic valve predominantly leaks blood back into the left ventricle. With this situation, a variable percentage of the blood that is pumped into the aorta with each beat leaks back into the left ventricle, necessitating a repeat handling of that volume of blood. When this is severe, the left ventricle will eventually enlarge in size, a dilatation of the left ventricle. Again, it can progress to only such a point before fiber stretch occurs, a point of no return by the left ventricle. If this dilatation is only modest, the ventricle has a remarkable capacity to reconfigure itself back to a normal size and, frequently, normal contractility will become reestablished. If, however, the left ventricle has dilated dramatically, especially if accompanied by reduction in the contractile function of the pump, it will no longer be capable of repairing itself. Timing is everything!

Just as the findings of aortic stenosis and aortic regurgitation are profoundly different, the symptoms are as well. With obstructive aortic stenosis, chest pain, blackout or dizziness, and shortness of breath are markers of a tight valve. With aortic insufficiency, severe shortness of breath, associated with evidence of congestive heart failure, are the presenting features.

An echocardiogram is the most important test in the evaluation of the severity of the aortic valve distortion and the degree of impairment it is imposing upon the proper handling of the blood. This is a great follow-up management tool, showing progression or lack thereof on yearly examinations. This test is also great because, unlike some, it causes no deleterious effects, such as radiation.

Before we replace the aortic valve, we perform cardiac catheterization, placing catheters to directly measure the degree of obstruction and leakage, the status of the left ventricle and perhaps just as importantly, the status of the coronary arteries.

One caveat is in order for individuals who have a bicuspid aortic valve. There is an association with problems within the *aorta* itself, out past the valve. The most common association is that of coarctation, a fibrous band constricting flow through the descending portion. These are almost always picked up in the young. The other association, fortunately much less common, occurs later in life. This is dissection of the ascending aorta, that portion just above the valve. I think this is largely due to the high velocity jet generated by the valve striking the wall of the aorta, inflicting decades of injury, thickening, and ultimate degeneration of the wall of the aorta. Thankfully, this is very uncommon.

Degenerative Aortic Valve Disease

These aortic valves are normal (three leaflet in construction) at birth only to degenerate progressively with each passing decade until they markedly alter hemodynamics. We are not sure why this occurs in some but not in others. It has to do with tendency of the valve structure to calcify—to form calcium deposits within the valvular tissue and between the leaflets—this closure point being called the commissure. This tendency is greater in the male sex, and is more common in those who have hypertension, resulting in greater hemodynamic stresses imposed on the valve; it is also accelerated in those with coronary artery disease.

We used to be sent patients with an aortic murmur and we would listen to them, perform an echo, which would invariably show some mild thickening, and we would then dismiss them as having *aortic sclerosis*, a harmless thing. We would usually reassure them that it would not cause trouble, as long as they took antibiotics when they got their teeth cleaned so as to prevent endocarditis, since these roughened valves are prone to infection. We have become aware of the fact, however, that commonly these valves eventually develop profound deterioration, with larger and heavier nodularity, until they become rigid. The alarming fact is that, under the microscope, the process looks just like arteriosclerosis: cholesterol plaques that form in arteries! These valves are *not* the benign, innocent structures we thought 30 years ago. We now have data showing an eventual 50% increase in cardiovascular mortality if you have a thickened aortic valve!

Finding this type of degenerative valvular process, seemingly artherosclerotic in nature, is strengthened by the finding, at least in my practice, that this is dramatically accelerated in those with metabolic syndrome. This is a syndrome marked by abdominal obesity, elevated triglycerides, insulin-resistance type diabetes, an increase in inflammatory markers, elevated LDL-cholesterol frequently of the dense particle type, and a low HDL-cholesterol. The finding of any three of these makes the diagnosis—and it is present in roughly 25% of the adult population in America. There is something about obesity, in that inflammation seems to be triggered, and this valve sometimes is the target structure—the heart the ultimate target organ—of this increasingly prevalent disorder. This is the reason the syndrome has morphed into the "cardiometabolic syndrome."

These abnormal valves seldom reach the stage of severity where replacement is considered prior to the sixth or seventh decade of life. Alas, such patients are frequently not ideal candidates for aortic valve replacement because of additional health problems.

I now treat all of these individuals (with this degenerative aortic valve that came normal from the factory) as though they have arteriosclerotic coronary artery disease, controlling their hypertension scrupulously, correcting any inflammatory markers or elevated cholesterol with statins. The aortic valve isn't really serviced by feeder arteries so this isn't the problem. We now believe that there must be inflammatory substances in the bloodstream to result in this strange disease. I personally think this sort of valvular degeneration is a red flag, pointing out the tendency to have a cardiac event due to an enhanced inflammatory state. As such, I treat it just exactly the same way I treat someone who has metabolic syndrome with a previous heart attack. My justification for this approach is that, when you look at the numbers, the incidence of cardiovascular death is about the same for the two.

II. Mitral Valve Disease

The mitral valve, remember, is the valve between the left atrium and the left ventricle, and the predominant cause of mitral valve disease and dysfunction has changed drastically during the last 30 years. Back then, at the tail-end of the rheumatic fever epidemic that raged during the 1930s through the 1950s, these valves were often terribly distorted from smoldering inflammation. This is what we call rheumatic heart disease. With the advent of penicillin in the early 1940s, "strep throat" caused by a streptococcus, could be readily treated. I have not seen a case of rheumatic fever for many, many years. Slowly, the patients with rheumatic heart disease are leaving us, not to be replaced by similar individuals. The rheumatic heart saga has almost reached its final chapter, at least in this country.

Now, mitral valve dysfunction is caused by one of two processes, almost equal in their contribution. One is caused by coronary artery disease, the other a primary degenerative process within the valve.

Mitral Regurgitation Associated with Ischemic Cardiomyopathy

With a heart attack, the mitral valve competency may be compromised due to infarction—injury from the heart attack—of the papillary muscle. This is the muscle protrusion from the wall of the left ventricle to which the thin strands attach to the valve tissue to the left ventricle insert. Another form of heart attack–induced mitral valve incompetence is that of progressive dilatation of the left ventricle, called an *ischemic cardiomyopathy*. In certain instances, the mitral valve ring may become so stretched out that the leaflets no longer grip against one another tightly enough to prevent escape of blood back into the left atrium when the left ventricle contracts in its pumping action. In this instance, mitral valve replacement should be considered. However, increasingly, we are using a rigid mitral valve ring to cause better apposition of the mitral valve leaflets, frequently along with endeavors to improve the geometry of the left ventricle, a feature that we have learned to be of great importance in function. In fact, we think the left ventricular geometry is of *paramount* importance in these sick ventricles.

Myxomatous Degeneration with Mitral Valve Prolapse

The other process that vies for dominance is that of mitral valve degeneration from a process known as *myxomatous degeneration*. This usually occurs in a valve that is quite redundant and frequently produces the diagnosis of mitral valve prolapse. This, however, is at the far extreme end of the spectrum of *mitral valve prolapse*, as this valve comes from the factory with an abnormal composition of the connective tissue frame on which the valve was constructed. As this degeneration progresses, the valve becomes more and more incompetent until it leaks profoundly. It may well have to be replaced or better yet, repaired, at that point. In circumstances of elongation of the mitral valve chordae, the support strands, or valve tissue redundancy, we now have very nice reparative procedures for these. In fact, at least 50% of these valves can be repaired.

Yet another variation on this theme is that of a mitral valve chordal rupture. The chordae tendinae are these 32 flimsy-appearing strands, like parachute cords, traveling from their insertion in the papillary muscle, a natural extension of the left ventricular muscle, to the valve tissue. In the event of myxomatous degeneration, these tiny chordae may become degenerative as well and one or more may rupture resulting in wide open mitral regurgitation. This causes florid congestive heart failure, as the lungs are flooded with blood that is leaking wildly back into the left atrium. This constitutes a medical and surgical emergency. Many of these valves can be effectively repaired, the preferred approach. If not, mitral valve replacement is done without delay.

In the past, we watched these myxomatous mitral valves carefully, as many of them leaked only moderately, and we were more casual in our approach. We have all been impressed that bad things seem to happen if you assume this watch-and-wait posture. Suggesting that these minimally symptomatic individuals go ahead and have their mitral valve either repaired or replaced is one of the hardest things to get across. This leakage increases slowly, the left ventricle slowly enlarging in lockstep, and the symptoms occur insidiously as well. People "accommodate" this subtle change and don't sense any urgency. I had one such patient in my practice recently. I had followed his degenerative myxomatous valve for years. Finally, the valve became thickened enough that it began to leak noticeably more, and his left ventricle was getting larger. I recommended valve replacement with a tissue valve, as he was 73 years old. He declined, saying he would get it done if he got short of breath. He died suddenly at home just two months later. These valves, previously thought to be fairly benign entities, more of academic interest than anything else, have taught us to intervene earlier than we habitually thought necessary.

III. Tricuspid Valve Disease

The tricuspid valve is the valve between the right atrium and the right ventricle and is somewhat similar in design to its counterpart on the left side, the mitral that we have been discussing. The tricuspid valve is not nearly as complex as the mitral valve, probably because it has much less importance, working as it does on the low pressure side of the heart. It rarely has to be replaced. It sometimes has to be repaired, since long-standing pulmonary hypertension, a high blood pressure in the pulmonary artery carrying blue blood to the lungs, will cause the right ventricle to become enlarged, the tricuspid ring patulous (enlarged and "sagging"), and the valve incompetent. We usually repair this valve with insertion of a ring, to which the tricuspid annular tissue is sewn, restoring once again a competent valve.

Carcinoid Syndrome

An unusual form of valvular dysfunction can result from a tumor. This tumor, called a carcinoid tumor, is primary in the colon. If it metastasizes to the liver, it can produce enough serotonin that the first valve the blood comes into contact with, the tricuspid valve, becomes markedly distorted resulting in severe regurgitation. This substance is secreted because this tumor is comprised of what is known as neuroendocrine tissue. The serotonin is secreted by the tumor. If it spreads to the liver, the serotonin enters the blood stream and causes symptoms—flushing and diarrhea—that flash a warning that something is severely wrong. We can find the tumor by doing a CT scan of the liver and we can determine that it is elaborating the chemical by measuring an end product of break-down, called 5-HydroxyIndoleAceticAcid (5-HIAA). This is treated by a combination of surgery and chemotherapy.

In large quantities, the chemical can also affect the next valve the blood comes into contact with, the pulmonic valve. This is less usual. By the time the blood gets to the left-sided heart valves, the substance has been rendered harmless by its pass through the lungs.

IV. Pulmonic Valve Disease

There are only a couple of ways that this valve warrants consideration. One of these is a congenital malformation, called valvar pulmonic stenosis. This is a congenitally abnormal valve and, if significant, is obvious at birth. I have seen a few of these just mildly deformed coming to attention in the middle years. Another way is to have the valve overwhelmed by dramatic elevation of the pressure in the pulmonary artery carrying blue blood to the lungs to pick up oxygen.

V. Endocarditis

Endocarditis is an infection, usually with a bacterium, on a heart valve. There are certain bacteria that have an amazing propensity to set up housekeeping on a heart valve. Two that come to mind are staphyolococcus aureus (on the skin) and the bacterium that commonly causes pneumonia, the pneumococcus—streptococcus pneumoniae. These can attack any valve, but are much more apt to land on a deformed valve, one that is thickened and produces turbulence. The tendency to do this is so great that, when we culture one of the organisms from the blood stream, we assume that it has formed a "culture" on a heart valve. This necessitates a longer course of antibiotics than would otherwise be required; however, you can't take a chance with one of these, as eventual valve destruction, causing the need for valve replacement, is often the price paid for a shortcut course of treatment. If there is widespread destruction of the valve tissue, or if part of the bacterial growth has fragmented, this valve should be replaced without delay, using a pericardial tissue valve.

Fungal infections can also develop. This usually occurs in immunologically compromised patients, such as those on immunosuppressants as protection against rejection of a transplanted organ, people using steroid suppression against a connective tissue disease, or HIV patients with faulty immune systems. It can also occur in individuals who have been treated extensively with broad-spectrum antibiotics.

Any physician in a big city hospital will have seen several cases of endocarditis from self-injection of drugs. Not only are the contents not sterile, the needle is often dirty, and the skin is never prepped. This is frequently tragic. It seems that normal valves are even susceptible if there is enough of a bacteria load injected. The most susceptible valve is the first the blood comes into contact with, the tricuspid valve. If someone comes in with lung abscesses (little pockets of infection in the lungs) one of the causes we think about first is injection of dirty material, resulting in tricuspid endocarditis, with embolization of some of this infectious culture to the lungs. The lungs tend to filter out bacteria so the other valves, the left-sided ones, tend to escape.

VI. Taking Care of Your Abnormal Valve

Lots of people know they have an abnormal valve. This ranges all the way from a deformed valve from birth to a valve that, with the passage of time, has thickened, calcified, and is now susceptible to infection if bacteria enter the blood stream. We know that a certain percentage of individuals will have bacteria that can be cultured from the blood as they exit the dental office after dental cleaning or manipulation. This percentage approaches 25%. Therefore, if you have a distinctly abnormal heart valve, be sure to obtain antibiotics to use as a prophylactic measure so that you can destroy the bacteria promptly as they enter the blood stream. You don't need to take an antibiotic for days before the procedure, just a couple of hours prior, so that you have a good blood level of the antibiotic when the procedure is done, and for a few hours following.

Valve Surgery

When a heart valve is diseased enough, we resort to some sort of valve surgery. This used to consist of replacement of the valve with either a tissue or a mechanical valve. We have used a tricuspid ring for a stretched-out tricuspid valve for decades, as we sorely hated to insert a valve of any kind in this low-flow right-heart position. Now, we use the ring for tightening up the mitral valve as well, especially in situations whereby the mitral valve problem is secondary to a severely impaired left ventricle—mitral valve repair and ventricular reconstruction together to restore the best contractile left heart pump possible after a devastating heart attack. In some circumstances, the surgeons are repairing the mitral valve. Certainly, over the last ten years, a great deal of creative energy has gone into reconstructing these valves in ways that we would not have thought feasible some few years ago.

REMINDERS

1. **The most common congenital heart problem in adults is a bicuspid aortic valve (it is two leaflets; it should be three).**
2. **Depending on the spatial orientation of the aortic bicuspid valve, predominant obstruction to flow, aortic stenosis, or predominant aortic insufficiency, a leakage, will result.**
3. **Timing of valve replacement is important. In aortic stenosis, we can**

usually judge appropriateness of valve replacement by the severity of the pressure drop across the aortic valve, the gradient, and the status of contractility of the left ventricular pump. You cannot wait on symptoms to tell you when to replace this valve!

4. Timing of aortic valve replacement with aortic regurgitation is much less important but should be done when the left ventricular pump starts to enlarge just slightly in size. If you wait too long, fiber slippage will have occurred and the pump will never return to its normal strength.
5. An infection of a valve is always serious. This is called endocarditis. A prolonged course of antibiotics is usually necessary to cure this. Sometimes the heart valve has to be replaced.
6. As with anything, it is better to prevent endocarditis than to treat it. The best way to do this is to use dental and surgical antibiotic prophylaxis if you have a markedly deformed valve, and to get in early for antibiotics if you develop pneumonia or a staph infection. Elderly people should get a pneumovac injection as a vaccine against acquired pneumococcal infection (the usual cause of pneumonia).
7. If you are told you need mitral valve surgery, make sure you obtain the services of a heart surgeon who is comfortable repairing the valve. For replacement choices, refer to Chapter 25 *Artificial Heart Valves Versus Tissue Valves*.

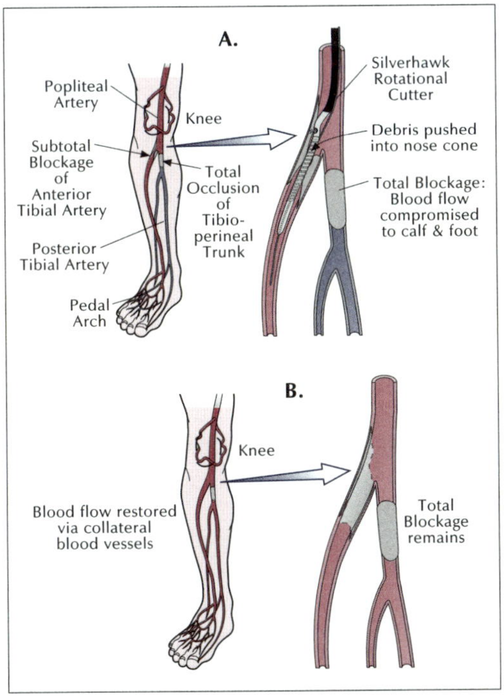

PERIPHERAL ARTERIAL DISEASE

Blockage of the Arteries to the Lower Extremities

PERIPHERAL ARTERIAL DISEASE (PAD) IS ATHEROSCLEROTIC plaque (cholesterol deposition within the wall of the arteries) in any of the arterial blood vessel branches to the lower extremities. It very seldom attacks the arm vessels except for the mouth of the subclavian artery. For practical purposes, I'll refer to that separately due to its unique presentation.

An Insidious Disease

There certainly is no more insidious disease than PAD. This disease cries out for regular exercise. If you are sedentary, arterial obstruction is frequently quite far advanced before you even become aware of it. By then, one of the predominant culprit vessels in PAD may well be totally occluded, with development of collaterals. These collaterals, tiny blood vessels that develop around a total blockage, are almost always adequate enough to prevent you from losing the limb with initial occlusion. However, they commonly do not provide adequate blood flow to prevent leg pain with exercise, called claudication, unless you really are quite sedentary. Subsequent to this, if any downstream vessel becomes compromised by a blockage (a common occurrence with this disease) the viability of the foot may become jeopardized and now we have no way to get to it, as the upstream vessel is totally occluded (blocked). We have seen many sedentary patients with treacherous blood supply to the leg and absolutely no leg pain—but they didn't walk much at all! In such instances, limb salvage becomes the immediate mandate. This is always terribly shocking to someone who until recently had no clue that a problem was brewing just beneath the surface. It is equally shocking to us, their doctors, that they were getting along with it. But, as George Bernard Shaw said so eloquently, "Custom will reconcile people to any atrocity."

The Epidemic

We have a huge job of education ahead of us, as PAD is becoming epidemic. The major reason for the emergence of this problem is diabetes, which is becoming much more prevalent. Since PAD is a frequent complication of not only Type 1 but also Type 2 diabetes, it stands to reason that PAD is not far behind. Type 2 diabetes is the form you acquire after reaching maturity. In the past, we knew that individuals who develop Type 1 diabetes were at high risk of premature circulatory problems in the lower extremities. The course with Type 2 disease is much more variable. However, this problem—frequently in conjunction with another known risk factor, such as smoking, elevated cholesterol, or hypertension—presents a huge risk for ultimate development of some degree of PAD. The diabetes epidemic is often and progressively part of the so-called metabolic syndrome. This is a makeshift moniker used to corral a host of problems that seem to mingle together anyway. They include abdominal obesity, hypertension, elevated LDL-cholesterol (frequently of the dreaded dense small-particle variety), low HDL-cholesterol, elevated triglycerides, insulin-resistant diabetes, and now an elevated high-sensitivity C-reactive protein (hs-CRP, an index of inflammation). Any three of these conditions make the diagnosis which now becomes cardiometabolic syndrome. This makes a bit more sense because the end product of this syndrome is the development of generalized arteriosclerosis, frequently involving the lower extremity arteries. The discussion of this syndrome is not so scary until you receive the statistics: Over 50% of American adults are overweight and fully 25% of American adults are thought to have metabolic syndrome!

Another factor makes this entire scenario more frightening. One of the major problems with preserving viability of the lower extremities has to do with small vessel disease. This is *always* associated with diabetes and not with the conventional risk factors such as high blood pressure, cholesterol and other lipids, smoking, or even inflammatory markers. These risk factors certainly aggravate and accelerate large vessel disease in the lower extremities; however, the small vessel problem is strictly due to diabetes. Consequently, when the person with altered tissue perfusion (blood flow, providing oxygen and nutrients) secondary to diabetic small vessel disease also gets large vessel disease, limb salvage becomes the order of the day. Unfortunately, this is not always possible because diabetes—in conjunction with the other known risk factors influencing large vessel disease—frequently results in what I call an *obliterative vasculopathy*. In this instance, there is virtual obliteration of the major vessels below the knees. The circulation is held together by a tenuous network of collateral blood vessels from one totally blocked artery to another in a desperate attempt to maintain limb-sustaining oxygen delivery. This process, widespread closure of the three major vessels below the knee, coupled with distal and small vessel disease, commonly leads to what we refer to as *critical limb ischemia* (CLI). Frequently with CLI, there is a non-healing ulcer of the foot, previously a prelude to almost certain amputation.

High Association with Coronary Artery Disease

Another reason to pay attention is the rather astounding association of this disease with arteriosclerosis of the coronary arterial circulation. Indeed, there is about a 5% yearly dropout of the PAD population each year due to coronary events. So when we make a diagnosis of PAD, we remain surveillant for the emergence of problems in the blood supply to the heart. The atherosclerotic risk factors are the same; therefore, attention to risk factors in treatment of one process treats the other as well.

Anatomy of the Circulation to the Lower Extremities

The anatomic arterial supply to the legs and feet is straightforward with little variation on the prototype. Basically, the abdominal aorta terminates in the lower abdomen, branching into the large iliac vessels, which continue to the groins where the femoral arteries begin. The major artery in the thigh is the superficial femoral artery. The other femoral branch, the profunda, may well save the leg in the event of superficial femoral occlusion, as the profunda will provide collateral vessels to bypass the obstruction so the downstream vessels can receive blood flow. The superficial femoral artery terminates at the knee level and transitions to the popliteal in the back of the knee. It, in turn, gives off the three branches below the knee, the so-called infra-popliteal arteries. These are the anterior and posterior tibial branches and the peroneal. These three vessels supply the foot. The anterior tibial comes off separately; the peroneal and posterior tibial come from the tibioperoneal trunk. The posterior tibial artery is the main artery to the calf muscles and foot; however, either tibial artery alone is usually sufficient to maintain tissue viability of the foot providing there is an adequate pedal arch communication in the foot.

Diagnosis of PAD

Since the toes are farthest away from the origin of arterial blood pumped by the heart, and since oxygen and nutrients are removed by the muscles all along the course of the arterial branches, it stands to reason that if there is obstruction at any level, the structures the greatest distance from the origin will suffer the most. Color, temperature, and ability or inability to grow hair are important observations when looking at the toes.

Actually, the ischemic (oxygen-deprivation) symptoms that limit activity are uniquely suited to the anatomic site of obstruction. For example, if the iliac artery is occluded, you get pain in that side of the buttock with walking. If, on the other hand, the superficial femoral is occluded, calf pain with exertion is more likely. If there is infrapopliteal disease (occlusion of the arteries below the knees) which is the type usually seen in diabetics, there may well be break down and ulceration in the skin of the toes. A good questioner and examiner can usually make a pretty good determination of the site of obstruction. This clinical impression is then corroborated by a Doppler exam. This is a test performed with an ultrasound machine that will tell us the direction and velocity of blood flow. It usually helps us decide whether or not further testing is necessary.

Of course, as in all cases of arterial obstruction, angiography is the gold standard. This is done by defining the wall of the artery with contrast material that stands out on x-ray film. In the past, this was entirely invasive, performed by introduction into the arterial system from the femoral artery. Now it can largely be handled on an outpatient basis, utilizing intravenous CT angiography. This will clearly identify the site(s) of obstruction and the status of collaterals, and will allow us to make a decision regarding the form of therapy most likely to be effective in each circumstance.

Treatment of PAD

In terms of treatment, surgical intervention was the only thing available for many years. Now we seldom refer a patient for surgery, though the problems are still just as difficult. They have just been, in large measure, transferred from the vascular surgeon to the interventional cardiologist.

The simplest vessel to work on is the largest vessel: the iliac artery. This vessel is so large and easy to get access to in most people, that we can usually convert a high-grade blockage to almost a normal appearance in about thirty minutes and can generally discharge the patient four hours later. This is exceptionally gratifying in that we can take patients who can barely walk from one room to another and render them totally asymptomatic with an iliac stent, a stainless steel mesh deployed by a balloon under high pressure. In deploying such a stent, we always incur some degree of damage to the inside of the artery when forcing the diseased wall outward to restore normal flow. Each artery will react uniquely to this damage. Some will react minimally; others will assertively increase scar-type tissue within the stent. The larger the artery, the more it can accommodate some degree of tissue proliferation within the stent and still retain a good opening for blood flow. These iliac arteries are usually so large that the stent deployment is satisfactory and the result is durable. Indeed, all but the most petite iliac arteries do well with stent deployment. These small vessels pose a larger problem, not only here, but also throughout the body.

Alas, iliac blockage is not common. The artery that most commonly becomes occluded in a non-diabetic patient is the superficial femoral just as it comes out of its muscular tunnel in the thigh, the so-called Hunter's Canal, in the region just above the knee. We all thought this would be a very easy vessel to treat when angioplasty balloons first came out. We quickly learned that it had an amazing tendency to re-block following angioplasty due to this injury-induced tissue build-up mentioned previously. When stents first came out, we certainly thought the problem was solved. To our dismay, these also reoccluded in a large percentage of patients. When Nitinol replaced stainless steel, our hopes again soared. In fact, the most aggressive tissue accumulation following stent-induced injury to the inside of a blood vessel is seen in the superficial femoral artery exactly at its emergence from this protective canal!

The most demoralizing thing in the world for the patient is to make repeated trips to the hospital or cath lab for the same problem, over and over. We make every effort not to stent the superficial femoral artery so we can avoid these repeat trips back for more work, as the incidence of restenosis (recurrent blockage) following a stent has to be in the neighborhood of 50%.

It would appear to me that currently the most effective and durable treatment for the superficial femoral artery is a cryoangioplasty system, utilizing a special balloon containing conduction coils. The balloon is inflated, at which time these coils are cooled dramatically with liquid nitrogen. This opens the artery wide but also creates an atmosphere, due to the cryo-injury, for subsequent cell death within the wall of the artery. We refer to this process as *apoptosis*. In the past, plain old balloon angioplasty caused injury to the wall and it responded with tissue accumulation that reblocked the artery. This balloon injury is different in that the cells in the wall of the artery drop out, with the subsequent fibrous tissue maintaining the integrity of the lumen (the central channel) of the artery. I've been able to achieve good long-term results in a large proportion of patients treated in this manner. (Figure 30)

If there isn't a great amount of calcium deposit in the plaque, another good approach is an athrectomy device: the SilverHawk. This device employs a rotational cutter and allows us to remove the inner core from the artery, concentrating on removing as much plaque as we can. This device offers the advantage of actually

Figure 30 Cryoangioplasty of the Femoral Artery

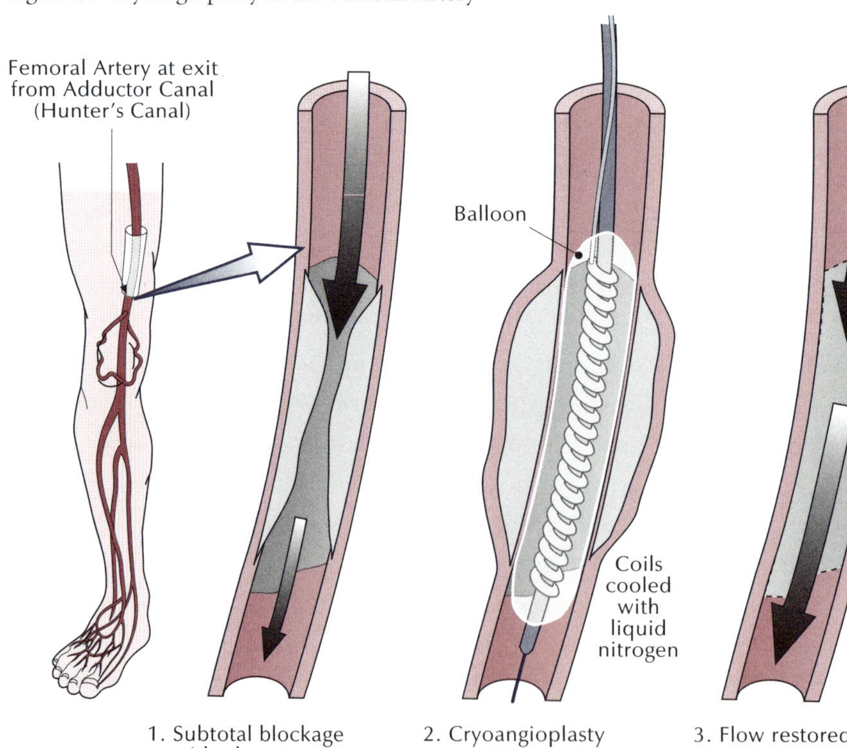

removing the arteriosclerotic plaque, cutting it away segment by segment, taking frequent angiograms to determine how much more work is necessary. It's very time-consuming, creates a good bit of radiation exposure to the patient as well as the interventionalist, and is frequently hampered by a dense deposit of calcium that seems to prefer the superficial femoral artery, especially in males.

Currently, these two procedures—cryoangioplasty and SilverHawk athrectomy—are the best approaches to effective treatment of high-grade superficial femoral artery blockages. They are much more durable than either the old-fashioned balloon angioplasty or stent deployment. Thus far, treatment of the superficial femoral artery has represented the most frustrating artery in the arterial circulation in terms of long-term results. We can make it beautiful by a variety of techniques. Getting it to remain wide open continues to be a major challenge for us.

The arterial branches below the knee, the infrapopliteal vessels, cause the most trouble *during* intervention. Like the limbs and branches of a tree, the farther you get from the trunk the smaller the branch. Think of the aorta as the main trunk, the iliac arteries as the major limbs, and the superficial femoral arteries as the large branches; then the infra-popliteal arteries are the small branches reaching the feet. These are frequently very small arteries and, particularly in diabetics, who make up well over 90% of patients with high-grade disease in these vessels, the disease is diffuse (scattered throughout). The athrectomy approach outlined above is rapidly gaining favor in these small arteries. (Figures 31a and 31b, page 414)

It is not too unusual to discover that an individual has closed off all but one infra-popliteal artery and, furthermore, the last remaining vessel is almost completely blocked off, frequently in multiple long segments. I refer to this as a lifeline artery, in that complete blockage of this last remaining artery will likely spell out eventual amputation of the limb below the knee. This represents, I think, a very challenging situation because many of these patients don't come in to see us until they've developed a non-healing ulcer on the foot. We then have to get to work on these leg vessels without delay in order to save the leg. There is a reason even more pressing than the obvious disability of amputation: When a leg is amputated, your mortality risk from a cardiovascular event increases. It increases even more with a second amputation. It's vitally important to hold onto these limbs.

If I see a lifeline vessel and it possesses only a single (or sometimes two) short, discreet blockage(s), I sometimes insert one or two of the drug-eluting coronary stents. These stents are impregnated with cancer drugs, either Taxol or Sirolimus. These drugs block the proliferation of cells. So while the stent is eluting the drug during about a

Figure 31a, 31b Infrapopliteal Disease & Silverhawk Repair

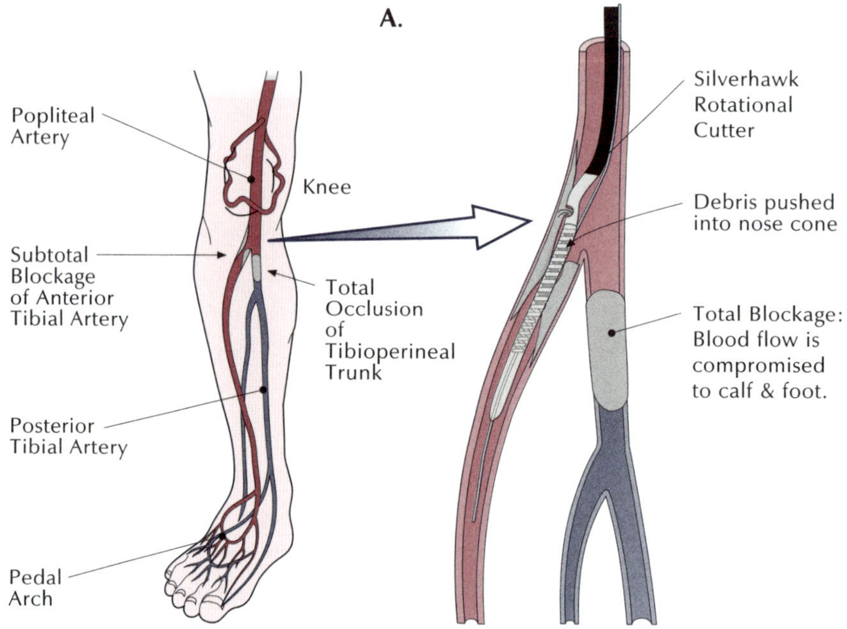

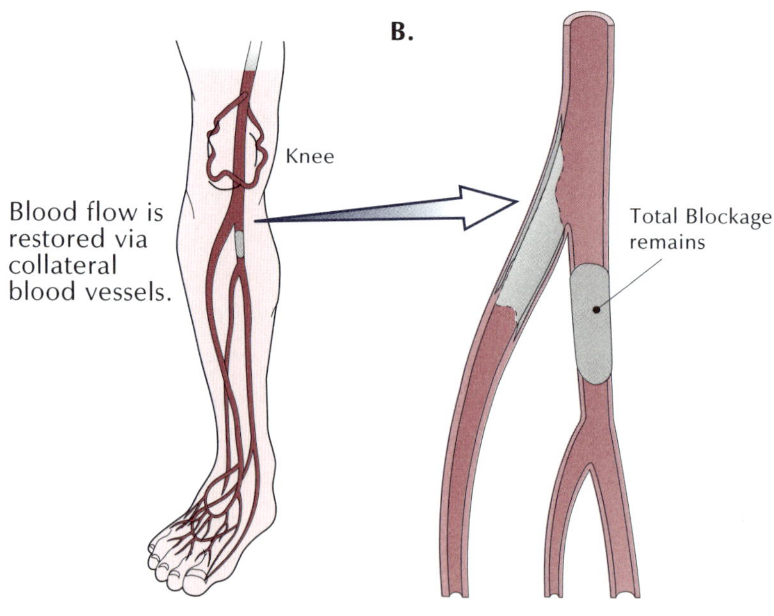

three-month period, the inside of the vessel, injured at the time of the deployment of the stent, is healing. This drug, then, prevents restenosis. This might seem expensive and drastic, but I assure you that it is usually much superior to other options and is much less expensive than repeated trips to the cath lab and perhaps eventual amputation. As in everything else in life, we need to fit the solution to the unique problem. The few patients who have received such treatment have all retained their limb and the artery is wide open. However, I make clear to the individual that this is an unapproved use. *Most* of these patients are not candidates for this anyway, as they have multiple, long segments of very high-grade blockage in the only remaining artery to the foot. We know that there is risk of delayed (late) closure of such stents months down the road. However, these patients with severe, diffuse peripheral arterial disease should receive indefinite treatment with platelet-active agents, aspirin and Plavix. If we are able to restore good flow, arteries treated in this manner should theoretically remain widely open.

Critical limb ischemia, usually from infrapopliteal disease, is so threatening that we may get only one shot at saving the limb. Because of this, we usually keep working assiduously on such a heavily diseased leg until we have at least one satisfactory straight line vessel from the knee to the foot and make sure that we have the most wide-open pedal arch communication possible. If we leave without at least one tibial open to the foot, there is overwhelming likelihood that the limb will eventually have to be removed. This vessel has to be one of the tibials, as the peroneal usually tapers off well shy of the foot. Occasionally, a large peroneal may provide enough collaterals to one of the tibial vessels that the limb can be salvaged; however, we usually must have at least one of the tibial arteries open in order to see wound healing of the ulcer that indicates successful limb salvage. This is now possible due to the long balloons, cutters, cold balloons, and drug-eluting stents in our ever-growing armamentarium. Sometimes we have to resort to a virtual storehouse of tools to get the job done and sometimes it takes a long, long time; however, we can usually provide a straight line artery to the foot. This procedure is not for everyone, as it takes a lot of commitment when the interventionalist could have done two other simpler cases in the same period of time. Be sure to choose as your interventionalist someone who does a lot of these and who is religiously and fanatically committed to keeping your leg just where it is.

Medical Treatment of PAD

So far, we have spent all of our time discussing intervention in PAD. There is a reason for this: We frequently don't see such a patient until the disease is so far advanced that we must intervene to improve the chances of limb salvage. In a busy cardiology practice performing peripheral intervention, we still amputate a large number of legs each year. It makes us sick at heart to have to resort to this, as it is life-changing and, with each amputation, life expectancy diminishes as well. In the past when we only had surgery to offer, we frequently treated PAD with medications until we had exhausted all efforts and then we performed surgery. It made no real difference whether the superficial femoral artery was 95% blocked or totally blocked. In either instance there was a variable degree of collateral development—small vessels "growing" around the total blockage as a God-given mechanism to retain the limb. Now, since we are intervening in most of these limbs with a catheter-based approach, it is *vitally* important that we retain an unblocked superficial femoral artery, as we have no other avenue to reach the vessels below it. Therefore, if the superficial femoral artery is 95% blocked, we feel a sense of urgency in preserving it as a pipeline to allow us to reach downstream branches when they become problematic.

There is no great pill to look to in treatment of PAD. We have some drugs that are widely touted to improve viscosity (like changing from 40 to 20 weight oil as winter approaches) and therefore enhance the flow of blood down partially blocked arteries. These are not terrific drugs and they do absolutely nothing to prevent progression of the disease.

We know that these vessels tend to remodel: Since flow down the smaller branches is frequently compromised, tiny clots frequently form, blocking off flow. Drugs that tie up clotting factors, such as Coumadin, are not terribly effective in these arterial branches. However, platelet-active drugs are quite effective. The old standby aspirin is one of them. A drug called Plavix is the strongest and the most effective drug in this regard, strongly exerting its action by preventing the attraction and aggregation of platelets in the blood stream. These microscopic elements, about a million or so per teaspoon, bring about the first stage in clot formation. If we can block platelets, we can interfere with clot formation and small vessel occlusion. These patients with PAD basically should *all* be treated with Plavix. These vessels also likely close because of the same plaque rupture that occurs within the coronary arteries. Additionally, they frequently possess sluggish flow. Plavix and aspirin help prevent the formation of clot in these zones.

Such patients should also be treated with drugs to prevent further progression of the arteriosclerotic process, including statin drugs for high cholesterol. These individuals deserve the same drastic reduction of LDL-cholesterol as those with coronary artery disease: levels in the 60–70 milligram per deciliter range. The statins are important for another reason: Plaques run in packs. This means that if one plaque has ruptured, paving the way for clot-formation and vessel closure, another is poised to do the same. The statins help to suppress this inflammation-triggered event.

These folks should also be urged to walk as much as possible as this will encourage the proliferation of collateral vessels. An aggressive walking schedule is probably the most important component of therapy, likely outweighing even the medication aspect. We have seen patient after patient with a number of totally blocked off arteries in the leg, yet due to an abundant proliferation of cascades of collaterals around total blockages, still have not only retained their limbs but also are actually capable of performing an extraordinary level of activity. There are two reasons: Collateral formation is especially prominent in the leg vessels and oxygen deprivation of the muscles in the legs promotes even further collateral formation. This is a unique situation. Of all the individuals who have coronary artery disease due to arteriosclerosis, some have absolutely no collaterals to the heart arteries as they close off and others have great collateral systems. However, *everybody* has the capacity to form collaterals in the lower extremity circulation. We need to engage this single plus and capitalize on it.

Obviously these individuals should be counseled to avoid tobacco. It is a vascular poison throughout the entire arterial circulation; however, it is a particularly bad with regard to PAD. We have seen many petite female smokers, for example, who have absolutely no evidence of arteriosclerosis in the coronary arteries, yet have terrible PAD. This doesn't happen in men, except as a very rare fluke. It does happen in women though. Continuation of cigarette smoking by those who have well-established PAD is a shortcut to amputation. It makes no sense to keep smoking, yet we see it every day! As doctors, we're committed to keeping your legs in their proper place: attached to your body. You must be, too. Don't throw away your life! As the Irish essayist George Bernard Shaw said, "Life is no brief candle to me. It is a sort of splendid torch which I have got hold of for the moment, and I want to make it burn as brightly as possible before handing it onto future generations." This is exactly the way I see it!

Finally, individuals with far advanced PAD, especially those with infrapopliteal disease, need to be educated in how to watch out for skin break-down over the toes. Once someone forms an infected ulceration on a foot, we have a horrible time salvaging the limb, especially if the infection has involved bony structures.

Surgery in PAD

If intervention via a catheter fails, many of the patients with above-the-knee problems can still be treated with surgical intervention. If surgery is required, it is usually for something like a total occlusion of a common femoral artery right in the groin or for a repeated failure in the superficial femoral artery. These can be bypassed using a procedure referred to as a femoral-popliteal bypass and, if there is good run-off distally down the infrapopliteal vessels, this is reasonably durable. If there is poor run-off due to diffuse disease in the small vessels downstream, it is generally a futile operation and one should search hard for an alternative answer.

We almost never refer a patient for a blockage in an iliac artery unless it becomes totally blocked before we see the patient and we are unable to find a freshly clotted channel through the total occlusion. Such surgery, an aortofemoral bypass, using a graft from the distal aorta to the common femoral artery, was common in the past. It is accessible only from an abdominal approach, and we can treat almost all blockages in the iliac artery with a stent if there is any passage at all for us to use for insertion of our tools.

REMINDERS

1. Pain in the buttock with walking may be due to obstruction of the iliac artery.
2. Pain in the calf with walking is likely due to blockage of the superficial femoral artery.
3. Skin breakdown and ulceration of the toes especially if you are diabetic, may well be a result of PAD, particularly in the vessels below the knee.
4. Early detection results in the most effective alteration of the course of the disease and the best treatment, usually without surgery.
5. Continued smoking in the face of established PAD is a sure path to serious problems, including potential amputation of the limb. Don't throw your life away!
6. Walking is the best exercise for individuals with PAD. It helps in the formation and proliferation of collateral vessels that can result in self-administered "bypass."
7. If your doctor wants to do surgery, ask if you can be treated via a catheter intervention instead.

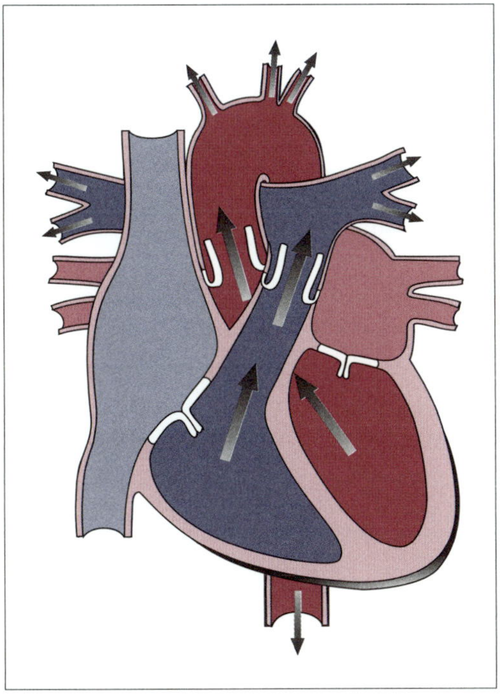

RHEUMATIC HEART DISEASE

A Heart Valve Problem Years After a Sore Throat

RHEUMATIC HEART DISEASE IS AN inflammatory process involving the valves of the heart. It originates from an infection with a bacterium, the ubiquitous streptococcus. The usual type of infection is *pharyngitis*, or the common "strep throat."

Almost everyone in life gets this at some point in time. If it is not eliminated but lingers on for months and months, the infected individual will build up antibodies against the bacterium, the organism causing the infection.

Unfortunately, due to some similarities between the composition of the bacterial cell wall and the protein in the valves of the heart, the antibodies that are formed against the bacterial invasion may cause considerable destruction of the heart valve tissue. This can smolder on long after the bacteria have been eliminated from the throat.

An acute episode of fever, joint pain, rash, and a new murmur all can derive from this initial event known as *acute rheumatic fever*. The major damage to the valves follows and is variable, depending on the intensity of the antibody production and the duration of the infection before intervention.

In the past, several rheumatic fever belts were identified. These existed in certain areas of the country where strep throat was particularly common—San Luis Valley of southern Colorado, parts of Wyoming, and some areas in the east. However, rheumatic fever could occur in any part of the world and did.

Thankfully, acute rheumatic fever is almost a thing of the past in many countries. We still see patients with the effects of rheumatic fever, expressed as valvular heart disease, but certainly not in the large numbers that were present in the '60s and '70s. When I was a cardiac fellow in Denver in the early and mid-'70s, I commonly saw these patients and it wasn't at all unusual to make a diagnosis of newly recognized rheumatic heart disease. I have not seen a new case in at least five years.

There is almost certainly a genetic predisposition to rheumatic fever. For example, in communities within streptococcus belts, virtually everyone contracted strep throat. However, only a sporadic case of rheumatic fever developed. When penicillin came along, it virtually eliminated this disease except in circumstances where careful monitoring of children's complaints were not carried out.

The most commonly afflicted heart valve is the mitral valve, the large valve between the left atrium, the holding chamber for oxygenated blood returning from the lungs, and the main pumping chamber of the heart, the left ventricle. It is extremely unusual to find a patient with a rheumatic aortic valve without even more severe damage to the mitral valve.

In the past, I would commonly be called by a referring physician who advised me that his patient had a loud murmur emanating from the aortic valve, and since the patient had a history of rheumatic fever, it might well be rheumatic aortic valve disease. It usually was; but in almost every circumstance, the mitral valve was much more heavily diseased. It is just more difficult to hear a rumble emanating from the mitral valve as opposed to the easily heard murmurs generated by the aortic valve. Since blood under high pressure is being pumped voraciously past this aortic valve, any obstruction or leakage is easier to detect. The aortic valve is the second most commonly involved valve in rheumatic heart disease.

Unless rheumatic fever existed for several years, it was extremely uncommon for the right-sided heart valves to be significantly involved in the rheumatic process. The tricuspid valve frequently leaked dramatically, but it was due to increased pressure in the pulmonary artery secondary to mitral stenosis (the scarring of the valve that prevents it from opening adequately) rather than from intrinsic pathology.

As would be expected from our knowledge of the process involved, the inflammation results in rather profound scarring of the valves with associated retraction of the valve tissue. In particular, the mitral valve apparatus becomes encased in scar, causing fusion of the little slender threads, the *chordae tendinae*, that anchor the valve to the underlying heart muscle. This pulls the valve downward and the valve tissue becomes tethered. The leaflets do not escape either and they become stuck in this mass of scar tissue, causing mitral stenosis (a stuck valve), also mitral regurgitation (leakage) as the elements allowing for adequate valve closure are deformed.

In the past, the initial operation for this mitral valve problem was mitral commissurotomy, a scalpel incision of the leaflets of the mitral valve. This was done because the mitral stenosis was almost always much greater than the regurgitation, or leakage. In fact, in many patients, the mitral stenosis was almost a pure process.

This operation was done in the days before the heart-lung machine had been invented, and it could only be performed well by a handful of surgeons around the country. It was not uncommon to see patients who had gone through three or four such procedures from doctors such as Lord Brock in London to Dwight Harken in Boston or Henry Swan in Denver. If you were a cardiac surgeon who had the *touch* in performing this delicate operation (sometimes separating these scarred-down leaflets with the tip of one's finger), you were well-known and your services were sought after. I remember when I was training in Denver, Dr. Swan's celebrity in the field was like a rock star. People with this now almost antique disease were simply desperate to gain relief.

We look back at some of this early surgery and it's easy to chuckle at the simplicity of it. However, it required incredible spirit and determination. For example, those early pioneers in heart surgery didn't have the great tools we have today nor was there good anesthesiology. To top it off, Dr. Harken in Boston lost six of the first group of patients he operated on for mitral stenosis. He would have given up, he felt terrible about it, but his colleagues knew of his passion (and compassion, a trait just as necessary) and urged him on. Remarkably, he lost only two of the next 15 patients he operated on! And these were all folks who were on death's door, very high-risk individuals for any operation, much less for a complex heart operation.

When heart-lung bypass support became available, this commissurotomy operation was still done in some instances but then valve replacement became a possibility. This procedure has been done for most of the patients in the civilized world who suffered from severe rheumatic heart disease.

By far the most devastating problem in rheumatic heart disease has been, and still is, stroke. With scarring of the mitral valve, it becomes relatively fixed in position and doesn't open appropriately. With this comes pronounced enlargement of the left atrium. When this happens, since the atrium becomes so large in this process, the individual is prone to develop atrial fibrillation—a chaotic, ineffectual electrical process.

Any patient who develops atrial fibrillation is at increased risk of clot formation within the left atrial appendage. However, the combination of mitral stenosis and atrial fibrillation is a particularly worrisome duo posing a huge risk for clot formation and subsequent embolization to the brain. Even if the patient is lucky enough for the clot not to travel the straightest route north but to turn the corner and go south, there is no good place for such a clot to land. The luckiest circumstance is for it to travel to the leg. Even there, it poses risk to limb viability and has to be removed.

Due to this markedly enhanced risk of devastating stroke with mitral stenosis-induced atrial fibrillation, each patient should be therapeutically anticoagulated with Coumadin lifelong. This is a drug, taken orally, that ties up the clotting factors in the liver. Though it's difficult to regulate, it's important in these patients with such a markedly enhanced tendency to form clot in their left atrial appendage to maintain their anticoagulation status at a fairly high level. For this reason, they should each have their own machine to measure this anticoagulation level.

REMINDERS

1. **Patients with rheumatic mitral stenosis and atrial fibrillation are particularly prone to develop an embolic stroke, and should always be anticoagulated. These patients should have a Protime machine at home to routinely check their blood for proper anticoagulation.**
2. **All rheumatic heart disease is caused by a prior infection with streptococcus, usually strep throat.**

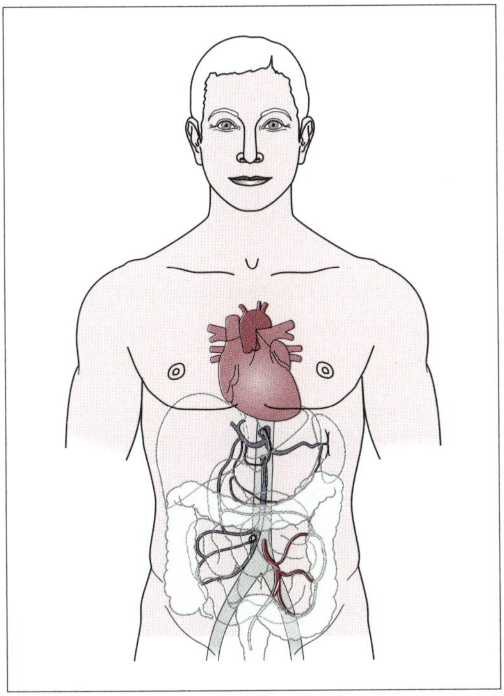

39 MESENTERIC INSUFFICIENCY

Problems with Blood Flow to the Gut

THE MEDICAL TERM FOR THE PROBLEM of inadequate blood supply to the gut is *mesenteric ischemia,* meaning intermittent or chronic oxygen deprivation of the structures within the abdomen. This is usually due to advanced arteriosclerosis: the ever-present cholesterol deposition within the wall of the artery. It may accumulate for years until it chokes down flow or worse, experiences disruption resulting in total occlusion from a clot forming on top of the ulcerated plaque.

There are basically two large arterial blood vessels supplying all of the organs within the abdominal cavity. The uppermost of these is the celiac axis, which gives off many branches to the liver, spleen, and stomach. The second, originating from the aorta just below the former, is called the superior mesenteric artery (SMA). It gives off the major branches to the gut.

The gut has been referred to by the functional medicine doctors as the "second brain." Functional medicine has become an interesting discipline, emphasizing the importance of individual variations in metabolism and bioavailability of necessary ingredients for health. These considerations are largely determined by the gut and it, in turn, is strongly influenced by genetic and environmental factors. They are likely correct. We make many decisions on "gut instinct." When the gut hurts, we are unhappy people. Not only that, but gut function is intimately involved with immune function—bad gut, bad immune system.

Almost always, only one of the two intra-abdominal arteries has to remain wide open for an individual to receive adequate blood flow to the gut, as there are a number of collateral systems that develop as a mesenteric vessel closes off. This is a built-in survival mechanism. In heavy smokers, especially women, and especially if there are other arteriosclerotic risk factors involved, we will occasionally find that one vessel has closed off and the remaining one is tightly blocked. This is a precarious situation.

The symptoms of mesenteric ischemia are usually fairly dramatic and consist of pain associated with oxygen deprivation of the wall of the gut. Those of you who have ever had a bloated feeling with cramping have experienced just a small measure of what these folks endure. This pain is brought on by eating. The gut requires only a modest amount of blood flow when not digesting food, but requires an immediate increase in blood flow following a meal to handle the extra work. However, if you have a limited amount of blood supply to the gut, are unable to increase it at all, and then eat a meal, the oxygen deprivation and lactic acid build-up in the tissues of the gut from insufficient blood flow causes a great deal of pain. We call this post-prandial (following a meal) pain. It is intense enough to convince the individual to eat frequent tiny portions of food—and in its most severe form, these folks come in looking starved. And they are.

In an individual who gives such a history or comes in with unexplained bowel problems, an abdominal or mesenteric Doppler examination can usually either dispel the notion or make a case for further evaluation. The next step used to be an invasive angiogram. Now using the 64-slice CT angiogram, a simple intravenous is started, contrast is injected, and we can frequently obtain prompt corroboration of the diagnosis.

If an abdominal problem is acute, then urgent measures are necessary to save gut viability and function. In other words, if a person with mesenteric ischemia comes into the emergency room with unremitting severe abdominal pain due to vascular compromise, he or she has most likely totally blocked a "lifeline" vessel to the gut. Since there are many causes for acute abdominal pain with an acute abdomen, this is merely one of several considerations in most people. However, if the person is elderly and has had other arteriosclerotic problems, mesenteric ischemia has to be thought of promptly, and either corroborated or ruled out quickly to get on with treatment. If this acute process is indeed due to vascular occlusion, there are only a limited number of precious minutes before the gut is irreversibly injured and long sections have to be removed. Like everything else, you want to keep as much of your gut as possible.

On the other hand, if this is an intermittent occurrence precipitated only by food, a CT angiogram is needed and one can go about the evaluation in a more leisurely fashion. I have not been able to do many of these evaluations very leisurely, however, as the patient is almost always in a bad way symptomatically. This, coupled with the fact that a person can usually get along quite well on just one mesenteric artery, tells me that the patient is likely living on just a tiny trickle of blood through only one artery. Since I am concerned about just when this last vestige of blood supply to the gut might fail, I go about this evaluation promptly, ready to intervene with stent deployment to the treacherously compromised vessel.

Unfortunately, the very type of person who is prone to develop this makes effective treatment difficult—the petite, heavy-smoking female. I have seen a number of these women, and they invariably possess quite small mesenteric vessels. Additionally, these vessels come out of the very front of the aorta, then turn down at a sharp angle and are very fragile. No matter the temptation, the doctor must not try to use a stent that is too large to increase the chances of keeping the small artery open. These vessels are prone to restenosis (blockage from scar tissue following stent deployment). Using an up-sized stent is always an allurement, since we know that the larger the stent, the less likely we are to see restenosis. The worst thing the doctor can do, however, is cause a disruption of this artery with copious blood loss. This can be fatal. It is exceptionally important that the operator has ample experience in deploying these stents. This is *much* more difficult than putting in a coronary artery stent.

Instead of over-sizing a stent within these vessels, I have started using a drug-eluting stent in these petite arteries. (Figure 32, page 426) This is the same stent that we use in the coronary arteries. In that location, we have shown a much lower restenosis rate than with the bare metal stent. It is an unapproved use, used in this instance as a humanitarian gesture. However, if this lifeline mesenteric artery closes without warning, the eventual mortality rate is almost 100%. It seems worth the extra money and the risk, even though use of these types of stents in the mesenteric arteries is not proven to be effective.

We know that late and sudden complete blockage can occur with these drug-eluting stents; however, in this instance we are trying desperately to provide a good blood supply to the patient's gastrointestinal tract, a life-saving procedure. Since this is usually the only remaining artery to the gut, such a patient should be on platelet agents (aspirin and Plavix) indefinitely. Still, this is an individual decision that must be made by each physician handling this delicate problem—not an enviable position of responsibility. It is important for the patient to remember that the doctor is trying every modality possible to preserve blood flow to the gut, as the consequences of removing a long segment of gut are drastic and unsavory.

If using a drug-eluting stent is too risky, we sometimes ask the vascular surgeons to take a look. They are not too eager to operate on these patients, as there is a very

Figure 32 Mesenteric Insufficiency

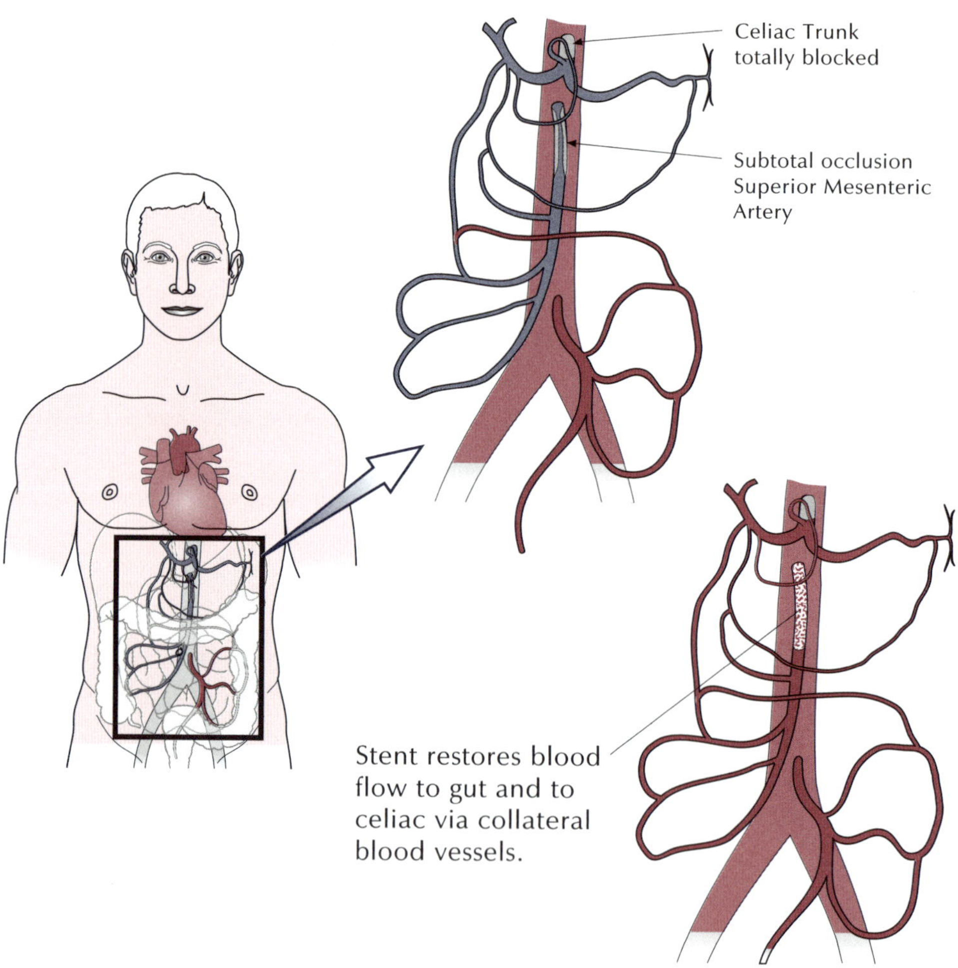

high rate of failure with bypass of the vessel or of reimplantation of the artery into the aorta. We, therefore, frequently find ourselves on our own in these precarious situations.

REMINDERS

1. Oxygen deprivation of the stomach and gastrointestinal tract, known as mesenteric ischemia, is produced by advanced arteriosclerosis involving the arteries supplying these intra-abdominal structures.
2. The pain associated with this is usually brought on by eating because the blood supply to the gut has to increase significantly to digest and handle this load. If the arterial supply to the gut is inadequate for the task, cramping pain will develop. These individuals frequently eat tiny meals in order to avoid the cramping. Consequently, they are often malnourished.
3. Stent deployment should be performed only by a seasoned physician. This is much more difficult and hazardous than deployment of a heart vessel stent. Do *not* assume that the person who implanted your coronary artery stent knows how to do this one.
4. Using stent deployment, we can usually achieve a good opening of one of the arteries leading to the gut. (Only one intra-abdominal artery is required for adequate gut function.) Stent deployment is usually vastly superior to surgical revascularization.
5. If you have this situation, stop smoking! If your one remaining mesenteric artery closes off, the mortality rate is extremely high—and if long segments of gut have to be removed, there is a distinct risk of "short gut" syndrome which is inadequate to satisfy your nutritional needs.

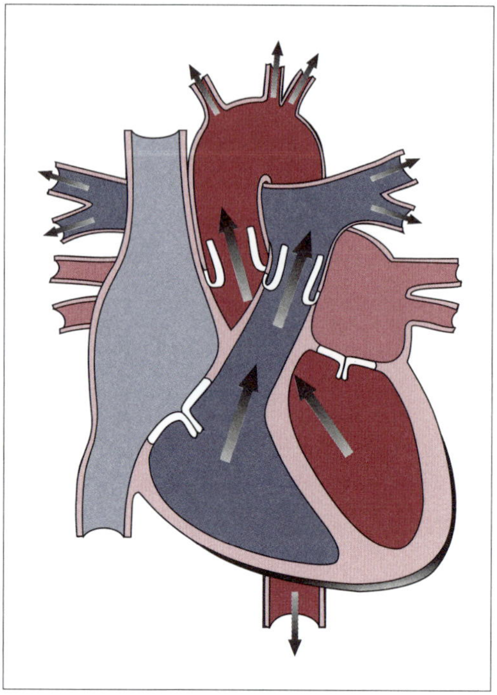

INFILTRATIVE HEART DISEASE

Abnormal Material within the Heart

INFILTRATIVE HEART DISEASE IS A RARE FORM of heart disease. I include it because I don't want you to get this book, only to find that it didn't mention your problem. Marked by diffuse deposits of some sort of material within the structure of the heart, it also makes for a difficult diagnosis in some instances. Treatment of each form is difficult and challenging. As the wonderfully perceptive physician, Sir William Osler, once said, "It is more important to know what patient has the disease than the disease the patient has."

Probably the most common infiltrative heart process is malignant spread of a tumor to the heart. We have to treat the underlying disorder. The most common cancers that spread to the heart are those involving organs contiguous to the heart. These are primary lung and breast tumors. They usually grow into the heart, involving the sac surrounding the heart, the pericardium. Lymphoma is a remote malignant process that can invade the heart. I have personally biopsied a mass in the right atrium that turned out to be lymphoma, which was previously unrecognized.

Amyloidosis is a condition of manufacture and distribution of an unusual protein, a so-called para-protein called amyloid. "Para" refers to a protein that is not normally found in the blood stream or anywhere else in the body. This is commonly a genetic problem but may be secondary to other chronic inflammatory processes. One of the structures that amyloid involves is the heart, usually the left ventricle. It causes a grotesque increase in wall thickness of the left ventricle. This increase is much greater than that which is commonly seen in hypertension.

This infiltration with amyloid causes a marked elevation of the left ventricular filling pressure, as this rubber-like material causes the left ventricle to become exceptionally stiff. The pressure has to increase in the left atrium in order to make the left ventricle stretch and accept the appropriate blood volume. Congestive heart failure and often atrial fibrillation develop. Amyloid can be found by doing a rectal mucosal biopsy. Unfortunately, there is no specific therapy at this time.

Sarcoidosis is also part of a diffuse process involving other organ systems. This is an unusual process marked by a specific type of inflammatory nodules called granulomas, scattered throughout the afflicted tissue. These granulomata are similar to the process that forms in tuberculosis. If the heart is involved, the lungs are almost always involved. If it invades the heart, it usually involves the mitral and aortic valves.

Sarcoid may invade the heart muscle directly and can cause life-threatening problems. Recently, a 40-year-old lady came into the hospital with *ventricular tachycardia* (VT), a life-threatening arrhythmia. Her coronary arteries were normal and her left ventricle contracted normally. The ventricle did seem thick, however, for the degree of hypertension she had. Still, no one thought of sarcoidosis even though there was mild leakage across the mitral and aortic valves. The cause of her arrhythmia was obscure until records from another hospital mentioned the possibility of sarcoidosis of the lungs several years before. We saw no involvement of the lungs so I did an endomyocardial biopsy of the lower septum of the heart. It showed typical sarcoid granulomata. Fortunately, sarcoidosis is treatable with steroid suppression. She did well but went home with an automatic implantable cardiac defibrillator (AICD) in the event that she developed another episode of VT.

Loeffler's eosinophilic endocarditis is a very rare infiltration of the right ventricle with esosinophils, a specific type of white blood cell that responds to allergic processes. This is a tough situation to treat.

In other parts of the world, a parasite can commonly infiltrate the heart and replace heart muscle with scar. The most classic is *Chagas* disease, prevalent in parts of Latin America. In fact, worldwide, this is the most common cause of congestive heart failure.

This should be considered in anyone who has a cardiomyopathy and congestive heart failure and also has a history of spending time in Latin America.

A very rare form of infiltrative heart disease is *hemochromatosis*. This is the deposition of iron salts within the heart. It is usually hereditary and associated with iron deposits in other organs as well. It infiltrates the skin, causing bronze discoloration; the liver, causing severe dysfunction; and the pancreas, causing diabetes. The only person I have seen with it came in because of congestive heart failure. He looked as though he'd been on a beach for two months straight. When I casually commented on it, he looked at me strangely and responded by saying he had never even been on a beach. He was an accountant who worked indoors. Finally, I connected the dots and made the diagnosis. The condition is treated with an agent that helps remove the iron from the bloodstream and tissues; it frequently only poorly responds.

REMINDERS

1. **Some infiltrative diseases of the heart are treatable. Many are not.**
2. **If you have traveled in South America and have congestive heart failure, you might have Chagas disease, which is treatable. Bring it up with your doctor if your travels make you a candidate for it.**

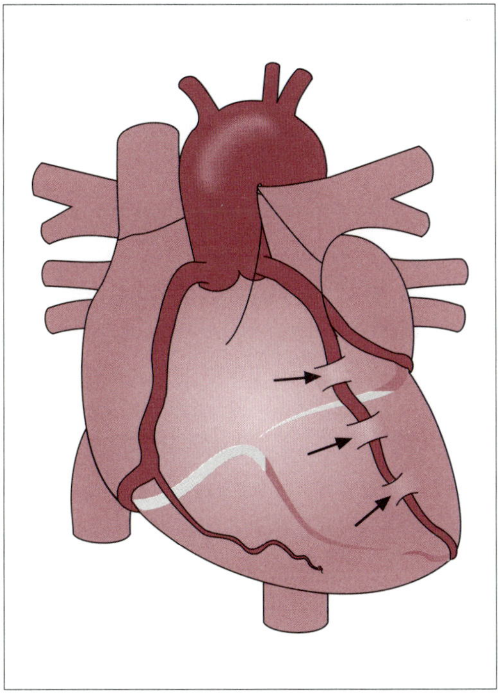

44 MYOCARDIAL BRIDGE

Bridge Over Troubled Heart

A *MYOCARDIAL BRIDGE* IS AN UNUSUAL ENTRAPMENT of one of the coronary arteries feeding the heart muscle underneath muscle fibers of the left ventricle. Entrapment is the common term we use when a nerve or artery becomes subject to pressure from adjacent structures. In this case, it is a coronary artery feeding the heart muscle. The entrapment is not rare; a problem with it is. Like many rare problems, it is not very important unless you have it. For those of you who do and for those of you who have a loved one with it, this is for you.

How Does It Develop?

As the protoplasmic jelly that will ultimately become the heart is firming, developing structure and form, the coronary arteries that come off the aorta and feed the heart muscle are also forming. The arteries wind up on the exterior surface of the heart, sending smaller and smaller branches of "feeder" vessels deep down into the muscle to provide oxygen and nutrients for the working pump. Therefore, heart muscle and heart arteries are developing just about simultaneously. The perfect end result is for all of the coronary arteries to course over the surface of the heart muscle.

However, if the embryologic precursors of the coronary artery get entrapped by one or more muscle cell fibers, it forms what is known as a myocardial bridge, or muscle bridge. Simply put, this is a bridge of heart muscle over a segment of the coronary artery, usually the vessel down the front of the heart, the left anterior descending.

The incidence of muscle bridges is by no means small. Many years ago, a pathologist in London looked at about 20,000 hearts and found a substantial occurrence of this anatomic variation. It makes all the sense in the world as—during embryonic life—the structure of the heart muscle, the valves, the coronary arteries, and the nerves that contribute to the formation of the heart, all develop about the same time from this protoplasmic "goo." Talk about choreography!

How a Muscle Bridge Causes Trouble

The muscle cells shorten during the cardiac phase known as systole. This synchronous cell shortening causes a reduction in cavity size of the pumps. Obviously, when the muscle cell that happens to be crossing over the top of the coronary artery contracts, it stands a potential for restricting blood flow through that artery.

This muscle bridge doesn't become important unless it significantly chokes off blood flow to the heart. The coronary arteries, and therefore the heart muscle, receive blood flow predominantly during diastole, when the heart is relaxed and blood can travel into the tissues without resistance. A muscle bridge tightens down on the coronary artery only during systole. Generally then, this is a pretty well-tolerated situation.

In certain instances, usually in a setting of high blood pressure which gives rise to hypertrophy (enlargement) of the heart muscle cells, this bridge may restrict the flow of blood to the heart muscle. This causes typical chest or jaw pain usually with exercise or other causes of increased blood pressure, heart rate, and attendant heart muscle energy requirements.

Medical Treatment

This situation can usually be treated with a drug to decrease the initial phase of contractility and the heart rate, the major determinants of myocardial oxygen requirement. Such a drug is a beta-adrenergic-blocker, such as Inderal. This (and reassurance) is usually all that is needed to maintain a happy heart. Most of these individuals do great.

Surgical Treatment Now Replaced by Drug-Eluting Stent Deployment

Very rarely, perhaps a half-dozen times in the last 30 years, I have been forced to send a patient to surgery to sever the muscle fibers overlying the left anterior descending coronary artery. This is not always effective, however, as a peculiar loss of elasticity in the wall of the coronary artery right at the site of the muscle bridge can develop due to aggressive, repetitive constriction of the coronary artery over many years.

The numbers are astounding. For example, a 50-year-old man with this problem, at a mean heart rate of 60 beats per minute, would have had 1,576,800,000 heart beats during his lifetime, each beat subjecting this poor coronary artery to the rhythmic lashing imposed by the heart muscle fiber contracting down on it. It is no wonder that the artery forms a thickening in its wall and narrows a bit. This thickening in the wall of the artery is similar to scar tissue.

Even when the bridge is severed with a scalpel, persistent deformity of the coronary artery may persist, a substantial narrowing that can limit flow down the artery. This is precisely the reason why a couple of my patients didn't have a great result from surgery and we wound up stenting them in order to pry this narrowed segment widely open. In other words, a stainless steel coronary stent was deployed by balloon inflation at high pressure, forcing this narrowed segment into the same profile as the contiguous segments. This is interesting, in that each one of these patients demonstrated a milking effect during systole. In other words, the coronary artery would narrow down severely during the phase of heart muscle contractility, but would open up a bit during diastole when the heart muscle relaxed. I thought severing of the bridge would do the job just as it had in the other patients I had sent for surgical correction of this problem, but it didn't. The reason was this scar-like deformity in the wall of the artery.

Personally, I believe in this age of drug-eluting coronary stents, the initial approach should be the deployment of such a stent. If effective, and it has been in a couple of my patients, this one-hour procedure obviates the need for open-chest surgery and the use of a beta-blocker, which is sometimes not well tolerated. These drug-eluting stents rarely restenose (narrow again due to scar tissue) because the cancer drug they are treated with prevents cell replication within the stent zone. The site where these myocardial bridges occur is almost always readily amenable to stent deployment. If the muscle bridge turns out to be so aggressive and strong that it deforms the stent significantly (which I have never seen but I suppose it could conceivably happen), no ground is lost and surgery can then be performed.

As with any use of the drug-treated stent, I recommend indefinite use of platelet drugs to prevent late clot formation. Your physician might actually want to use a plain non-drug-treated stent in this instance—a decision between you and your doctor.

REMINDERS

1. A muscle bridge over the left anterior descending coronary artery is common.
2. It only causes trouble if the muscle fibers bridging the artery start to enlarge or if the individual participates in some activity that is exceptionally strenuous.
3. Surgery is not necessarily the answer. If your doctor recommends open-chest surgery for this, get another opinion.
4. In my opinion, a muscle bridge is better managed through deployment of a coronary stent.

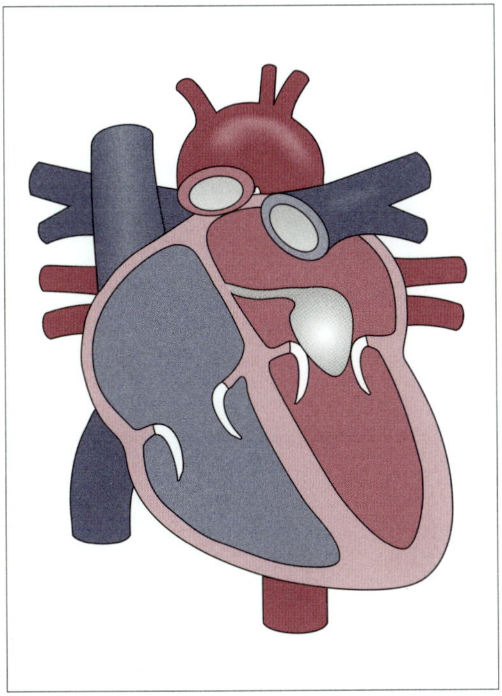

42 TUMORS OF THE HEART

Many Types, Different Symptoms

BY FAR THE MOST COMMON TUMOR of the heart is one that has originated elsewhere, such as a tumor of the lungs or breast, and which has metastasized (traveled) directly to the heart muscle. These tumors have to traverse the sac surrounding the heart (the pericardium) first and, in so doing, usually produce a collection of fluid in the pericardium. We can withdraw a sample of this fluid and make the diagnosis promptly. Treatment is unique to the underlying cell type, and surgical drainage of the pericardium is frequently necessary.

There are, however, certain tumors that originate in the heart and blood vessels as a primary process. These are all somewhat uncommon, but it is very important to diagnose them early.

Figure 33 Pedunculated Left Atrial Myxoma

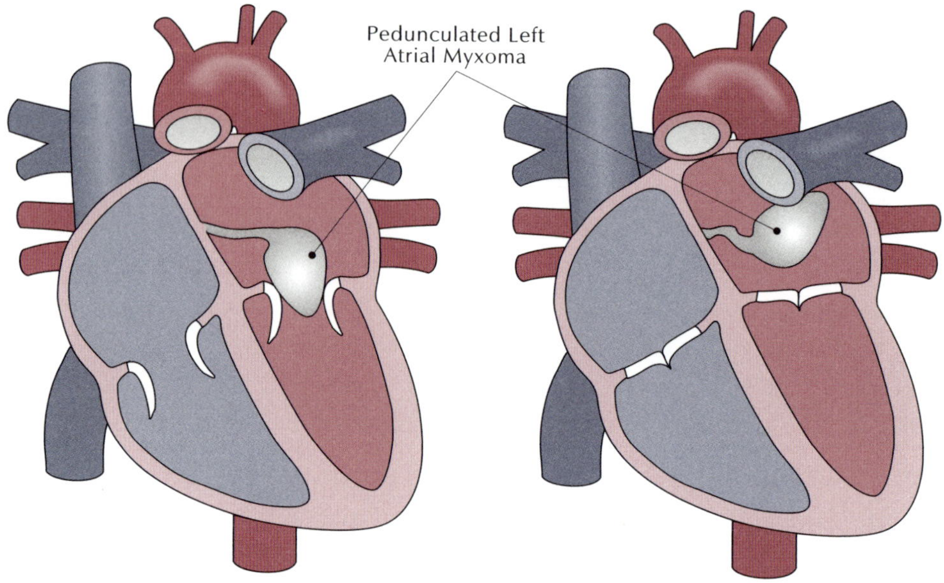

Left Atrial Myxoma: A Benign Primary Tumor of the Heart

By far the most common primary heart tumor is the *atrial myxoma.* These are almost all benign and almost all originate from the left atrial side of the inter-atrial septum, the barrier between the right and left upper chambers of the heart. Utilizing echocardiography, these myxomas are very characteristic in appearance, as they are attached to the septum by a stalk (pedunculated) and possess a somewhat rounded tip. (Figure 33) In fact, the mace-like tip may be formed from its repetitive projectile motion against the mitral valve annulus. They may appear somewhat similar to a morel mushroom.

Benign? Yes, but they do not always behave in a benign fashion. For example, they can exist within the heart for a very long time without causing any symptoms whatsoever and then, inexplicably, cause a major problem. They can be so silent for so long that no one has a clue that the tumor is in there. For all I know, there's one inside me at this moment; I would have no symptoms of its presence. Plato once said, "Ignorance, the root and the stem of every evil." And he was surely right, for one of these silent tumors may suddenly explode onto the scene with delivery of an ominous symptom!

Occasionally a good examiner with extremely good ears is able to hear a "tumor plop" through a stethoscope. This isn't a very reliable means of detection, as I have gone back and listened to every single one of these I have found and I couldn't even talk myself into hearing a plop or any other unusual sound.

At some point and for no obvious reason, a platelet aggregate (platelets are tiny elements in the blood stream that initiate the clotting process by clumping together) may form on the hammer-like end of the tumor and when this platelet clump is ultimately flung off, a stroke or *transient ischemic attack* (TIA) may occur. A TIA is a reversible neurological deficit. In this case, the platelet clump, thrown to the brain, will block off a small artery, causing symptoms of a stroke. Then, as the clump is dispersed by the circulating blood, the symptoms reverse. If this embolus (a clot formed in one place—in this case the heart—and tossed into the blood stream to land in another place) is more mature, it may not become dispersed and a stroke will ensue.

These atrial tumors are usually obvious on an echocardiogram and the technician is usually very excited about finding one. They are easily cured by surgical resection.

I have personally seen one large left atrial myxoma that was causing obstruction to left ventricular filling. The patient, a lady of about 60, had been treated for asthma for years at a leading university. She did not have asthma, though her symptoms mimicked it. She was cured by resection of the large left atrial myxoma.

This underscores the extreme need for obtaining an echocardiogram to clear the heart of wrongdoing before making the diagnosis of asthma. Usually asthma is really asthma, which is caused by the intermittent narrowing of the small air passages in the lungs. Air forced out through these narrowed channels produces the characteristic wheezing of asthma. Sometimes, however, the wheezing is due to pulmonary water secondary to a cardiac condition, known as *cardiac asthma*. Obviously, it is very important to make this distinction.

This woman, for example, had been treated with experimental asthma drugs, at some risk, for several years before she stumbled into the hospital after blacking out. The reason for the blackout spell was that the tumor had gotten so large and the stalk so long, it was completely closing off flow of blood into the left ventricle temporarily. It turns out that the stalk was long enough and the ball-like projectile end was large enough that it was plopping into the mitral valve annulus, the ring holding the mitral valve tissue between the left upper and left lower chambers. For a time, it blocked the flow of blood from the left atrium into the left ventricle and she didn't get enough blood to her brain. The tumor would unstick itself and life would go on. This is exactly the same process that had caused her "asthma" for the last ten years! When she was brought into our hospital after she had blacked out, she said, "Oh, it's just my asthma again." The tumor filled almost the entire left atrium and had obviously been there for a long, long time.

Occasionally, these myxomas can originate from the right atrial side of the inter-atrial septum. These are rare. I have seen two individuals, both Native American, who had tumors in both atria.

Heart Valve Tumors

The most common tumors affecting the heart valves are the *fibroelastomas*. They are usually on the mitral or aortic valve and account for about 8% of all benign primary tumors of the heart, almost always occurring in men.

Rare Heart Tumors

One tumor that can involve the right heart predominantly is an *angiosarcoma*. (As Plato so wisely said, "They certainly give very strange names to diseases." Medical names usually try to identify—frequently using Latin or Greek roots—the why and the where. For example, *angio*, in a blood vessel; *sarcoma*, the cell type.) This tumor usually involves the superior vena cava and grows into the right atrium. I published an article on one of these that originated from the left side of the heart, starting off life in the pulmonary veins, and it ultimately mimicked a mitral valve problem by causing an increase in pulmonary water.

I will make one comment to those who might be dealing with a rare cardiac tumor or may have a family member with such an entity. Any well-trained cardiac surgeon can remove one of the tumors from the atria that I have discussed above, the myxomas. They can be removed in less than an hour and a prompt recovery is predictable. The same is true of a tumor limited to a heart valve.

With these other rare tumors of the heart, I firmly believe that a surgeon in a large referral hospital should be selected. This is doubly true if we are talking about one of the rare primary tumors affecting the heart muscle. A place such as that will take a multi-disciplinary approach to the problem and involve a cardiologist, a cardiac surgeon, oncologists, and well-versed pathologists. These more exotic conditions should simply be referred to a huge referral hospital where the surgeon has operated on similarly affected hearts and knows how the team is going to reconstruct the heart when the tumor is excised. Like all things, there is no substitute for experience, and you gain this only from a high volume of work.

REMINDERS

1. Asthma is not always caused by a primary pulmonary process. Sometimes it is "cardiac asthma."
2. A benign atrial myxoma or a heart valve tumor can be removed by any good cardiac surgeon with a predictable good outcome.
3. Exotic cardiac tumors, especially those involving the heart muscle, need to be excised by a surgeon especially skilled at these procedures.

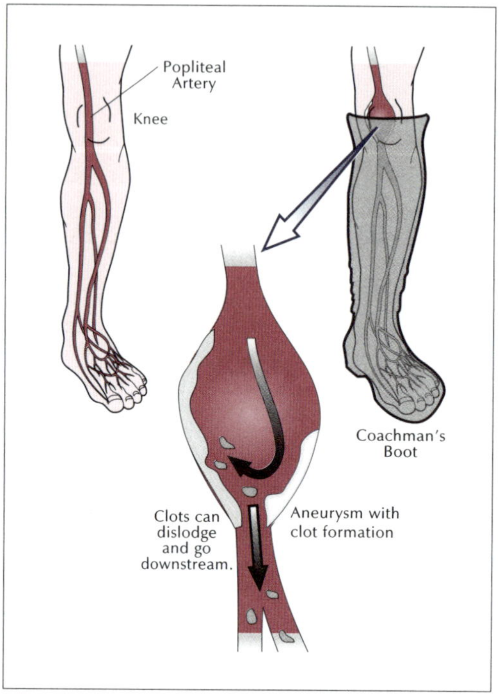

UNCOMMON ARTERIAL ANEURYSMS

Ballooning of the Arteries in Unexpected Places

ANY BALLOONING OF A STRUCTURE CONTAINING blood is called an aneurysm—no matter where it is located. The most common site of aneurysm formation is within the aorta, the giant blood tube carrying red blood to all parts of the body. The most common site for aneurysm formation within the aorta is the area just below the take-off of the renal (kidney) arteries. This commonly involves the large arterial branches, the iliac arteries, leading to the legs. We now generally repair these aneurysms by endoluminal stent-graft techniques, utilizing a tube graft inserted via a catheter from a groin artery in order to seal off the aneurysm, protecting its owner from catastrophic rupture.

There are also aneurysms that form in uncommon sites. These uncommon aneurysms usually occur in one of three zones:

1. Arteries leading to the extremities.
2. Arteries leading to the organs within the abdominal cavity.
3. Arteries within the cranium, carrying blood to the brain.

Lower Extremity Arterial Aneurysms

The lower extremity arteries seem to be more readily involved than the upper. Interestingly, trauma often plays a role in both. When not due to trauma, they are almost always secondary to arteriosclerosis from long-standing deposition of cholesterol within the wall of the artery and, when caused by arteriosclerosis, there is almost always widespread involvement of the entire arterial circulation, especially the heart vessels.

The superficial femoral artery, residing within the thigh, is the major artery to the leg. The term superficial is misleading, as it tends to make one think that this artery is less important. Nothing could be further from the truth. It is the kingpin vessel supplying blood to the lower extremity. It almost never develops an aneurysm unless it has received a severe blunt or penetrating trauma. The reason is that is it protected as it travels through the fleshy thigh, a very vulnerable area were it not for a canal. This canal, anatomically named the adductor canal due to the muscle protecting it, is commonly referred to as *Hunter's canal.*

Dr. John Hunter was a British surgeon who was obsessed. He performed extensive dissection on cadavers throughout the autopsy suites in London at a time when doing so was exceptionally dangerous. His main interest was the artery just below Hunter's canal, the popliteal. While the most common aneurysm of the lower extremity arteries, the popliteal behind the knee, was identified by Greek physicians in about 200 B.C., it was Dr. Hunter who recognized the pathophysiology and treatment of this problem.

It was common for carriage drivers to develop a popliteal aneurysm. Apparently these coachmen wore knee-high boots. The roads were pitted and rough. This bouncy ride resulted in repeated irritation from the top edge of their boots, chafing the kinked popliteal artery in its most vulnerable area just behind the knee. In some of these individuals, a popliteal aneurysm would form and with repeated insult, would enlarge. (Figure 34, Page 442) This posed the risk of rupture. It also posed the more likely risk of clot formation within the aneurysmal sac, setting the stage for dislodgement and embolization (travel to another spot) of clot material to the downstream arteries. Such a blockage would result in oxygen deprivation of the distal tissues and threaten the viability of the lower leg, including the foot. Frequently, amputation (and loss of their livelihood) was the only option.

We still see traumatic popliteal aneurysms. However, the majority of the ones we see today are arteriosclerotic. As previously mentioned, an aneurysm usually develops in a predisposed artery. In other words, while all aortas are subjected to the tangential wall

Figure 34 Popliteal Aneurysm with Clot

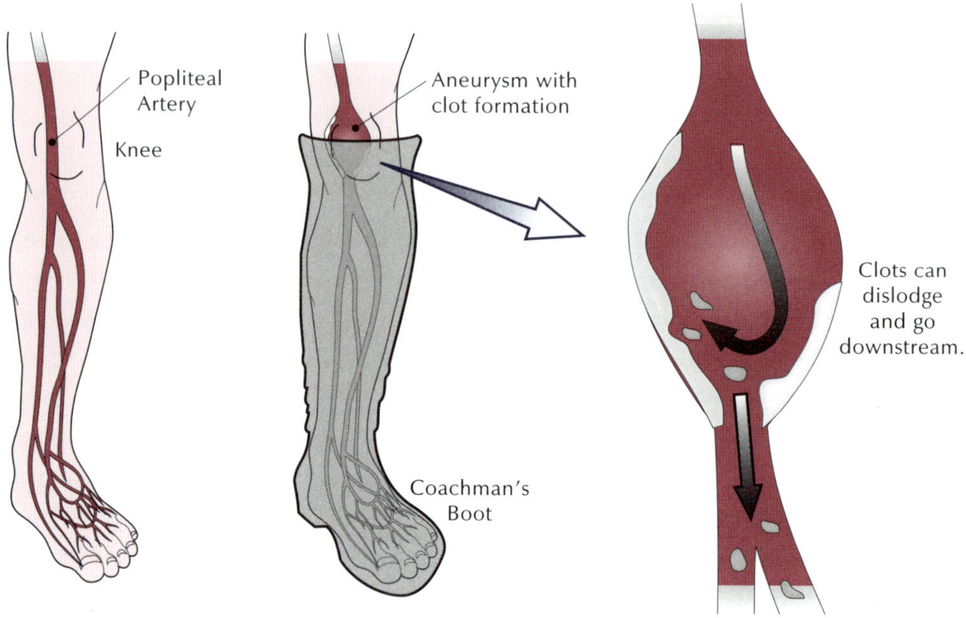

stress of blood pressure, only a few develop an aneurysm. We know there is a fairly strong hereditary influence as well. The same is true of these popliteal aneurysms. In my experience, one-half of these develop in individuals who have had or will develop abdominal aortic aneurysms. Additionally, if you develop one on the left, there is at least a 50% chance of also developing one on the right.

The presentation of one of these is just as it was with the coachmen. A partial clot usually forms, is swept off, and lodges in one of the distal arteries choking off blood flow to that segment. The individual comes in with a painful lower leg and foot, usually with pallor (paleness), and with decreased skin temperature. If complete occlusion of the popliteal artery develops due to a clot, saving the leg is of the essence and this constitutes a medical and sometimes a surgical emergency.

In the past, the only treatment we had for a popliteal aneurysm was placing a bypass graft from the proximal vessel to the distal, tying off the artery in between so it could not rupture. Now, we almost always handle these with a covered stent delivered via a groin catheter, and the individual can go home the same day. Vice President Cheney recently underwent such a covered stent exclusion of his popliteal aneurysm.

Upper Extremity Arterial Aneurysms

If aneurysms of the lower arterial circulation are rare, the ones involving the upper extremity branches are rare as hen's teeth. Like aneurysms elsewhere, the *proximal* aneurysms involving the upper extremity arteries are usually arteriosclerotic. Again, they probably develop only in predisposed arterial walls and are aggravated by hypertension. However, the more *distal* ones frequently involve trauma and are also frequently present in a congenitally predisposed zone of artery. I don't mean just an artery that is genetically predisposed by virtue of a weak wall. I mean one that, due to anatomic reasons (entrapment of the artery within an unyielding canal), is prone to aneurysm formation from repeated trauma to the wall of the artery.

The proximal arteries leaving the aorta, carrying arterial blood to the upper extremities, are the subclavian arteries. At the armpit, this subclavian artery transitions into the axillary artery. Just past this is where the bulk of upper extremity aneurysms form, and they usually become apparent in fairly young people.

At this subclavian-axillary junction, the artery and the major nerve (the brachial plexus) have to traverse a canal formed by muscle and bone. The muscle is the scalenus muscle inserting into a rib and leading into the neck to the jaw bone. The bone forming the boundary of the canal is usually the first rib. This area is called the thoracic outlet, the exit from the thorax (chest). In about one-half of 1% of all of us, a developmental holdover, the cervical rib, is present. In thin individuals with a cervical rib, the canal can become compromised, leading to potential aneurysm formation in the subclavian-axillary artery.

Usually the symptoms in these individuals are due to compression of the brachial plexus. This encroachment on this very large nerve induces numbness and pain of the upper extremity. Occasionally, however, the first symptom is from development of an aneurysm within the artery that is traumatized by this tight canal.

The last one of these I saw was in a college senior. He was a superb athlete, a professional-level tennis player. He was committed to the sport and his own improvement and practiced his serve incessantly. He developed pain in his serving hand and finally came in with pallor of that hand, as well as an absent pulse at the wrist. He had a subclavian-axillary arterial aneurysm with clot material within it. Some of this had become dislodged and washed downstream, obliterating blood flow to the hand.

This young man was treated with infusion of a clot-buster, a thrombolytic drug, within the artery to salvage the hand. We then repaired the aneurysm. However, since the primary problem was a cervical rib with a very small thoracic outlet, we did that repair at the same time, resecting the unneeded and unwanted cervical rib so this wouldn't happen again. Despite this, his career was lost, as he had irreparable damage before we ever saw him.

Another congenital anomaly that can result in aneurysm formation is the anomalous (wrong place) take-off of the subclavian artery—the artery that serves the arm and hand. Due to the intense hemodynamic stress imposed as it twists around to get to the area that it was meant to serve, it can develop an aneurysm. This is repaired only by surgical techniques.

An even less common form of aneurysm involving the upper extremity arterial circulation is one from recurrent trauma caused by use of a hammer or a jackhammer. This involves the distal portion of the ulnar artery in the hand and has to be repaired by microvascular techniques.

Aneurysms Involving the Mesenteric Arteries

The most common artery involved in aneurysm formation within the circulation of the gut, liver, and spleen is clearly the splenic artery. This is sometimes secondary to trauma or infection, but also occurs as an isolated phenomenon due to arteriosclerosis. In the past, this was handled surgically. If it involves the proximal portion, and the artery is large, I see no reason why a competent interventionalist could not deploy a covered stent within this artery.

Splenic infarction is the way some of these are picked up. In other words, clot material, formed within this aneurismal sac, washes downstream and a portion of the spleen loses its blood supply. Pain in the left upper quadrant of the abdomen develops. We also pick these up accidentally with abdominal CT or MRI done for other reasons.

The aneurysms that form in the mesenteric arteries supplying the intestinal tract, the superior mesenteric and celiac axis, are almost always due to tight chronic occlusive plaque, creating a jet of blood that causes erosion of the wall of the vessel distal to this plaque. They pose a problem only from the standpoint of stent deployment within the arteriosclerotic lesion.

Aneurysms within the Brain Circulation

These aneurysms, sometimes called *Berry aneurysms*, are due to a fault within the arterial wall that is present from the time of birth, which is true for quite a percentage of all aneurysms but especially important in these frequently silent aneurysms.

In the early years of life, these arteries look normal and if an angiogram were performed to outline the wall of the arteries, they would still look normal. At some point, due to the unrelenting burden of blood pressure imposed against the wall of the artery, this abnormal zone allows for gradual aneurysm formation. While these develop in individuals who have perfectly normal blood pressures, they will likely develop at an earlier age in those who have high blood pressure, as this just increases the tangential wall stress against the "weak" segment of the artery.

The lucky ones with this phenomenon show up with a headache secondary to enlargement of the aneurysm or with a very limited bleed into the brain tissue. This poses a medical emergency and should be addressed by a team of doctors headed by a neurosurgeon and an interventional radiologist. Vascular coiling—the insertion of a small coil within the aneurysm, inserted through a catheter—is frequently used to treat these intra-cranial aneurysms, usually with an excellent outcome.

Since there is a hereditary component to the ultimate development of these aneurysms, close relatives should be counseled. I am never sure how far to take the screening procedure, for these individuals are not easily screened with any degree of durable reliability. The only thing worse than failure to screen is a poorly performed screening test. Since these unusual aneurysms develop at different stages in different people, we might screen you, and declare you healthy, only to have you show up with one eight years later. I just mention the hereditary aspect to relatives so they know to ask for early evaluation in the event of a vascular headache.

Other Vascular Aneurysms

We can see aneurysm formation within any blood vessel that has arterial characteristics. However, the ones above are the most common of these rare aneurysms. Aneurysms in the coronary arteries are usually the result of a viral invasion of the arteries, called *Kawasaki's disease*. The ones in the pulmonary arteries (to the lung) are usually secondary to a very high pressure within the pulmonary circulation—pulmonary arterial hypertension. The ones in the carotids (going to the brain) and the renals (going to the kidneys) are usually secondary to arteriosclerosis.

We occasionally see an individual with aneurysms virtually in every part of his arterial circulation. I recently saw a 55-year-old laborer who came into the hospital with chest and abdominal pain. By angiography, we determined that he had saccular aneurysms in his coronary circulation. I thought he might need to have bypass surgery and checked his subclavian artery leading to the left arm to be sure that a branch off it, called the internal mammary, could be used as a bypass conduit. He had a giant aneurysm in the subclavian, too. This alerted me that this might be a systemic problem so I studied the mesenteric arteries leading to the gut, the renals leading to the kidneys, and the leg vessels. This relatively young man had aneurysms everywhere! He obviously was one of those rare individuals born with an inherited disorder, leading to multiple faults within the circulatory system. This defect is in the underlying matrix of the arterial wall—the support structure.

REMINDERS

1. Any pain involving a foot or hand—especially if associated with pallor and inability to use the fingers—could represent aneurysm formation within the arteries serving them. They are rare.
2. Most of these aneurysms in the extremity arteries can be managed by covered stent deployment without the need for surgical intervention.
3. There is definitely a hereditary influence in aneurysm formation. If a parent had one, you are possibly predisposed to one.

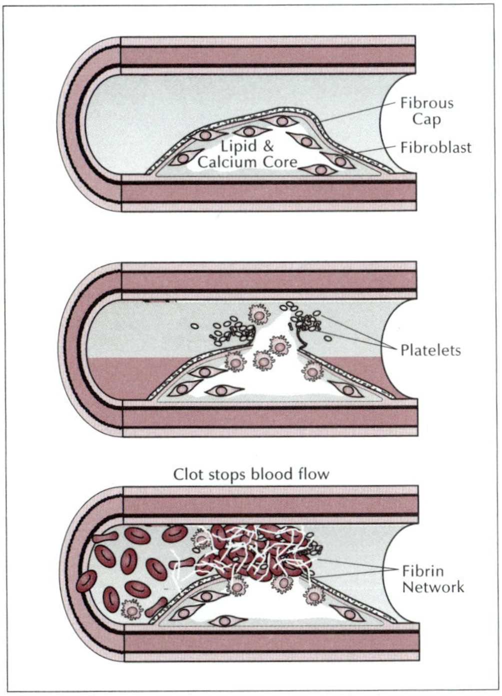

44 HOMOCYSTEINE

An Amino Acid Can Harm You

I ALMOST CONSIDERED THE PROBLEM OF EXCESS homocysteine under the "lipids" chapter, as we so often draw a homocysteine level when we perform a lipid analysis as part of the coronary risk factor screen. However, homocysteine is not a lipid; it is an amino acid. It just happens to be an amino acid that can seriously influence your lipids, as well as other physiologic factors.

We all carry around a certain blood stream level of homocysteine. Normal levels do no harm to the arterial wall. However, homocysteine is converted to other amino acids and several vitamins must participate in the chemical pathway to make this conversion occur. These are folic acid, Vitamin B6, and B12. A high level of homocysteine, then, should point to a possible relative deficiency of these vitamins within the blood stream. This is frequently the case. Homocysteine can also be elevated by a low thyroid level or renal disease and, in certain instances, by a medication. Whatever the cause, it can promptly be restored back to normal by taking a supplement of these three vitamins for just pennies a day. They will see to the channeling of much of this homocysteine into the formation of the other amino acids that depend on this one for their creation.

While this situation was very controversial for many years, there is now convincing data to show that too much homocysteine is detrimental to the wall of arteries—mostly by an indirect action. While normal homocysteine levels do nothing deleterious, a significantly elevated level seems to promote not only the oxidation of low-density lipoprotein which, in turn, is deposited within the wall of arteries, it also seems to promote aggressive clotting as well. With these events, it helps set the stage for the "perfect storm," the injurious arterial wall problem leading to occlusion and heart attack. In ultra-high levels, homocysteine can really wreak havoc on the arterial wall throughout the body.

After this has been treated, a repeat blood test needs to be performed to be sure the level of homocysteine has fallen into a non-harmful range. Measurement of this pesky amino acid is sometimes overlooked as relatively unimportant. However, remember, arteriosclerosis risk factors are additive. Therefore, if this is added to others like smoking, elevated LDL-cholesterol, and high blood pressure, it serves as yet one more problem promoting the aggressive laying-down of plaque within your circulatory system. It needs to be treated!

REMINDERS

1. **Homocysteine is an amino acid and is present in all of us.**
2. **If you become deficient in the vitamins, folic acid, B6, and B12, you may develop high blood stream levels of homocysteine.**
3. **High levels of homocysteine promote the oxidation of the harmless LDL-cholesterol, converting it to the harmful variety that is deposited within the walls of arteries in arteriosclerosis.**

GLOSSARY

Abdominal Aortic Aneurysm (AAA) The most common aneurysm, an outpouching of the aorta just below the takeoff of the renal arteries carrying blood to the kidney.

Acute Coronary Syndrome An unstable situation, with chest pain or other symptoms at rest, usually with electrocardiographic changes, implying a threatened, or an on-going, heart attack.

Automatic Implantable Cardiac Defibrillator (AICD) Implanted device that emits an electrical shock when a fatal rhythm disturbance of the heart is recognized.

Alcohol Septal Ablation The injection of pure alcohol into the first septal perforating artery to cause a therapeutic heart attack of the unwanted muscle bulge that can cause a large pressure gradient between the left ventricle and the aorta and can cause sudden death.

Alveolus A functional air pocket where oxygen is exchanged for carbon dioxide in the lungs. Pl: Alveoli.

Amaurosis fugax Transient loss of vision in one eye due to debris in the retinal artery.

Amiodarone A potent antiarrhythmic drug. Complication is pulmonary fibrosis.

Amyloid An unusual form of protein, called paraprotein, not normally found in the body.

Aneurysm Any outpouching of a structure, usually an artery but sometimes a heart chamber, such as a left ventricular aneurysm occurring after a heart attack.

Angina The clinical syndrome of pain secondary to a narrowed coronary artery.

Angioplasty The opening of an artery by expansion of a balloon.

Angiotensin Produced by a pathway in the kidney in regulation of water and the correct tone within the small muscular arteries of the body in modulation of blood pressure. Angiotensin I is converted to II by an enzyme, Angiotensin Converting Enzyme.

Angiotensin Converting Enzyme-Inhibitor (ACE-I) A drug that blocks an enzyme, reducing the amount of an end product that increases blood pressure.

Angiotensin Receptor-Blocker (ARB) Works at the tissue level to block the effects of Angiotensin II, a vasoconstrictor compound.

Anomalous A structure that is in the wrong location.

Antibody A defense protein manufactured by the body to combat an antigen.

Antigen A protein foreign to the body, usually looked upon as an invader.

Antioxidant Any compound that lends an electron to a free radical, converting it from an injurious compound known to accelerate aging and disease to a harmless one.

Aorta The giant blood tube carrying oxygen-rich blood to all organs in the body.

Aortic Aneurysm An outpouching in the wall of the aorta.

Aortic Dissection A separation of the wall of the aorta. A tear, usually brought about by a dissecting hematoma, a collection of blood, driven along by pressure. Many times, the aortic wall is made of abnormal matrix, allowing the dissection to start; others result from a plaque rupture in the wall of the aorta.

Aortic Valve A three-leaflet valve between the left ventricular pump and the giant blood tube, the aorta. Its main function is to prevent blood that has been pumped from leaking back into the pumping chamber.

Apoptosis Programmed cell death, perhaps due to aging of cellular machinery.

Arginine An amino acid necessary for production of nitric oxide, responsible for relaxing the tone of an artery.

Arrhythmia Any variation from the normal sinus rhythm. Can be dangerous, or not.

Arteriole A small muscular walled artery, used in regulation of the resistance against the arterial blood flows.

Artery Any blood vessel carrying blood away from the heart.

Arteriosclerosis Formation of cholesterol deposits within the wall of arteries.

Atheromatous The deposit of lipid within the arterial wall.

Athrectomy The removal of the inside of an artery at the site of a plaque system, using a rotational cutting device. The major one is called the SilverHawk Athrectomy Device.

Atrial Fibrillation Irregular, chaotic electrical activity in the upper heart chambers.

Atrial Flutter Rapid, organized electrical activity within the upper heart chambers.

Atrial Septal Defect (ASD) A communication between the two upper cardiac chambers, a congenital defect.

Atrium One of the upper chambers of the heart. A reservoir.

Autoimmune Cardiomyopathy Due partially to the destruction of heart muscle antibodies. The heart muscle is a sequestered protein, kept out of the bloodstream, unless there is widespread destruction of muscle, as by a virus invasion. Then, as the muscle protein is released into the bloodstream, the body recognizes this as foreign protein that is potentially dangerous, and, consequently, forms antibodies against it.

Autoinfarction The blood supply becomes lost (blocked) and the organ it supplied becomes irreversibly damaged.

AV Node The electrical node of cells between the upper and the lower heart chambers, where the electrical conduction is slowed. This prevents the ventricular response to atrial fibrillation from being conducted so rapidly that it would be fatal.

Berry Aneurysm A small aneurysm in the brain.

Beta Blocker A drug that blocks a certain type of stimulus to a cell. Decreases heart rate and blood pressure.

Bicuspid Aortic Valve An aortic valve that has only two leaflets instead of the requisite three. It is prone to be silent at birth, then produce a murmur. It will either become obstructive to blood flow into the aorta, or will leak blood back into the left ventricle, or both, as it becomes more degenerative.

Bioavailability The presentation of a particular mineral, vitamin, or food to the bloodstream as a consequence of the function of the gut, perhaps largely influenced by the bacterial and yeast population within the gut.

Bioprosthesis Any tissue heart valve, usually either from porcine or bovine source.

Biventricular Pacemaker A device used to synchronize the two ventricles. One lead goes into the right ventricle and the other into the coronary sinus to stimulate the left ventricle.

Bradycardia Any slow heart rate.

Brain Natriuretic Peptide (B-Peptide) The substance produced when the atrium is stretched. Roughly correlates with the degree of congestive heart failure.

Bronchitis An inflammatory narrowing of the bronchi, the air passages in the lungs.

Brugada Syndrome An inherited sudden death syndrome, due to an abnormality in its ionic channel, leading to a potentially fatal cardiac arrhythmia. It can usually be found by electrocardiographic analysis. Sudden death may occur at rest or during sleep, as well as with activity.

Capillary The tiny, maze-like vessels that connect the smallest artery to the smallest vein, leaving off oxygen to the tissues, taking up carbon dioxide by the hemoglobin molecule in the red blood cell.

Cardiazem A calcium-blocking drug, particularly useful for slowing the heart rate in the event of a rapid arrhythmia originating in the upper chambers.

Cardioversion The process of shocking the heart from an arrhythmia so that it can restart in normal sinus rhythm.

Carotid Artery The artery carrying blood to the brain.

Carotid Endarterectomy The operation used to "apple core" the carotid, removing plaque obstruction.

Celiac Axis The large trunk giving arterial branches to the liver, spleen, stomach, and part of the gut.

Cellular Integrity The proper composition and function of the cell.

Cerebellum The portion of the brain responsible for balance and equilibrium.

Cerebral Cortex The portion of the brain responsible for motor movements.

Cerebrovascular Accident (CVA) A stroke, caused by damage to brain cells.

Cholesterol A blood lipid that is comprised of good (HDL) and bad (LDL) fractions. Deposited within the wall of an artery in formation of a plaque.

Chordae Tendenae The 32 thin connective tissue strands connecting the mitral valve to the protrusion of left ventricular heart muscle, called papillary muscles, holding the valve in place when the ventricle contracts.

Chronic Limb Ischemia (CLI) Rest pain from insufficient arterial blood flow to the leg. Usually associated with severe disease below the knee as well, frequently accompanied by a non-healing ulcer of the foot. Often associated with diabetes.

Chronotropic The effect of speeding or slowing heart rate. Ex: A negative chronotropic drug will slow the heart rate or conduction of electricity in the heart.

Circadian Rhythm A term to describe the 24-hour cycling of hormones and substances that ready us for the day. If stressed, they can be harmful and possibly trigger early morning heart attack, stroke, and high blood pressure crises.

Circle of Willis The anatomic circle at the base of the brain, variable in completeness, connecting the two sides of the circulation to the brain. May prevent a large stroke.

Clot A network of fibrin as a defense mechanism against injury. Often formed within a blood vessel when the covering of a plaque has become ruptured or eroded.

Clot-Buster My term for a thrombolytic drug, one that disperses clot.

Coarctation of the Aorta A congenital stricture of the descending aorta within the chest. Frequently associated with a bicuspid aortic valve.

Collagen The main protein within connective tissue, which provides structure and support.

Collaterals Tiny arteries connecting one artery to a tightly, or completely, blocked artery in an effort to keep the tissues served by the blocked artery viable.

Commotio Cordis Sudden death resulting from ventricular arrhythmias caused by a blow to the chest, usually from a baseball.

Communication An abnormal connection between chambers of the heart or blood vessels.

Compliance A term denoting elasticity of a heart chamber or an artery.

Congenital Abnormality An abnormal structure from birth.

Congestive Heart Failure (CHF) A condition resulting from a high pressure within either atrium so that blood is backed up and water is pushed into tissues.

COPD Chronic obstructive pulmonary disease, usually the 4th leading cause of death in the United States, 90% of which is caused by cigarette smoking.

Coreg The beta-blocking "miracle drug" used in treatment of congestive heart failure. The best drug to reclaim, or prevent loss, of heart muscle and ventricular configuration.

Coronary Angiogram The outlining of the wall of the coronary artery with contrast material that stands out on x-ray.

Coronary Artery One of three arteries supplying blood to the heart muscle.

Coronary Artery Disease The deposit of blood fats within the wall of the heart artery.

Coronary Calcium Score The measure of the quantity of calcium within coronary arteriosclerotic plaques. Roughly correlates with the severity of the coronary disease.

Coronary Occlusion The blockage of a coronary artery, expressed as a percentage.

Cor Pulmonale Right heart failure due to pulmonary artery hypertension.

Cortisol A substance necessary for life. Thought of as a stress hormone, as excessive amounts are associated with stress and depression.

Coumadin The only long term anticoagulant, works by tying up clotting factors manufactured in the liver.

Continuous Positive Airway Pressure (CPAP) Used to treat sleep apnea and also very useful in treatment of pulmonary edema, when the lungs are flooded with water.

Cryoangioplasty The use of liquid nitrogen to cool the coils within a balloon when the balloon is dilated at high pressure to open a plaque system in the leg arteries. The cold helps induce apoptosis, cell death, within the layers of the artery, helping it to maintain this open lumen.

Cryptogenic Of unknown cause. Ex: A cryptogenic stroke.

CT Angiogram A relatively noninvasive way to obtain a good angiographic picture of the arterial circulation throughout the body. Currently done with a 64-slice tomogram, making the invasive coronary angiogram largely obsolete.

Cutting Balloon A balloon containing blades, used to cut scar tissue in restenosis lesions following insertion of a stent in an artery.

Cytokine A compound, likened to a hormone, in that it can signal for a particular process. Usually referred to as an inflammatory cytokine, initiating the cascade of events that leads to a heart attack.

Decussation The crossing over of nerve fibers in the brainstem, on their way to the spinal cord. A problem in one cerebral cortex of the brain will, therefore, affect the motor function on the other side of the body.

Deep Venous Thrombophlebitis (DVT) for on of patho gic clot within the deep drainage veins, most commonly those in the lower extremities.

Diastole That phase of heart action when the pumping chambers are relaxed, taking in blood from the atria.

Digoxin An ancient drug, still used to slow the ventricular response to atrial fibrillation.

Dilate To enlarge.

Dilated Cardiomyopathy A large left ventricle, which can be due to a variety of problems from volume overload to destruction of muscle.

Dissection When applied to a blood vessel, the separation of its layers.

Diuretic A drug that promotes elimination of water by the kidneys.

Dominant Cerebral Hemisphere The side of the brain that controls speech.

Doppler A noninvasive tool which measures velocity and direction of blood flow, useful for determination of the severity of a plaque within an artery.

Doxorubicin A chemotherapeutic agent that can cause destruction of heart muscle cells.

Drug-Eluting Stent A stent impregnated with a cancer drug, either taxol or sirolimus, which leaches out over a three month period, preventing cell replication that could cause the artery to become blocked with scar tissue.

Dyspnea Air hunger.

Echocardiogram The transmission of sound waves into the heart. Different tissues have different echo-absorption and refractoriness, generating an architectural form of the heart structures and any unusual material on the valves or in the heart structures. Color flow and Doppler will give information about pressures within the heart, function of the muscle, and valve leakage or shunts.

Edema Water in the tissues. Peripheral edema is water in the leg tissues.

Effusion Development of a pathologic collection of fluid.

Ehlers-Danlos Syndrome An uncommon collagen problem marked by elastic skin, heart block, and tendency to have a painless aortic dissection.

Eisenmenger's Physiology A situation that exists when the pulmonary artery pressure, in response to a cardiac shunt, becomes equal to the systemic pressure feeding the brain, limbs, kidneys, and gut.

Embolism The movement of a clot from the site of formation. To embolize.

Embolus A clot that has formed in one area and travels to another.

Emphysema Destruction of lung tissue, usually from smoking, with coalescence of air pockets into large, useless air-containing structures, called bullae.

Endoluminal Stent-Graft The tissue-covered stent device placed in the aorta or other arteries to wall off an aneurysm.

Endothelin A strong vasoconstrictor substance, probably one of the substances responsible for pulmonary hypertension.

Endothelium The diaphanous inner lining of arteries responsible for the health of the artery. Nitric oxide, a vaso-relaxant, is manufactured here.

Enzyme A molecule that causes a chemical reaction to proceed.

Epinephrine One of the "fight or flight" substances released when we are frightened or angry. Also released in the early morning hours as a natural cycle.

Erythropoietin A substance produced by the kidney that brings about production of red blood cells, also known to lend protection to the heart muscle against damage.

Esophageal Spasm Contraction of the smooth muscle in the wall of the esophagus, resulting in a forceful esophageal squeeze. Can mimic the pain of a heart attack.

Etiology The cause.

Fibroblasts Cells that form scar tissue. Reinforce the fibrous cap, covering a cholesterol plaque.

Fibromuscular Hyperplasia (Dysplasia) The "string of beads" narrowing of an artery, usually in a renal artery supplying the kidney, less commonly involves the carotid artery to the brain. Cause unknown. Usually in young women.

Fibrosis Scar formation.

Fibrous Cap The thin scar-like covering of a plaque within an artery. Protects the plaque from splitting open, causing a complete thrombotic occlusion of the artery.

Free Radical An end product of metabolism, increasing with age, thought to be responsible for some of the degenerative diseases because of cellular damage.

French Paradox The fact that the French, who eat foods rich in saturated fats, also have a low incidence of coronary artery disease, thought to be due to their increased consumption of wine, high in concentrated tannins.

Genome The nucleic acid, determining the characteristics of the organism. Ex: Viral genome, evidence of the previous presence of a virus in the tissues.

Heart Attack Damage to the heart muscle, usually as a result of a closed coronary artery.

Heimlich Maneuver The encirclement of one's arms around another, fists in the upper abdomen, with a sudden tightening in hopes of forcing air upward with enough energy to loosen and expel an object lodged within the throat, blocking the airway.

Hematoma A collection of blood.

Hemoglobin The molecule within each red blood cell that has the capacity to carry either oxygen or carbon dioxide, one at a time. It leaves off oxygen to the tissues, taking up carbon dioxide in the swap. At the lung level, it leaves off carbon dioxide, taking up oxygen.

Heparin A drug used to prevent clot proliferation.

Heparin-Induced Thrombocytopenia A drop in platelet count, sometimes associated with an increased tendency to clot, brought on by repeated exposure to Heparin, in unusual circumstances in which antibodies to Heparin have been formed. Must be thought of in any usage of Heparin complicated by enhanced clot formation.

High Blood Pressure Generally thought of as systolic pressure exceeding 140 mmHg or diastolic pressure above 90 mmHg.

High Sensitivity C-Reactive Protein (hsCRP) A marker of inflammation.

Holter Monitor A 24-hour recording of the heart rhythm.

Homeostasis Balance between opposing forces, such as balance between clot formation and clot dissolution.

Homocysteine An amino acid that, in excess, can damage the inside of arteries.

Hypertension High blood pressure. Unless specified, that within the general arterial circulation, called "systemic" hypertension.

Hypertrophic Cardiomyopathy A usually inherited condition marked by the pathologic accumulation of muscle, frequently disorganized. The most common is IHSS.

Hypertrophy An increase in the size of muscle fibers.

Hypoxia A low blood oxygen level. Also hypoxemia.

Idiopathic Hypertrophic Subaortic Stenosis (IHSS) A form of hypertrophic cardiomyopathy in which there is proliferation of abnormal heart muscle in the left ventricular outflow tract. As such, it frequently prevents flow of blood past the muscle bulge and may cause blackout spells or sudden death if severe and untreated.

Idioventricular Rhythm When the top two pacemakers built into the heart, the sinus and the junctional, fail for some reason, usually degeneration of the electrical system, an electrical focus within the ventricular muscle will emerge. Its rate is very slow, usually about 25-30, but it is enough to keep one alive until an artificial pacemaker can be installed.

Iliac Artery The large limb, coming off the terminal aorta, leading to the legs.

Immunosuppression Any medication or condition that prevents the immune system from functioning in a protective role.

Infrapopliteal Arteries The three arteries supplying the calf and foot. Typically involved in obliterative vascular disease in diabetes.

Inferior Vena Cava (IVC) The giant blood tube carrying blue, oxygen-depleted blood back from the legs and lower trunk to the heart.

Inferior Vena Cava Filter A device deployed in the vena cava through a catheter so clot from the leg and pelvic veins on their way to the lungs can be caught.

Inflammation A tissue response to injury.

Inflammatory Cytokines Proteins secreted that bring about erosion of tissue and clotting and clotting of an artery. There are also "protective" cytokines within the body.

Inflammatory Molecules Usually referring to cytokines that are a result of inflammation.

Insulin Resistance A condition marked by normal levels of insulin, but tissue resistance to its effects. Usually part of the metabolic syndrome, of which obesity is a large part.

Internal Carotid Artery The branch of the common carotid that supplies blood to the brain.

Interstitium The area between cells.

Interventional Usually means work on the heart or any artery or vein through a catheter-based system.

Intra-Aortic Balloon Pump (IABP) A device inserted from the groin artery, the femoral, to a position within the thoracic aorta, inflating when the heart is relaxed, deflating when the heart is contracting, to displace blood that the heart will not have to pump. To unload the heart in the event of injury, such as a large heart attack, or to reduce the amount of backward flow of blood, as in mitral regurgitation, the leaking back across the valve.

Intracranial Hemorrhage A bleed into brain tissue.

Ischemia Oxygen-deprivation, usually due to a blocked artery.

Junctional Pacemaker The subservient pacemaker just below the AV node. In the event of failure of the sinus node pacemaker within the heart, the junctional area possesses electrical cells that will depolarize at a rate of about 40, enough of a rate to provide good cardiac output.

Lactic Acid The end product of metabolism that causes muscle burning.

Lacunar Stroke The small stroke resulting from closure of a small blood vessel in the brain, usually caused by hypertension.

Left Atrial Appendage The little outpouching off the left atrium where clot can form. Of no known use except as a trouble-maker.

Lipid A blood fat. A catch-all term for any blood fat.

Long QT Interval Syndrome An inherited condition, due to an abnormal ion channel, that may predispose one to sudden cardiac death due to an arrhythmia.

Lovenox A fraction of Heparin, used to prevent clot formation. Can be injected under the skin.

Lumen The inside channel of a blood vessel, where blood is carried.

Macrophages Large cells within a plaque that secrete enzymes that can cut through the protective fibrous cap, allowing for plaque erosion and arterial occlusion with clot.

Mallory-Weiss Syndrome A tear of the wall of the esophagus, the symptoms of which can mimic a heart attack or an aortic dissection. Always caused by intense vomiting.

Marfan's Syndrome A congenital syndrome marked by tall, skinny habitus, spidery fingers, a high, arched palate, high arches of the feet, and abnormal heart valve and blood vessel tissue. The aorta is more apt to tear relatively painlessly and the mitral and aortic valves are apt to become floppy and leak.

Matrix Composition of a structure, such as the network of an arterial wall.

Mechanical Valve A replacement heart valve. These are usually of a tilting disc variety, made of pyrolytic carbon to provide durability and to reduce clot formation.

Metabolic Syndrome A poorly named syndrome marked by trunkal obesity, insulin-resistance, elevated triglyceride levels, inflammation, and elevated LHL-cholesterol levels.

Metabolism The processing of foodstuffs and compounds in the production of energy.

Metalloprotease One of the enzymes that can cut through the fibrous cap.

Microflora A collection of bacteria of a certain type. Ex: microflora of the gut.

Migraine Syndrome Headache, frequently associated with visual disturbances, which is at least partially due to vasomotor instability.

MiniMaze The use of laser to inscribe burns within the left atrium to re-establish normal sinus rhythm in someone who has atrial fibrillation.

Mitochondria Cellular energy-producing packets.

Mitral Regurgitation The leakage of blood back across the mitral valve into the left atrium.

Mitral Stenosis Caused only by rheumatic fever, the scarring down of the mitral valve.

Mitral Valve The valve between the left upper and left lower chambers of the heart. The most complex valve in the heart. Prevents blood from leaking back into the left atrium when the main pumping chamber is contracting, pushing blood into the aorta.

Mitral Valve Prolapse The protrusion of tissue of the mitral valve back into the left atrium when the left ventricle contracts. Usually due to redundant tissue or elongated chordae, the support structures. May cause atypical chest pain and palpitations. Frequently harmless but can be serious if the valve is degenerative.

Morphology Composition and Structure.

Myocardial Bridge A muscle bridge over a coronary artery, which can restrict flow down the coronary during systole, when the muscle is tensed.

Myocardial Infarction (MI) A heart attack, usually caused by closure of a blood vessel supplying the heart muscle. Destruction of heart muscle.

Myocardium The heart network of muscle fibers.

Natrecor A drug used to vasodilate blood vessels, promote diuresis, and treat severe CHF. The best drug for acute treatment of intractable CHF.

Neurocardiogenic A reflex from the brain to the heart.

Nitric oxide A potent vaso-relaxant manufactured in the endothelium of any artery. Responsible for the tone within the wall of the artery and, therefore, the blood flow.

Nitroglycerin (NTG) A potent relaxant of the wall of blood vessels, particularly those of veins. Used in treatment of angina, as it relaxes the wall of the veins, reducing the work of the heart, allowing it to re-establish equilibrium between blood supply and demand. Can also be used to acutely unload the heart in the event of heart failure. Will drop the blood pressure.

Occlusion To block, usually with clot in the case of the circulation.

Oxidative Stress The damage imposed by the end products of metabolism, brought about by the formation of free radicals. These increase within cells with age.

Pacemaker An electrical device inserted within the heart to maintain heart rhythm.

Pacemaker Syndrome A drop in blood pressure caused by the insertion of only a single ventricular lead, resulting in a loss of the atrial contribution to the total cardiac output. Also, sometimes a pulsatile rush sensed when the atria contract when the tricuspid and mitral valves are closed. All symptoms can usually be addressed with a dual-chamber pacemaker system.

Palpitations An awareness of rapid or irregular heart action.

Paradoxical Embolus A clot that has formed elsewhere and has traveled, but has crossed over from the venous circulation to the arterial circulation, implying a shunt between the two circulations, which should, under normal circumstances, be isolated from each other.

ParaValvular Leak The leak around the main body of a heart valve that has been installed, either due to a stitch pulling through thin tissue or an infection. Can cause CHF if great enough and can cause hemolysis, the breakdown of red blood cells.

Paroxysmal Supraventricular Tachycardia (PSVT) A rapid rhythm within the upper cardiac chambers.

Patent Foramen Ovale (PFO) Persistence of an embryonic communication between the upper chambers of the heart. May be responsible for a paradoxic embolus and stroke.

Pathologic Any deviation from normal structure and function. A disease state.

Pericardial Effusion A collection of fluid brought about by some sort of pathologic process that involves the pericardial sac.

Pericarditis Inflammation within the pericardial sac.

Pericardium The connective tissue covering of the heart.

Pheochromocytoma A tumor, usually benign, of the adrenal gland that pumps out large quantities of excitatory substances, epinephrine and norepinephrine, which cause the heart to speed up and raise the blood pressure. They may also cause diarrhea, shakiness, and weight loss. To be looked for in any case of refractory high blood pressure.

Phlebitis An inflammatory process within a vein.

Plaque A deposit of fatty material within the wall of an artery, usually also containing some calcium.

Plaque Rupture Splitting of the fibrous cap covering a plaque, opening the plaque and exposing its contents to the circulating blood elements.

Platelet Agent Any medication that will block platelet aggregation.

Platelets Tiny, microscopic elements within the bloodstream that serve as the first line of defense against injury, clumping in the initiation of a clot.

Pleuritic Pain aggravated by breathing due to inflammation of the connective tissue covering of the pleural around the lungs, or the pericardium, surrounding the heart.

Popliteal Aneurysm An out-pouching of the popliteal artery. In the past, these were usually traumatic, the Coachman's Curse. Now, they are usually arteriosclerotic.

Popliteal Artery The artery just behind the knee.

Post-Partum Cardiomyopathy Weakness of the heart muscle after delivery of a baby, thought to represent invasion of the heart muscle by a virus during a time of increased demands of the heart muscle.

Post-Viral Cardiomyopathy Heart muscle weakness thought to be secondary to invasion of the heart muscle by a virus that has tropism (affinity) for the muscle.

Premature Atrial Contractions (PACs) Extra beats originating within one of the two upper heart chambers. They are harmless but may cause one to be very symptomatic.

Premature Ventricular Contractions (PVCs) Extra beats originating from the ventricles.

Prinzmetal Angina Also called variant angina, caused by spasm within the wall of the artery. Much more common in women, influenced by hormones. As contrasted to the usual angina, this comes on at night or at rest.

ProAmatine A drug to use in providing tone in the small arteries throughout the body, particularly in the legs, when the automatic reflexes to make this adjustment so you will keep a normal blood pressure when rising, have failed.

Prothrombin Time (Protime) Measurement of anticoagulation with Coumadin.

Pulmonary Artery The artery carrying blue blood from the right ventricle to the lungs.

Pulmonary Embolus A blood clot, formed elsewhere, that has traveled to the lungs.

Pulmonary Hypertension A high blood pressure within the pulmonary artery.

Pulmonic Valve The valve between the right ventricle and the pulmonary artery. Its job is to prevent blood that has been pumped into the pulmonary artery from leaking back into the right ventricle.

Pulmonary Vascular Resistance The pressure against which blood flows in the small vessels in the lungs.

Radiofrequency Ablation The use of energy of radiofrequency waves to burn unwanted electrical circuitry within the heart.

Raynaud's Phenomenon Tendency toward vasospasm of a digital artery, leading to cold, white fingers when exposed to cold temperatures.

Renal Artery The artery leading from the abdominal aorta to the kidney, carrying blood to be filtered by the kidney, removing waste products from metabolism.

Renal Artery Stenosis The blockage of a renal, or kidney, artery. May cause hypertension.

Renin Manufactured by the kidney to determine the amount of salt and water to be kept within the blood vessels. May be excessively manufactured when the kidney feels it is cheated for blood, such as when the renal artery is blocked.

Renin-angiotensin-aldosterone System (RAAS) The blood pressure and volume regulatory mechanism in the kidney, over-stimulated in congestive heart failure and when the renal artery is blocked.

Renovascular Hypertension High blood pressure partially caused by a blocked kidney artery, causing the kidney to put out too much renin, as the kidney simply reads that it is receiving inadequate amounts of blood. Sometimes partially resolves when the renal artery is opened by a stent.

Resistance The pressure against which blood has to flow, regulated by the tone within small muscular arterioles throughout the body. This is determined by need for more blood pressure, as in shock, and is inappropriately elevated in several pathologic states, including congestive heart failure and when too much renin is put out by the blood-starved kidney in response to a blocked artery.

Restenosis The recurrent blockage, by a type of scar tissue, after an artery has been opened by angioplasty or by stent deployment. It is caused by a reaction of the arterial wall to the damage imposed by the high pressure used to open the artery.

Rheumatic Heart Disease A valvular disorder brought on by a Streptococcal infection, usually sore throat, as a child.

Rhythm The cadence, or repetitive action of the heart, established by the prevailing electrical activity.

Rhythmol A drug used to maintain the God-given rhythm.

Sarcoidosis An infiltrative process, whereby granulomata are laid down within tissue, usually lung but may also affect the heart.

Scleroderma A collagen vascular disease that can cause severe pulmonary hypertension.

Septal Myomectomy Surgical removal of a muscle bulge in the outflow tract of an individual with IHSS.

Septum The partition between two chambers. Ex: Atrial septum or ventricular septum.

Shunt The passage of blood from one chamber or vessel into another where it was not intended, in the natural form of things, to be.

Sick Sinus Syndrome A degeneration of the sinus node, frequently associated with other electrical problems within the heart.

Silent Coronary Artery Disease Arteriosclerosis within the coronary arteries supplying the heart muscle with blood, with no symptoms. This silent aspect can be secondary to abnormal nerve receptors, caused by diabetes, inadequate investment with nerves from birth, or may simply mean that the blockage is not causing enough oxygen-deprivation of the tissues to cause pain.

Silent Ischemia Oxygen-deprivation of the heart muscle that fails to bring about bothersome symptoms, such as pain. Usually detected by electrocardiographic changes in absence of pain.

SilverHawk An athrectomy device, using a rotational cutter to open critically narrowed arteries in the lower extremities.

Sinus Node The node of cells in the upper heart that have special electrical characteristics, spontaneously leaking ions across their cell membranes to initiate an electrical spark to be carried throughout the heart, cause muscle contraction.

Sinus Rhythm The God-given rhythm, originating from the sinus node within the right upper cardiac chamber.

Sirolimus A cancer drug used to treat stents to prevent cell replication within the stent due to damaged intima, the inside of the blood vessel, when the stent is deployed under high pressure.

Sleep Apnea A condition of suspension of breathing during deep slumber, usually associated with some degree of obesity, especially fat deposit within the neck. A frequent accompaniment of both congestive heart failure and atrial fibrillation.

Sotalol A drug used to control arrhythmias.

Stenosis Any blockage, usually expressed as a percentage. A 75% stenosis of an artery would mean that it is three-quarters closed off.

Stent A stainless steel circular device crimped onto a balloon to be deployed within a blocked artery under high pressure.

Stroke Damage to brain tissue, due to blockage of a blood vessel feeding that brain tissue or by a bleed within the tissue.

Subclavian Artery The large artery carrying red blood to the arm. Each subclavian artery gives off a small branch, the vertebral artery, that travels up the neck to feed the cerebellum, the base of the brain controlling equilibrium and balance.

Subclavian Stenosis The blockage of the subclavian artery, usually right in the mouth of the artery. This can cause the arm to become desperate for blood, stealing it from the base of the brain via the vertebral artery.

Suffused Tissue flooded with blood.

Superficial Femoral Artery The main artery within the leg, sending red blood on its way to the foot. It is prone to close off painlessly, as there is usually a network of collaterals that will provide enough blood to maintain viability to the lower leg and foot. However, once this closes off, there is no access to the leg arteries below it.

Superior Mesenteric Artery The artery feeding the gut.

Superior Vena Cava (SVC) The venous drainage of the head and arms into the right heart.

Syncope A blackout spell, frequently brought about by inadequate blood supply to the brain because of an arrhythmia or heart block.

Syncytium The spiraling network of heart muscle fibers.

Systemic Vascular Resistance The tone within arteries throughout the body.

Systole The contractile phase of the heart.

Tachy-Brady Variant of Sick Sinus Syndrome Fast, alternating with slow, rhythm. Usually the fast limb is atrial fibrillation, while the slow is a sluggish sinus node.

Tachycardia A rapid rhythm.

Tachycardia-Related Cardiomyopathy Weakness of heart muscle, stunned due to a very rapid heart beat that has gone on undetected for days, weeks, or months.

Tamponade A fluid accumulation within the heart sac, strangulating heart action.

Taxol A cancer drug used to treat stents placed in coronary arteries. This drug helps prevent restenosis due to scar tissue by blocking cell replication in the area of the stent, the portion of the artery that has been injured by the high pressure used in stent deployment.

Thallium Scan A scan of the heart, using radioactive material, trying to sort out whether a blockage exists within a coronary artery supplying heart muscle, whether it has resulted in heart damage or supplies normal muscle.

Thrombolytic A drug with capabilities of dispersing, or lysing, clot.

Thrombophlebitis Clot formation within a venous structure, usually one of the deep veins draining the legs or pelvis.

Thrombophilic Disorder A disorder marked by enhanced clot formation. It can be due to a variety of syndromes, such as Protein C or S deficiency, anti-phospholipid antibody syndrome, antithrombin III deficiency, Leiden Factor V mutation, and lupus anticoagulant. Any one of these can lead to greatly exaggerated clotting properties and have to be thought of in instances of clot formation when it is unexpected.

Thrombotic A closure of an artery or a vein by clot formation.

Thrombus Blood clot formed anywhere in the body within either vein or artery.

Thumpversion The conversion of a potentially fatal ventricular rhythm, usually ventricular tachycardia, by a forceful blow to the chest.

Tikosyn A medication used to hold the heart in sinus rhythm, rather than atrial fibrillation.

Tone The tension within the wall of a muscular artery, determining size and, therefore, flow.

Transesophageal Echocardiography (TEE) The advancement of an echo probe down the esophagus to a position behind the heart to obtain details of heart structure and aorta.

Transient Ischemic Attack (TIA) A reversible neurologic deficit, caused by transient blockage of a blood vessel supplying the brain with red blood.

Tricuspid Valve The valve between the right upper and the right lower heart chambers. As the blood traverses the heart, it is the first valve the blood encounters. Its function is to prevent blood from leaking back into the right atrium when the right ventricle pumps its contents into the pulmonary artery on its way to the lungs.

Trifurcation Arteries The three small arteries below the popliteal artery in the leg, supplying the foot. Either one of the tibial arteries can maintain tissue viability of the foot.

Triglyceride A blood fat, manufactured in response to ingestion of sugars.

Tropism An affinity for a certain type of tissue or cell. Ex: Viral tropism.

Unstable Angina An unstable process, frequently leading to a heart attack if not interrupted, due to plaque rupture within a coronary artery, threatening to clot. An acceleration of pain, frequently at rest or nocturnally, heralding a heart attack.

Vagus The nerve that supplies both the heart and part of the gastrointestinal system, slowing the heart, frequently in response to distension of the stomach or bearing down.

Varicosity A dilated segment of a large superficial vein, due to degeneration of the valve structures within the vein.

Vascular Resistance The tone within the small muscular arteries.

Vasoactive The ability expressed by an artery to enlarge or become smaller, usually in response to a nerve-transmitted signal or a chemical.

Vasomotor Instability The reactivity of an artery. Any artery that possesses a ruptured plaque may become unstable, with spasm contiguous to the plaque. All arteries have the ability to dilate, or constrict; this is more pronounced in vasomotor instability.

Veins Thin-walled structures carrying blue blood from which oxygen has been extracted by the tissues, back to the heart. Easily collapsed, very low pressure environment, slow flow. Major disease is thrombophlebitis.

Venous Valves Chevron-shaped structures within the large veins, opening to allow blood to be milked back toward the heart, closing to prevent blood from leaking back down to its previous level. Broken down to form varicosities.

Ventricular Fibrillation A chaotic, very rapid rhythm coming from the lower heart chambers, always fatal unless interrupted by electrical shock.

Ventricular Septal Defect (VSD) A communication between the two lower cardiac chambers, the ventricles, usually from birth though it can be created by a heart attack.

Ventricular Tachycardia A rapid rhythm coming from a focus within the heart muscle of one of the lower heart chambers. Frequently secondary to oxygen-starvation of the heart muscle, or previous damage of muscle. Usually life-threatening.

Venule The smallest vein down the branching network. The first vein picking up blue blood from the tissues.

Vertebral Artery The artery coming off the subclavian artery that goes up the neck to supply blood to the cerebellum.

Viability Alive and able to function.

Vulnerable Plaque One that is lipid-laden, has a thinned-out fibrous cap, and is ready to rupture.

Wolff-Parkinson-White Pre-Excitation An anomalous tract of electrical conduction tissue that brings about rapid arrhthmias within the upper chambers of the heart. Can sometimes cause a fatal arrhythmia. Usually treated with radiofrequency ablation.

Zaroxolyn A potent diuretic used primarily as a "bail-out" medication when conventional diuretics aren't removing fluid.

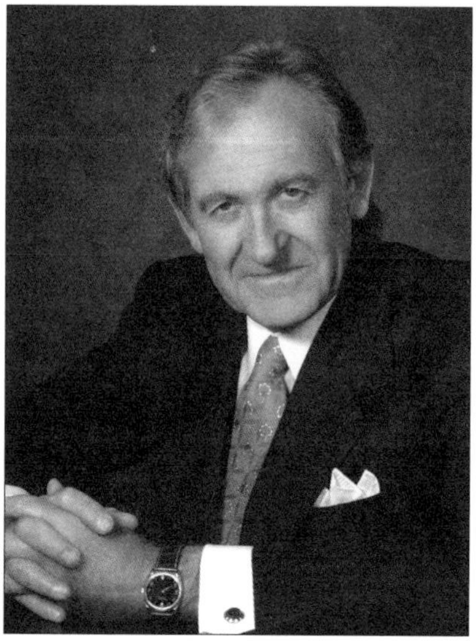

Dr. Gerry L. Maddoux is a board-certified cardiologist who has practiced cardiology for the last 30 years. Involved primarily in interventional cardiology, he has become increasingly interested in patient education for prevention and care of heart disease. *Your Heart, Treat It Like You Love It* is the result of requests by hundreds of patients that he write a book on the information he provides them to help keep them informed on their conditions and care.

Dr. Maddoux is a Fellow of the American College of Cardiology and the American College of Chest Physicians, and a Member of Alpha-Omega-Alpha Honorary Society.

Dr. Maddoux has published articles in medical journals on unique cardiac situations and clinical research information. He has brought these cardiac experiences together in *Your Heart, Treat It Like You Love It* in an effort to combat the rise of heart disease and to educate the patient in all of us.